The Nature and Treatment of Hypothermia

Publications in the Health Sciences

Publication of this book was assisted
by a grant from the McKnight Foundation
to the University of Minnesota Press's program
in the health sciences, and by grants from
the Minnesota Sea Grant Program
[Project Contribution No. 120 (R/S-1)] and the
Department of Physiology, School of Medicine,
University of Minnesota at Duluth.

The Nature and Treatment of Hypothermia

edited by *Robert S. Pozos, Ph.D.,*
and *Lorentz E. Wittmers, Jr., Ph.D.*

University of Minnesota
Continuing Medical Education
Volume 2

University of Minnesota Press ☐ Minneapolis

Published by the University of Minnesota Press,
2037 University Avenue Southeast, Minneapolis, MN 55414
Printed in the United States of America

Library of Congress Cataloging in Publication Data
Main entry under title:

The Nature and treatment of hypothermia.

(University of Minnesota continuing medical education; v.2)

Includes index.

1. Hypothermia. I. Pozos, Robert S. II. Wittmers, Lorentz E. III. Series. [DNLM: 1. Hypothermia—Congresses. 2. Hypothermia—Therapy—Congresses.
W1 UN944T v.2 / WD 670 N285 1981]
RC88,5.N37 1983 616.9'89 82-23909
ISBN 0-8166-1154-8

Contents

Contributors

G. A. Barker, M.B., Department of Anaesthesia, University of Toronto, Toronto, Ont.

D. J. Bohn, M.B., Department of Anesthesia, University of Toronto, Toronto, Ont.

K. J. Collins, M.B., B.S., D.Phil. (Oxon.), Department of Geriatric Medicine, School of Medicine, University College, London, London, UK

A. W. Conn, M.D., Intensive Care Unit, Hospital for Sick Children, University of Toronto, Toronto, Ont.

K. E. Cooper, M.B., B.S. (Lond.), M.A., D.Sc. (Oxon.), Department of Medical Phsyiology, Faculty of Medicine, University of Calgary, Calgary, Alta.

J. F. Edmonds, M.B., Department of Anaesthesia, University of Toronto, Toronto, Ont.

A. V. Ferguson, B.Sc., Ph.D., Department of Medical Physiology, Faculty of Medicine, University of Calgary, Calgary, Alta.

Ralph Francesconi, Ph.D., Heat Research Division, U.S. Army Research Institute of Environmental Medicine, Natick, Mass.

Frank St. C. Golden, M.B., B.Ch., Ph.D., Institute of Naval Medicine, Gosport, Hants, UK

Murray P. Hamlet, D.V.M., Experimental Pathology Division, U.S. Army Research Institute of Environmental Medicine, Natick, Mass.

J. S. Hayward, B.Sc., Ph.D., Department of Biology, University of Victoria, Victoria, B.C.

Milton J. Hernández, Ph.D., Department of Physiology, Howard University College of Medicine, Washington, D.C.

W. C. Kaufman, Ph.D., Department of Human Biology, University of Wisconsin, Green Bay.

Donald W. Kerr, M.S., Experimental Pathology Division, U.S. Army Research Institute of Environmental Medicine, Natick, Mass.

Loren A. Kuehn, Ph.D., Defence and Civil Institute of Environmental Medicine, Downsview, Ont.

Ian McA. Ledingham, M.D., Department of Surgery, Western Infirmary, Glasgow, Scotland

G. Patrick Lilja, M.D., Department of Trauma and Emergency Medicine, North Memorial Medical Center, Minneapolis, Minn.

Peter Lomax, M.D., D.Sc., Department of Pharmacology, University of California at Los Angeles School of Medicine, Los Angeles, Calif.

Milton Mager, Ph.D., Heat Research Division, U.S. Army Research Institute of Environmental Medicine, Natick, Mass.

Keith H. Marks, M.B., Department of Neurology, Milton S. Hershey Medical Center, Pennsylvania State University, Hershey, Pa.

William J. Mills, M.D., Department of Medical Education, University of Alaska, Anchorage, Alaska

Martin C. Moore-Ede, M.D., Ph.D., Department of Physiology, Harvard Medical School, Boston, Mass.

Bruce C. Paton, M.D., Department of Surgery, University of Colorado Health Sciences Center, Denver, Colo.

John F. Patton, Ph.D., Experimental Pathology Division, U.S. Army Research Institute of Environmental Medicine, Natick, Mass.

R. S. Pozos, Ph.D., Department of Physiology, School of Medicine, University of Minnesota at Duluth, Duluth, Minn.

Donald E. Roberts, Ph.D., Experimental Pathology Division, U.S. Army Research Institute of Environmental Medicine, Natick, Mass.

Barbara B. Tabeling, M.D., Department of Anesthesiology, College of Medicine, University of Florida, Gainesville, Fla.

L. E. Wittmers, Jr., Ph.D., Department of Physiology, School of Medicine, University of Minnesota at Duluth, Duluth, Minn.

Richard S. K. Young, M.D., Department of Neurology, Milton S. Hershey Medical Center, Pennsylvania State University, Hershey, Pa.

Preface

Controversies concerning the nature and treatment of hypothermia continue. A limited amount of research has been done on humans, but anecdotal stories abound with respect to various aspects of this complex topic. This book is a collection of papers and discussions presented at the symposium "The Nature and Treatment of Hypothermia" held in Duluth, Minnesota, June 1-3, 1981. The emphasis of the symposium was on human responses to acute and chronic cold stress. The authors presented the "state of the art" in their area of expertise. The discussion is included since it provides further information on hypothermia and highlights the areas of continued controversy.

The symposium approach to the topic of hypothermia was multidisciplinary. Both the clinical and basic science staffs presented their data, experiences, and speculation with respect to the problem of humans in the cold, the prevention and treatment of hypothermia. Spirited discussion resulted from questions dealing with the efficacy and safety of cardiopulmonary resuscitation of the hypothermic victim. Much research needs to be done concerning hypothermia. We hope these proceedings will give some sense of direction for those interested in this area.

The editors acknowledge the following groups and foundations for their financial support of the conference: The Duluth Clinic Education and Research Foundation; Miller Dwan Medical Center Foundation; Reserve Mining; St. Luke's Hospital; Minnesota Sea Grant Program; UMD School of Medicine; Undersea Medical Society; The Upjohn Company; and Mobil Oil Company.

The authors have acknowledged their own support in their chapters.

R. S. P.
L. E. W.

Introduction

Lorne A. Kuehn, Ph.D.

This book will come as a pleasant surprise to researchers engaged in the practical and clinical aspects of rewarming human victims of accidental hypothermia. Although the field has been the subject of intense study for over three decades, there are as many differences of opinion expressed today as there were in the reports and documentaries about hypothermia and cold injury published shortly after the Second World War. Molnar's article on immersion hypothermia (1), written in 1946, and Burton and Edholm's book *Man in a Cold Environment* (2), written in 1955, are still considered classic works on the subject and mandatory reading for any neophyte beginning studies in the field. A more recent classic reference is Keatinge's *Survival in Cold Water* (3), published in 1969. Although an elegant treatise on the subject of immersion hypothermia, Keatinge's work is not a complete review of hypothermia encountered in other and more diverse cold-inducing environments.

Until now, there has been no single publication that embodied all the current approaches to accidental hypothermia in humans. This volume is the result of a workshop whose subject was the nature and treatment of hypothermia. Under the chairmanship of Dr. Robert Pozos and Dr. G. Cotton of the University of Minnesota-Duluth School of Medicine, the workshop was held in June 1981. Recognized experts on hypothermia and rewarming informally presented their findings and opinions over three days, and the collected presentations plus edited discussions have been summarized for this volume by Dr. R. Pozos and Dr. L. E. Wittmers of the University of Minnesota-Duluth School of Medicine.

Accidental Hypothermia

Accidental hypothermia and the resuscitation of humans affected by it have been a problem for centuries. Hypothermia has long been a factor in military operations and civilian life in the Northern Hemisphere. In Chapter 16, Dr. Frank St. C. Golden describes the history of hypothermia and its treatment, emphasizing the early development of some of the rewarming methods now commonly accepted. Golden also describes the types of hypothermia and the various methods of treatment.

Several definitions of "accidental hypothermia" exist. Gregory and Doolittle (4) defined it as a series of physiological events associated with reduction of body temperature in an uncontrolled manner in which any associated disease present in the victim does not require a specific aggressive therapy during rewarming to a normothermal state. It has been defined more simply (5) as the unintentional lowering of body-core temperature below 35°C in an otherwise healthy individual.

Most students of this subject recognize three general types of accidental hypothermia that correspond to the environmental circumstances of the accident. The most rapidly involved and dangerous form is termed "immersion hypothermia." It occurs as the result of brief exposure to very cold water in which the thermal demand of the environment is significantly greater than the capacity of the victim's body to produce heat. The victim may lose consciousness and drown in less than 20 minutes. Shivering is extensive and very uncomfortable. Chapter 12 by Dr. R. Pozos and Dr. L. Wittmers discusses shivering and its relationship to metabolism. Internal fluid shifts are not prominent, and blood glucose and cortisol are maintained at high levels. In Chapter 1, Dr. John Hayward reviews the major physiological events in humans during the initial period of accidental hypothermia when the body is still attempting to defend itself against the intense cold insult before becoming unconscious. Pertinent to body-core temperatures as low as 33°C, this chapter reviews the extent of knowledge that can be obtained from human subjects in ethical experiments.

A less severe but equally dangerous form of accidental hypothermia is called "mountain hypothermia" or "exhaustion hypothermia." It is the result of prolonged exposure to cold-air environments, especially when the victim is physically tired or hungry. The body's usable energy stores are depleted. The victim shivers much less than the victim of immersion or may not shiver at all. The onset of hypothermia and exhaustion is slow and may involve changes in mood and personality. Changes take place in fluid and electrolyte balances, with increases or reductions in blood glucose and cortisol levels. This particular malady has been reviewed by Dr. W. C. Kaufman in Chapter 4, which also contains many practical suggestions on preventing and alleviating this condition in hostile environments.

The third form is the slowly evolved "subclinical hypothermia" or "chronic hypothermia." It occurs after the victim's lengthy exposure to a cool-air environment and is often associated with inadequate clothing and food intake. It is commonly considered to be a problem of the elderly. Though body-core temperatures are normal, chronic cold stress results in considerable intercompartmental fluid shifting. Of increasing concern for the aging population in the developed world, geriatric hypothermia is becoming a common malady aggravated in part by the economic recessions and uncertainty that now trouble the developed and developing worlds. Chapter 3, by Dr. K. Cooper and Dr. A. Ferguson, details the environmental and physiological conditions that predispose the elderly to hypothermia.

Three chapters (Chapter 5 by Dr. Milton Hernández, Chapter 7 by Dr. Peter Lomox, and Chapter 9 by Dr. Milton Mager and Dr. Ralph Francesconi) review the basic physiology of the thermoregulatory process and its control and dysfunction. These chapters provide the information readers need to appreciate the subtle deterioration of the body's mechanisms and functions during heat loss and subsequent hypothermia. Dr. Murray Hamlet, Dr. Bruce Paton, and Dr. Frank St. C. Golden (in Chapters 8, 11, and 16, respectively) describe the physiological changes concomitant with lower body temperatures and internal fluid shifts.

In general, the order of physiological events that occur at various body-core temperatures during the cooling process are experienced in reverse order upon rewarming. Death due to accidental hypothermia is interpreted as a failure to revive the victim and should be pronounced only after efforts at resuscitation, including rewarming, have failed. With the application of proper rewarming procedures, victims have been revived from hypothermic states with core temperatures as low as 18°C.

The degree of accidental hypothermia can be categorized into two types: acute and subacute. Victims of acute hypothermia are those who have core temperatures of 30°C or lower and who have lost consciousness or are in a comatose state. Golden (5) also describes victims of acute hypothermia as those who have become hypothermic in less than 6 hours. Subacute hypothermia victims have core temperatures above 30°C and are conscious and able to assist their rescuers during rescue and subsequent rewarming. Their hypothermia may have taken between 6 hours and 24 hours to develop. Chronic hypothermia usually occurs over a period in excess of 24 hours.

Death in accidental hypothermia usually results from cardiac arrest or ventricular fibrillation, a subject treated at length in Chapter 11. Selective cooling of the endocardium and subendocardial conducting system in relation to the myocardium increases the risk of ventricular fibrillation, particularly for tissue temperatures below the 25°C-to-30°C range. Cardiac massage, use of various anesthetic agents, and changes in hydrogen-ion concentration or carbon dioxide level also increase the risk of ventricular fibrillation. Prolonged hypoxia has been discounted as a primary cause because the oxygen present in the hypothermic circulation is considered sufficient for the reduced myocardial work. A sudden onset of hypoxia or an increased cardiac demand may bring about ventricular fibrillation, however.

A major hazard in the rewarming process is the rapid infusion of cold blood into the heart; such an infusion may cause ventricular fibrillation. Actions leading to the rapid infusion of cold blood into the heart include manhandling the victim in the rescue process or in the application of antidrowning therapy and perhaps the injudicious application of surface-supplied heat (causing vasodilatation of the extensively vasoconstricted peripheral tissue with a resulting surge of cold blood into the heart). It has been postulated that this surge causes a precipitous drop in heart temperature of 1°C to 2°C, termed "afterdrop," which can trigger ventricular fibrillation. It should be noted that there is no hypothermic core temperature from which recovery is impossible if sufficient medical resources are used in a timely fashion; however, given the ineffectiveness of defibrillation techniques for victims with core temperatures of less than 30°C, great efforts must be made to prevent the onset of fibrillation, especially in the field environment where defibrillation equipment is rarely available.

Atrial fibrillation is commonly observed in victims of hypothermia and does not require any specific treatment. The temperature at which ventricular fibrillation occurs during progressive hypothermia is not fixed but probably has a wide range depending on biological variation and, in some instances, concomitant use of drugs. Factors that tend to aggravate the tendency toward ventricular fibrillation in cold hearts are hypotension, stimulation of the throat, barbiturates in the blood, abnormal levels of blood calcium, and disturbed blood pH and pCO_2.

Associated with the afterdrop phenomenon in hypothermia victims or with the rewarming of chronic or subacutely hypothermic victims is the phenomenon of rewarming collapse. Rewarming collapse is a type of shock phenomenon, the causes of which are unknown. It may be due to a further afterdrop, peripheral vasodilatation drawing extensively on the cold heart's output, or even release into the general circulation of the stagnant blood with concentrated metabolites that was held out in the vasoconstricted tissue.

Jessen (6) reported that, even when plasma electrolytes are normal when the rewarming treatment begins (even after near-drowning), a severe fall in potassium ions (hypopotassaemia) may develop as a delayed stress reaction in the pancreas, with an increased outflow of insulin resulting. This increase in combination with the necessary glucose infusion transports potassium ions into cells at an accelerated rate. The phenomenon could explain the deaths that sometimes occur after active rewarming has been stopped and the body-core temperature has almost returned to normal.

In order to avoid the problem of ventricular fibrillation, rewarming treatments should involve rapid rewarming, preferably in the central regions of the body. Rapid correction of electrolytes should take place throughout the rewarming process along with concurrent symptomatic treatment, such as artificial ventilation, external cardiac massage, and defibrillation as required.

Rewarming

Chapters 12 and 15 (by Dr. G. Patrick Lilja and Dr. William J. Mills, respectively) are concerned specifically with rewarming techniques for the emergency treatment of hypothermia. As these chapters show, the optimal type of rewarming regimen applied to a victim depends to some extent on the type of accidental hypothermia—immersion, mountain, or chronic—as well as on the degree of hypothermia—acute or subacute. The history of the hypothermic process in the victim seems to be as important in determining the success of the rewarming as the type of rewarming itself.

Many advances in rewarming therapy have been made during the last two decades, but a definitive plan for the treatment of accidental hypothermia has not yet been accepted by the majority of investigators in the field. Several key issues remain unresolved, namely, the optimum rate of rewarming, the need for intravenous fluids, the role of oxygen administration and positive-pressure ventilation, and the involvement of drugs. Arguments about the value of rapid versus slow rewarming have not been entirely settled, but it is known that during rewarming there is no need for overly aggressive treatment of hypotension, bradycardia, or hyperventilation since these problems resolve themselves as normothermia is approached. The complex interaction between drugs and hypothermia suggests that the use of all drugs should be restricted during rewarming; yet, some researchers maintain that the application of steroids may be useful for treating victims of mountain hypothermia but of little benefit to elderly victims of chronic hypothermia.

The rewarming therapies of choice have not been definitely documented, and more effective treatment techniques need to be developed. Progress can only come about through carefully conducted clinical and experimental studies on animal models; since ethical considerations limit experiments on humans to hypothermic states with core temperatures of 34°C or higher, levels at which many of the important physiological changes associated with hypothermia are not apparent.

Concern has been expressed about the problem of determining when rewarming is complete for victims who have undergone intense hypothermic exposure. Rewarming is conceptually complete when the whole body's heat content has been restored to its precooling level, but this state is difficult to recognize. Webb (7) warned that individual rectal, esophageal, tympanic, subcutaneous, and skin temperatures or combinations of these temperatures restored to predive values do not correlate reliably with calorimetric determinations of restored body heat. The simplest indicator that the rewarming procedure has been carried on long enough may be the onset of sweating, which is a sign that the state of thermoneutrality has been attained and that the body is beginning to enter hyperthermia.

Unfortunately, subjective thermal sensations are not reliable indicators in this regard. Webb (7) reported that his subjects felt warm soon after they stopped shivering; this took place before the rewarming was considered through calorimetric determinations to be half-complete. Similar observations were reported by Collis, Steinman, and Chaney (8), who described the hot-bath rewarming of nine subjects cooled in 7.5°C water to hypothermic states associated with rectal temperatures of 35°C. Abrupt cessations of shivering occurred during rewarming in hot-water baths when the skin temperatures were warmed to values of 33°C, and core temperatures were at their lowest values during the core-temperature afterdrops. Subjective feelings of warmth persisted throughout the subsequent rewarming even though rectal and tympanic temperatures were at or below 35°C. These observations were also made in another experiment involving the hot-bath rewarming of eight hypothermic subjects by Hayward, Eckerson, and Collis (9). Such experiments demonstrate that thermoregulatory heat production in humans depends on an interaction of signals from peripheral and central receptors. Rapid peripheral warming of the skin in hypothermic subjects effectively shuts off shivering in a short period of time.

Surface Rewarming

Historically, surface methods of rewarming have been the easiest to effect, particularly in the field, and have had an advantage in that extensive training is not necessary for rescuers to apply many of these techniques. Furthermore, the equipment required is often available in or near the field. These methods have in common the direct provision of heat to the external body surface only, and they rely on internal heat conduction and blood flow to convey the heat into the colder body core.

Nearly all methods of surface rewarming suffer from the problem of accentuated afterdrop. As the peripheral tissues are warmed or disturbed, vasodilatation reappears in the vasoconstricted tissue and releases pooled peripheral blood into the heart, thereby lowering its temperature and perhaps triggering ventricular fibrillation. Cardiac failure may also occur as a result of the cold myocardium's inability to compensate for the increased cardiac output required. It is also possible that in the rewarming of slowly cooled victims the fluid shifts induced by the hypothermia are quickly reversed; fluid shifts result in a relative hydremia and failure of the cold heart due to its having a low output as a consequence of high fluid overload and high peripheral resistance.

Rewarming shock is also produced during the treatment of victims who have experienced a slow onset of hypothermia in which the intravascular volume is decreased secondarily to fluid shifts. Rewarming shock is a form of hypodemia secondary to a diminished central blood volume. Neither cardiac failure nor rewarming shock can be well managed in a nonhospital setting. The application of surface rewarming techniques also tends to reduce the magnitude and extent of shivering, thereby removing one intrinsic avenue of rewarming for the body.

Most experts now agree that surface-deployed techniques are optimally applied to subacutely hypothermic victims with core temperatures between 32°C and 35°C for whom the risk of ventricular fibrillation is not great. In order to reduce further the chances of filbrillation presumed to be brought on by afterdrop, optimal surface techniques involve the application of heat only to regions of high heat transfer, such as the head, neck, trunk, and groin; the patient's limbs should not be actively warmed. Such techniques include passive reclination in a blanket; direct transfer of heat by body-to-body contact; hot-tub bathing; use of hot-water suits, blankets, and mattresses; use of the radiant heat cradle; showering and use of electric blankets and heat packs.

Core Rewarming

Core rewarming methods provide heat directly to the "core" of the body, which is usually considered to be the contents of the trunk beneath the skeletomuscular and adipose shell. The application of heat to the core does not greatly disturb the state of peripheral vasoconstriction in the extremities and body-surface layers; thus, the problems of afterdrop and possible fibrillation and cardiac arrest, as well as rewarming shock, are avoided. Internally applied heat also significantly improves the cardiovascular functioning of the cold heart.

The literature is somewhat divided on the efficacy of core rewarming techniques. Some experts claim them to be relatively simple methods available in most hospitals or even in minimally equipped medical outposts. Others claim that, despite their theoretical advantage in rewarming, they have limited applicability because the equipment and skilled medical teams needed to attend the victim take time to assemble and any delay in providing treatment could result in a fatality. In addition, most of the core warming methods involve a risk of infection and other damage for the patient, particularly when the treatment is under field conditions. Consequently, the rise of core warming methods is not recommended for stable patients.

Core warming methods include respiratory heating, peritoneal dialysis, mediastinal irrigation, extracorporeal circulation, hemodialysis, intragastric lavage, colonic lavage, and various forms of diathermy. The usefulness of one of these methods, respiratory warming, has attracted considerable attention recently, and it is the subject of Chapter 17, by Dr. Donald E. Roberts, Dr. John F. Patton, and Donald W. Kerr.

Comparisons of Methods of Rewarming

There are many conflicting reports in the literature on the efficacy of various rewarming techniques. In one recent review (10), it was stated that there is no statistical evidence that the death rate is lower with any one method of rewarming as compared to another. In fact, it has been claimed that all have a poor success rate.

There has been a gradual improvement in most, if not all, rewarming techniques over the last two decades. In 1961, Duguid, Simpson, and Stowers (11) stated that of 23 elderly chronic hypothermia victims only 3 survived treatment and another 4 were brought to normothermia only to die of other diseases. Of the others, 16 died during rewarming, 13 in the first day of treatment. Such poor rates of success were confirmed by other workers (12) in 1964. Of 15 chronic victims spontaneously rewarmed, only 3 survived rewarming, 1 of them dying within a week after treatment.

During the early 1970s, greater success was reported. Ledingham and More described the rewarming of 30 patients in 1972 (13), with rewarming to normothermia achieved in 28 and an overall survival rate of 76%. In 1980 (14), they reviewed their success rate again for the period of 1963 to 1978. Of the 44 cases of drug-related hypothermia, rewarming to normothermia was achieved in all cases, with the subsequent death of 12 people. When an additional 77 cases of other types of hypothermia were included in the evaluation, the overall mortality rate was about 60%.

In another instance, Bowman (15) stated that the risk of fatality for treatment of mild hypothermia was 25%; for moderate cases, 52%; for severe cases, 66%; and overall for all cases, 49%.

The fatality rate appears to be highest for elderly victims (about 80%) as compared with very young victims (about 10%) (16). It is about 30% for those patients with core temperatures in the region of 33.9°C to 35°C. Accidental hypothermia as a percentage of all hospital admissions in various hospitals in North America and Great Britain appears to be quite high, approximately 1% to 2% of all admissions, the majority of those being elderly victims of chronic hypothermia with disease- and drug-related complications.

An extensive review of the statistics on rewarming is Gregory and Doolittle's 1973 report pertinent to Alaska (4). Of 201 treatment cases studied, 103 (51.2%) survived rewarming and 98 (48.8%) died. All cases were characterized by firm diagnosis and treatment, the vast majority (194 of 201) being treated by external means. The method of rewarming did not appear to be as important to success in the treatment of moderate hypothermia as compared to severe hypothermia. In patients treated by surface means, the success rate decreased in correlation to the body temperature of the victim at point of initiation of treatment. The mortality rate for passive surface techniques was lower (44.6%) than for active surface techniques (60.3%). All patients (7) rewarmed by core-temperature rewarming techniques survived. Peritoneal dialysis seemed to be particularly useful for managing renal insufficiency as well as certain drug-related problems. All core-temperature techniques reviewed except peritoneal dialysis were criticized as being too slow to implement and as requiring expensive medical teams and equipment.

The comparative speed of rewarming and ease of application in either the field or the hospital for the various methods are shown in Table I-1, which is based on information from a number of different studies.

Table I-1
Comparison of Methods of Rewarming

Method	Rate of Core-Temperature Increase (°C per hour)	Ease of Implementation	
		Field	Hospital
Surface Techniques:			
Blanket insulation in warm room	0.5-1.0	Good	Good
Body-heat rewarming	Low	Good	Superfluous
Radiation treatment (heat cradle)	0.5-1.0	Poor	Good
Hot-bath rewarming	3-4	Good	Good
Hot-water suit, blanket, mattress	1-2	Good	Good
Hot-water showers	1-2	Good	Superfluous
Electric blanket, heat pack	Approx. 1	Good	Good
Core Techniques			
Respiratory rewarming	0.5-2.0	Good	Good
Peritoneal dialysis	0.5-4.5	Poor	Good
Mediastinal irrigation	8.0	Poor	Good
Extracorporeal circulation	7.0-10.5	Poor	Good
Hemodialysis	0.5	Poor	Good
Intragastric lavage	2-3	Poor	Good
Colonic lavage	Low	Good	Good
Diathermy (microwave)	4.7	Poor	Good
Food and Drink	Negligible	Good	Good

Near-Drowning

As Dr. Barbara B. Tabeling points out in Chapter 18, drowning and near-drowning complicate the treatment of acute immersion hypothermia. Simultaneous cardiac and respiratory arrest may take place when water enters the nose and ears of the victim, precipitating a vagal reflex that causes cardiac slowing and minimal inhalation of water. The heart is then submitted to hypoxia, ever filling, with an excess of potassium ions and a deficit of sodium ions. The low temperature of the environment protects the brain against anoxic inury from the prolonged cardiac arrest so that, if proper treatment is applied within a certain period after the incident, resuscitation from the drowning and hypothermia with minimal neurological damage is possible. The small body mass of children accentuates the possibility of survival compared to the chances for older and more massive individuals since children experience more rapid and severe hypothermia. This topic is explored by Dr. Richard S. K. Young and Dr. Keith A. Marks in Chapter 2. The body-core temperature of a naked anesthetized infant can be lowered to 24°C or 25°C in little more than 30 minutes with ice-water cooling. Cardiac arrest, not fibrillation, occurs in such cases.

Initial resuscitation measures include ventilation with 100% oxygen via an endotracheal tube and intravenous administration of sodium bicarbonate, epinephrine, and calcium carbonate. Surface warming can be done with hot, wet towels and hot-water bottles; core warming can be carried out with hot-water enemas and gastric lavage. Postive-pressure respiration assists breathing.

Descriptions of many cases, particularly children, treated this way have appeared in the literature. The majority of the patients have survived without serious neurological deficits. No correlation has been demonstrated between postimmersion intelligence quotient and either estimated survival time or water temperature. No long-term emotional or personality disorders have been manifested, even in cases involving several hours of cardiac arrest. However, in cold-immersion experiments on dogs (17), it was shown that multiple focal areas of necrosis of varying size were distributed throughout the brains of the animals. These areas were related to the presence of blood in the brain during hypothermia and were reduced in dogs receiving low-molecular-weight dextran after circulatory arrest. No cerebral lesions were found that could be ascribed to exhaustion of metabolites or to profound hypothermia without circulatory arrest.

Questions That Remain to be Answered

Despite the comprehensiveness of the chapters comprising this volume, it is clear that more experimental work must be done to resolve certain troublesome questions. When is fast rewarming contraindicated? When are surface techniques more suitable than core-rewarming techniques? What combinations of surface and core rewarming techniques are compatible, and to what degree of benefit?

One important modifying parameter often neglected in hypothermia studies is the importance of circadian rhythm as it effects the disposition of humans to this malady. This topic is elegantly discussed in Chapter 6 by Dr. Martin C. Moore-Ede, who further points out that dissociation between thermoregulatory circadian rhythms might be a particular problem for the elderly that leaves them more vulnerable to hypothermia than are younger individuals. This is an important area for future research.

Ethical considerations quite rightly limit experiments on human volunteers to mild hypothermia associated with core temperatures of 35°C. Animal experiments can provide some guidance for treating moderate and severe hypothermia, and case histories of accidental victims who are admitted to hospitals can also provide some clues to the most efficacious techniques in specific cases. It is not inconceivable that the mathematical modeling of the rewarming process might be able to provide answers for these questions.

References

1. Molnar G: Survival of hypothermia by men immersed in the ocean. Jour Amer Med Assoc 131:1046-1050, 1946.
2. Burton A, Edholm O: Man in a Cold Environment. London, Edward Arnold 1955.
3. Keatinge W: Survival in Cold Water. Oxford and Edinburgh, Blackwell Scientific Publishing, 1969.
4. Gregory R, Doolittle W: Accidental hypothermia: Part II. Clinical implications of experimental studies, Alaska Med. 15:48-52, 1973.
5. Golden F: Accidental hypothermia, Jour Roy Nav Med Serv *58*:196-206, 1972.
6. Jessen K: Central rewarming technique in the treatment of profound accidental hypothermia, AGARD Conference No. 286 on Aircrew Safety and Survivability (Limited to Combat Aircraft), May 1980.
7. Webb P: Rewarming after diving in cold water. Aerospace Med *44*:1152-1157, 1973.
8. Collis M, Steinman A, Chaney R: Accidental hypothermia: Experimental study of practical rewarming methods. Av Space Environ Med *48*:625-632, 1977.
9. Hayward J, Eckerson J, Collis M: Treatment of accidental hypothermia: An experimental study of inhalation rewarming. Univ. of Victoria Report (U.S. Coast Guard Contract 09-7025-75), June 1975.
10. Anonymous: Rewarming for accidental hypothermia. Lancet *1*:251-252, 1978.
11. Duguid H, Simpson R, Stowers J: Accidental hypothermia, Lancet *2*:1213-1219, 1961.
12. McNicol M, Smith R: Accidental hypothermia, Brit Med Jour *1*:19-21, 1964.
13. Ledingham I, Mone J: Treatment after exposure to cold. Lancet *1*:534-535, 1972.
14. Ledingham I, Mone J: Treatment of accidental hypothermia: A prospective clinical study, Brit Med Jour *2*:1102-1105, 1980.

15. Bowman W: Comments made in "Medical aspects of mountain climbing." Jour Winter Emerg Care *2*:31-47, 1977.
16. Vaisrab S: Accidental hypothermia in the elderly. Jour Amer Med Assoc *239*:1888, 1978.
17. Edmunds H, Folkman J, Snodgrass A, Brown R: Prevention of brain damage during profound hypothermia and circulatory arrest, Annals Surg *157*:637-649, 1963.

PART I. The Diagnosis of Hypothermia

CHAPTER ONE

The Physiology of Immersion Hypothermia

J. S. Hayward, B.Sc., Ph.D.

The physiology of hypothermia in humans can be divided into three categories related to the stage or circumstances of cooling. One is the condition of induced hypothermia in a clinical setting, in which anesthetized patients are cooled in order to reduce the oxygen demand of tissues during certain brain and heart operations. In this situation, the hypothermic physiology is passive and poikilothermic in nature. The second category of hypothermic physiology is also passive; it pertains to the comatose victim of accidental hypothermia. The important difference between the first and the second categories is that the comatose state in the second often has been preceded by an initial period of active physiological regulation in the body's attempt to defend normothermia. As a result, such a comatose victim exhibits a number of physiological features that are a legacy of the previous defensive phase.

The third category of hypothermic physiology is the initial defensive phase just mentioned. For those concerned with the treatment of victims with severe hypothermia, it is important to appreciate the physiological features of conscious persons attempting to thermoregulate their bodies during the period of cooling to the poikilothermic level. This presentation attempts to review the major physiological attributes of humans during the defensive phase, with cold-water immersion used as the example. As could be expected, the responses are essentially those of a specialized case of stress physiology, and they mimic, at least initially, intensive sympathetic stimulation. The results presented here are derived from experimental studies on humans during cooling to levels as low as 33°C to 34°C core temperature. They are derived from the work of several researchers over about the last two decades.

Respiratory Responses

A conspicuous reflex response to sudden immersion in cold water is hyperventilation (1, 2, 3). Cold receptors in the deep skin provide a massive drive to the respiratory control system during the first few minutes of immersion. The pulmonary ventilation rate during the first minute increases to approximately five times the level of preimmersion rest as a result of increases in both respiratory frequency and tidal volume. End-tidal pCO_2 falls to 20 to 25 torr. Typical results are shown in Figure 1-1. Recent findings in the author's laboratory for subjects suddenly immersed in 0°C water show similar magnitudes of ventilatory responses. The respiratory quotient (RQ) was also measured and gave values of 1.4 to 1.7 commensurate with the high rate of $C0_2$ release. The hyperventilation response is greatest during the first minute or two, and by 5 min the ventilation rate is reduced to a level more dependent on metabolic rate.

The practical consequences of this hyperventilation are several. The initial gasping facilitates aspiration of water and the likelihood of drowning. Some individuals are much more responsive with hyperventilation than others; this results in prolonged reduction of arterial pCO_2, which can lead to reduced cerebral blood flow with clouding of consciousness or to muscular tetany with reduced swimming ability (1). A number of factors attenuate the hyperventilation response. These include protective clothing, preheating in a sauna, and habituation to cold-water immersion. There is also evidence that the response of females is less than that of males and is independent of differences in subcutaneous fatness.

This respiratory stimulation also has an effect on breath-hold duration during submersion in cold water. A recent study in the author's laboratory showed maximum breath-hold time during submersion in 0°C-to-15°C water of only 15 to 25 sec.

Cardiovascular Responses

It is well known that the primary physiological defense against cold is peripheral vasoconstriction. This certainly applies to cold-water immersion, although no thorough study of the change in total

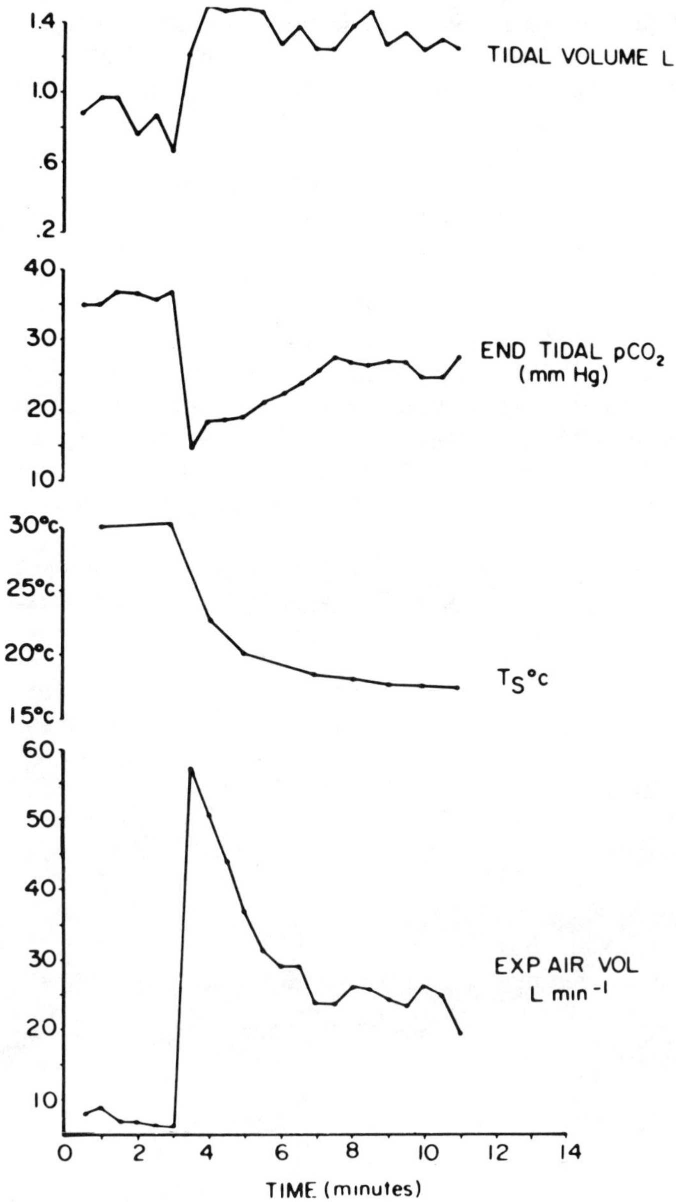

Figure 1-1. Ventilatory responses in relation to skin temperature (T_S) of a subject immersed (at minute 3) in 15°C water. (From Cooper et al. [1].)

peripheral resistance during cold-water immersion is presently available. Many studies on limb blood flow show great reduction in perfusion and shift of venous return to deep vessels, which potentiate countercurrent heat exchange. This relative ischemia of the limbs, which is so important to peripheral tissue insulation, has metabolic consequences, such as acidosis and electrolyte changes, that are important to the management of the hypothermia victim after rescue.

In very cold water (e.g., less than 10°C), cold-induced vasodilatation due to cold paralysis of vascular smooth muscle (4) is a possibility. This condition is very obvious from the reddening of the skin of subjects during prolonged immersion in cold water. However, this author has not observed sudden increases in core cooling rate commensurate with skin vasodilatation. It is probable that constriction of deeper vessels in warmer tissues is being maintained such that skin blood flow is negligible despite skin dilatation. Cyanosis could be avoided because of the higher solubility of oxygen in cold blood and skin, together with the insignificant oxygen consumption of the cold skin.

The heart rate increases greatly during the initial shock of cold-water immersion and subsequently depends on changes in metabolic

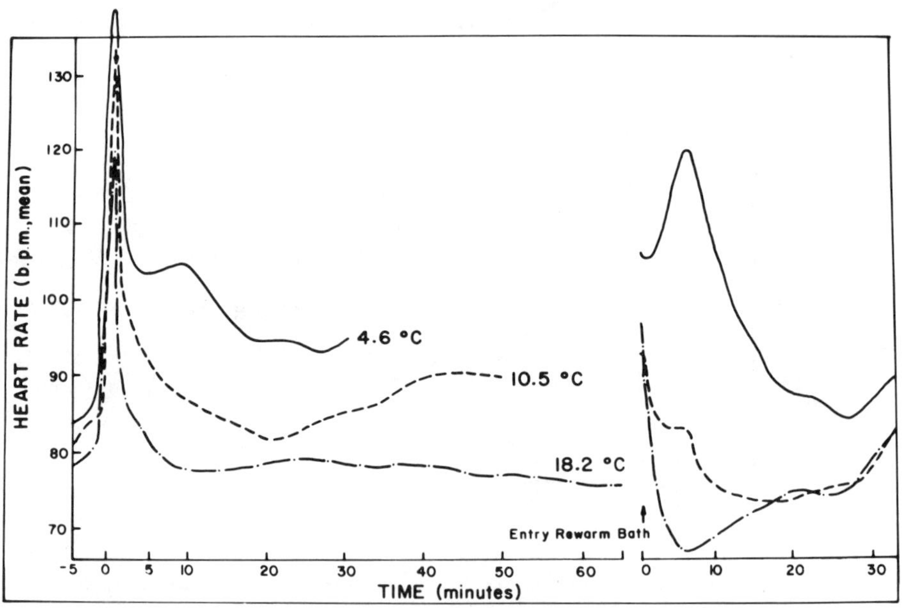

Figure 1-2. Mean heart-rate response for subjects at three water temperatures and during rewarming in a 42°C bath. (from McKay [5].)

rate (5). Typical results at three water temperatures are shown in Figure 1-2. If immersion is prolonged until maximum shivering thermogenesis is attained (see later section), the heart rate of nonexercising subjects can rise as high as 130 to 140 beats per minute.

A recent study in the author's laboratory monitored arterial pressure and cardiac output during immersion in 10°C water. Systolic pressure rose from a preimmersion level of about 130 mm Hg to 180 to 190 mm Hg during most of a 2-hour immersion. Cardiac output by Swan-Ganz catheter increased from 5 to 6 L perminute to 8 to 10 L per minute.

Electrocardiographic recordings during cold-water immersion show several characteristics. During the early, shock phase, occasional atrial and ventricular extrasystoles and sinus arrhythmias are observed (4, 5). It is likely that cardiac dysfunction is one of the factors contributing to occasional sudden deaths in cold water (4). With progression into mild hypothermia, there are small but stastically significant increases in the QT interval and in the amplitude of the T wave (5). J-point deflection and ST-segment elevation or depression are rarely seen in mild hypothermia down to 34°C in conscious subjects (5).

A victim's submersion in cold water while he or she is holding his or her breath illicits the well-known bradycardia of the dive reflex. Recent results in the author's laboratory show that the bradycardia is only about 15% greater in water of 25°C or less than it is in warm water of 30°C to 35°C. There is no significant increase in the bradycardia below 25°C water temperature. This suggests that the enhanced resuscitatability of cold-water near-drowning victims is due to the effect of lowered temperature on the tissue's oxygen demand rather than to significant improvement in the dive reflex in cold water.

Endocrine Responses

Typical of stress physiology, cold-water immersion stimulates catecholamine and adrenal steroid output. Catecholamines have received the most study. Urinary levels of epinephrine and norepinephrine increase (6). Plasma norepinephrine increases to approximately three times the preimmersion level (Figure 1-3) and is directly correlated with metabolic rate (7).

Diuresis

It is well known that humans suffering from hypothermia as a result of exposure to cold, dry air (e.g., during a mountaineering accident)

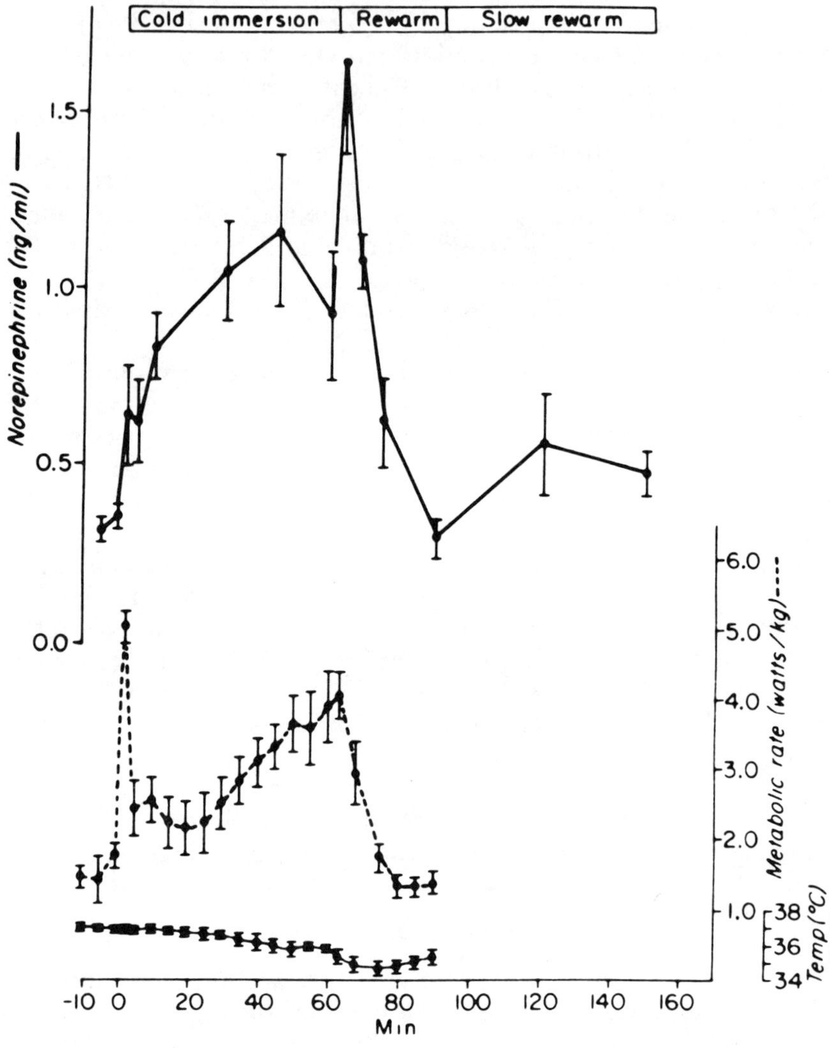

Figure 1-3. Plasma norepinephrine, metabolic rate, and rectal temperature during cooling in 10°C water followed by rewarming in a 42° bath. (From Johnson et al. [7].)

are frequently hypovolemic due to water loss via several routes and to inadequate water intake. For this reason, therapy calls for fluid restoration as well as rewarming. During cold-water immersion, fluid loss is also increased due to the combination of immersion and cold-induced diuresis (8, 9). Figure 1-4 shows that urine flow rate doubles with immersion in thermoneutral water and is increased 3.5-fold when the water is cold. Water pressure and peripheral vasoconstruction combine to increase central blood volume, causing reflex diuresis. The results in Figure 1-4 also show that alcohol inhibition of vasopressin secretion causes a further increase in diuresis when combined with cold-water immersion. Prolonged immersion in moderately cold water could readily lead to a level of fluid loss that warrants the same remedial attention directed to those suffering from air-exposure hypothermia.

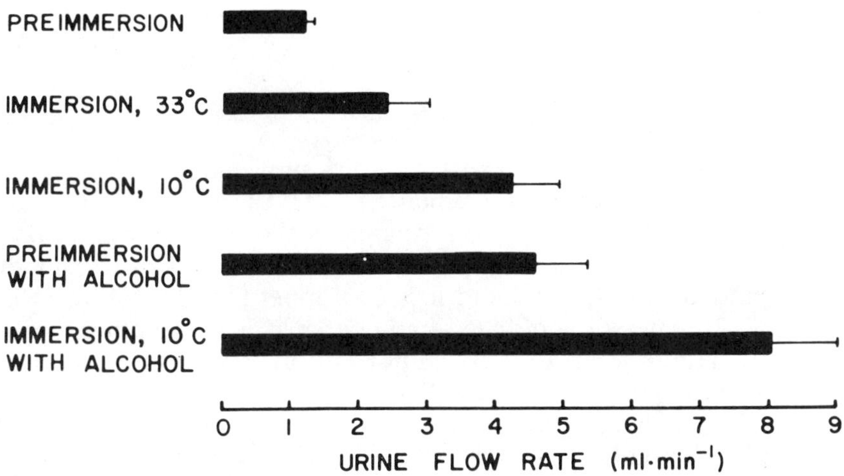

Figure 1-4. Effects of immersion, temperature, and alcohol on the urine flow rate of humans. (From Cupples et al. [8].)

Neuromuscular Effects

As a consequence of the strong peripheral vasoconstruction that defends core temperature during cold-water immersion, the temperatures of limb muscles and nerves fall considerably. Limb strength, coordination, and response time deteriorate accordingly. A study of seminude subjects in 10°C water found that after the first 5 min of immersion grip strength began to fall at a rate of approximately 1.8% per minute (1). There was also a considerable decrease in conduction velocity in the large fibers of the peripheral nerves and an increase in twitch time in response to direct stimulation of the muscles. Such cold-induced decrement in the performance of limb musculature is a major contributing factor to cold-water fatalities in cases in which victims need to swim or to pull themselves out of the water.

Study of the electroencephalogram (frequency-components, amplitudes, visual-evoked responses) of conscious subjects cooled to 33°C to 34°C in 10°C water showed that only very minor changes in brain function occur with mild to moderate hypothermia (10). Apparently, an even lower brain temperature is required to cause significant impairment of conscious, integrative function. This does not mean that a mildly hypothermic brain is always able to control behavior in a rational, survival-oriented manner. There are many tragic examples of victims who must have suffered only mild brain cooling but who "gave up," panicked, or otherwise showed disorganized mental activity under conditions of intense peripheral discomfort, alarm, and fear, which accompany cold-water accidental immersion.

Heat Loss

The high rate of heat transfer from the skin of immersed humans to cold water has been well documented (11, 12, 13). The resultant cooling of various body regions is related to the extent of blood-flow reduction and to the surface-volume relationship of the segment. Fingers and toes and arms and legs cool most rapidly, followed by the trunk. In cases of prolonged immersion, it is the cooling rate of the trunk region that is most important in determining survival. Thermographic evidence (Figure 1-5) has been presented to indicate some variation in the rate of heat loss from various regions of the trunk (14). Normally, personal flotation devices should keep the head and most of the neck out of the water. When these areas of high levels of heat loss are also underwater (e.g., in "drownproofing"), the body's total heat loss and cooling rate are greatly increased (15).

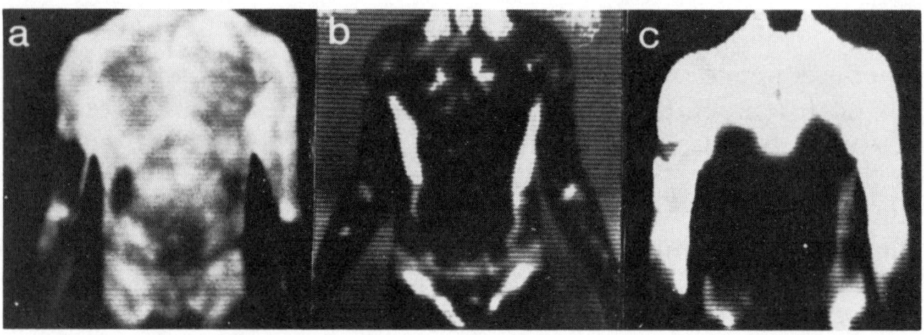

Figure 1-5. Thermograms indicating relative heat loss areas of humans (a) before immersion in 7.5°C water, (b) immediately after holding still in the water for 15 min, and (c) after swimming for 15 min. (From Hayward et al. [13].)

Despite the obvious and critical problem of high heat loss in humans immersed in cold water, no adequate, quantitative assessment of total body heat loss (e.g., but direct calorimetry) at various water temperatures is available.

Metabolic Heat Production

The metabolic response of humans to cold-water immersion has been studied by several researchers (12, 16, 17, 18). The initial response (e.g., at 15 min of immersion of a lightly clothed, nonexercising human) is a function of water temperature, $Hm = 4.19 - 0.11T_W$, where H_m is metabolic heat production in kilocalories per minute and T_W is water temperature in degrees Celsius (12). It has been shown (12) that the initial response is similar in magnitude to that of a nude human in cold air of the same temperature with a wind speed between 5 and 10 miles per hour. The thermogenic response evolved as a response to skin temperature (in air), not to the rate of heat loss in water. During prolonged immersion, the metabolic response is augmented by core cooling (Figure 1-6) according to a multiplicative relationship between skin and core thermal signals (18). The thermoregulatory heat production of a human in cold water is highly correlated with the electrical activity of shivering muscles (EMG) (18). Maximum shivering thermogenesis in humans is approximately 4.5 times the resting rate of heat production. Figure 1-6 also shows that in the absence of a cold skin (10 min of bath rewarming) metabolic heat production above the resting level is not stimulated in spite of considerable core hypothermia.

It is not known how long individuals can maintain an elevated shivering level or at what core temperature shivering fails. Various evidence suggests that shivering does not fail completely until unconsciousness occurs at a brain temperature near 30°C or below. Hypoglycemia induced by fatigue, and especially in conjunction with alcohol intoxication, can reduce metabolic heat production during entry into hypothermia (19).

Cooling Rate

Despite the thermoregulatory responses of immersed, unprotected humans in water temperatures lower than about 25°C, heat loss overwhelms heat production and core cooling results (Figure 1-6). In lightly clothed, nonexercising young men and women, cooling rate (C, in degrees Celsius per minute) is a function of water temperature (T_W, in degrees Celsius) according to the equation $C = 0.0785 - 0.0034T_W$,

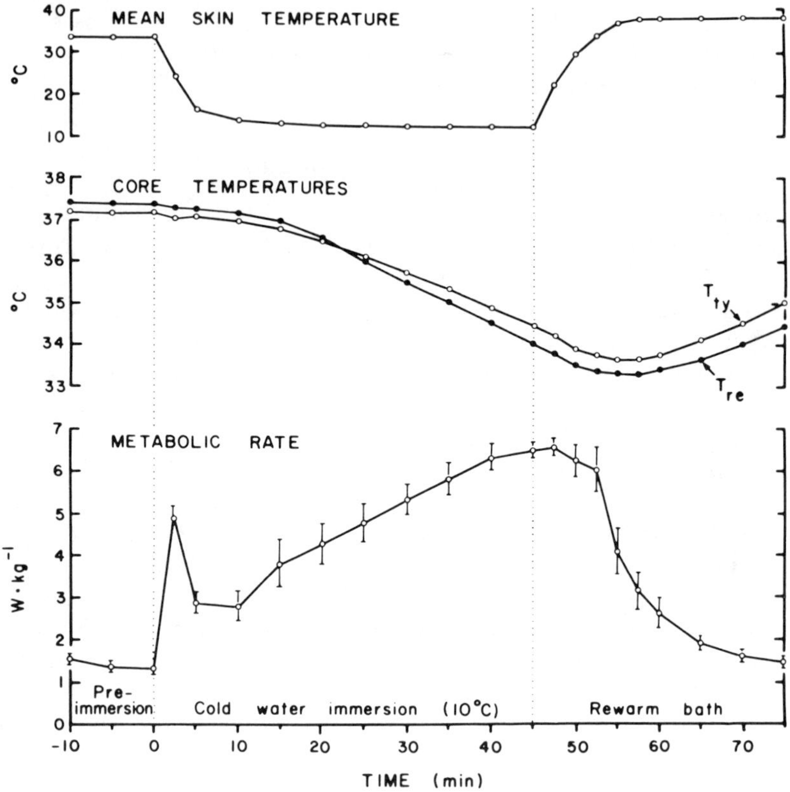

Figure 1-6. Metabolic heat production of nonexercising male during cold-water immersion and bath rewarming in relation to skin and core (tympanic [T_{ty}], rectal [T_{re}]) temperatures. (From Hayward et al. [17].)

which describes the line shown in Figure 1-7. Based on such cooling rate data, it is possible to estimate survival time in cold water. When a core temperature of 30°C is chosen as a point of "incipient death" (when the victim is likely to become semiconscious and drown or to have cardiac problems), a generalized graph such as Figure 1-8 can be constructed. This graph represents a central tendency, but the shaded area around the line representing the mean attempts to indicate a portion of the *large* amount of individual variation that exists in cooling rate and predicted survival time. A recent study performed in the author's laboratory on 10 male and 10 female subjects (all of

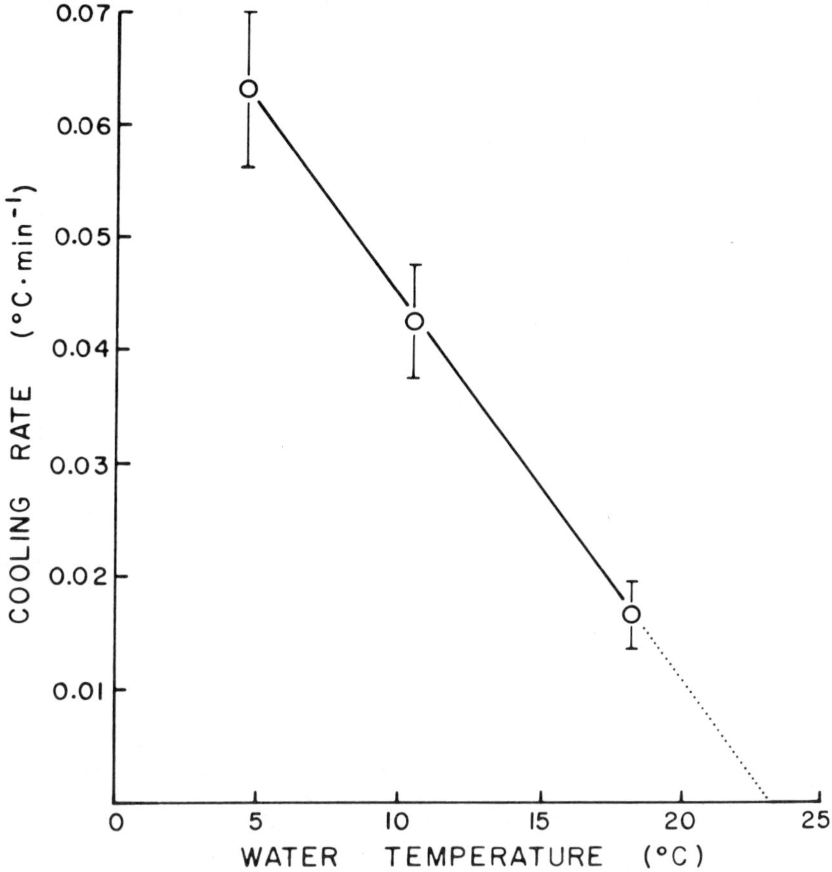

Figure 1-7. Mean rectal cooling rate of nonexercising, lightly clothed males and females during immersion in seawater at different temperatures. (From Hayward et al. [11].)

whom were lightly clothed and who were immersed in 0°C water) confirmed cooling rates and led to the prediction of an average survival time at this water temperature of about 1.5 hr, as indicated in Figure 1-8.

It is important to consider the major factors that are known to influence the cooling rate of humans under any specific set of cold-water conditions. The following outline briefly describes these factors.

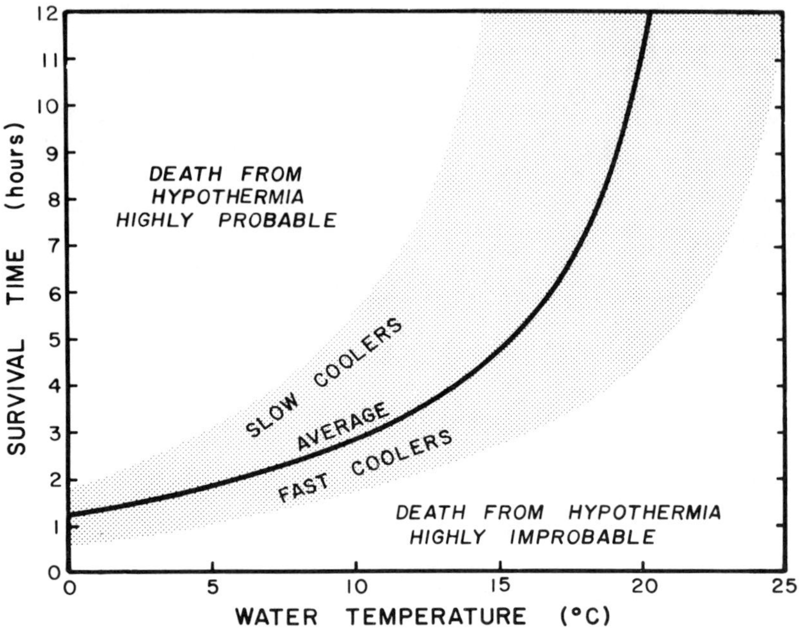

Figure 1-8. Predicted survival time of lightly clothed, nonexercising humans in cold water based on the time required to cool to 30°C core temperature. The graph shows a line for the average expectancy and a broad zone that indicates the large amount of individual variability associated with different body size, build, and fatness. The zone would include approximately 95% of the variation expected for adult and teenage humans under the conditions specified. The zone would be shifted downward by physical activity such as swimming and upward slightly by thermally protective behaviors and heavy clothing. Specialized survival suits and jackets are capable of increasing survival time from 2 to 10 times (or more) the basic duration shown here. In the zone where death from hypothermia is highly improbable, cold water greatly facilitates death from drowning, often in the first 10 to 15 minutes, and especially for those not wearing a PFD.

A. Individual Differences

1. *Subcutaneous Fatness:* The amount of subcutaneous fatness is the most important variable determining cooling rate through its effect on tissue insulation (20, 21, 22, 23).
2. *Body Size:* Larger body size is accompanied by a reduction of the surface-to-volume ratio and core cooling rate (22, 24). Children cool faster than adults for this reason and because they generally have less fat than adults (23, 25).

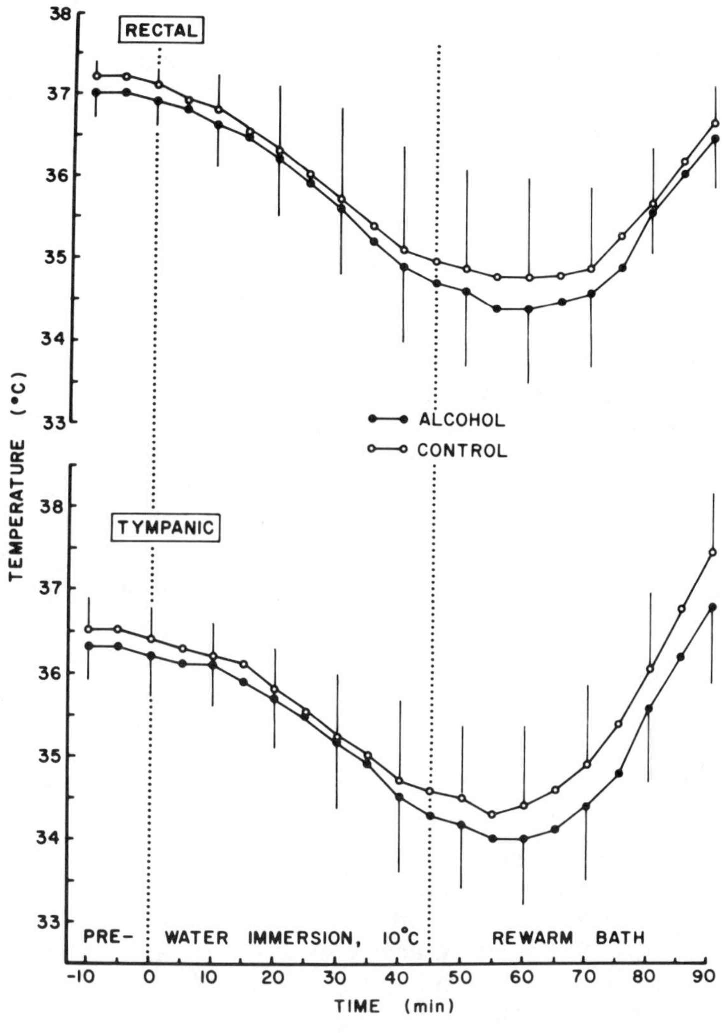

Figure 1-9. Core cooling rates with and without alcohol intoxication (70 to 85 mg%) during cold-water immersion and bath rewarming. (From Fox et al. [26].)

3. *Body Build (Somatotype):* For any one body weight and fatness, mesomorphs cool more slowly than ectomorphs (again, due to differences in surface-to-volume ratio (22, 26).
4. *Shivering Response:* There are substantial differences among

individuals in their shivering response (12). Good shiverers tend to cool more slowly.

5. *Alcohol Intoxication:* High doses of alcohol impair thermoregulation. Doses of alcohol in the range of legal impairment (80 to 100 mg% or less) do not significantly affect the cooling rate in cold water (27, 28) (Figure 1-9).

B. Behavioral Effects

1. *Activity:* Gross physical activity (e.g., swimming) especially activity involving the limbs, counteracts peripheral vasoconstriction and increases tissue conductance and heat loss to a greater extent than any increase consequent in heat production (28). Core cooling is about one-third faster when an unprotected human is moving than when he or she is holding still and shivering in cold water (12).
2. *Posture:* Any posture that reduces the amount of the body's surface exposed to the cold water reduces heat loss (15). Assuming a curled-up, arms-close-to-the-chest, and legs-together posture is an instinctive aspect of behavioral thermoregulation. The cooling rate can be reduced by a small (but often important) amount. The huddling of two or more persons with maximum body contact is an example of the same principle (15).

C. Technological Factors

The "behavioral physiology" of humans includes their technological capacity, which provides the greatest scope for variation in the cooling rate in cold water.

1. *Regular Clothing:* The more clothing worn, the less heat loss (29, 30). This tends to have only a minor effect on the cooling rate since regular clothing is not designed to be effective when submerged in water.
2. *Special Survival Garments:* A variety of suits and jackets that provide a wide range of thermal protection in the event of accidental immersion in cold water are now available (31). The special garments keep the wearer dry beneath the garments and/or surround the wearer's body with closed-cell foam. Dry, foam suits (e.g., Figure 1-10), especially when combined with thick clothing worn beneath them, can provide insulation that rivals the blubber of marine mammals.

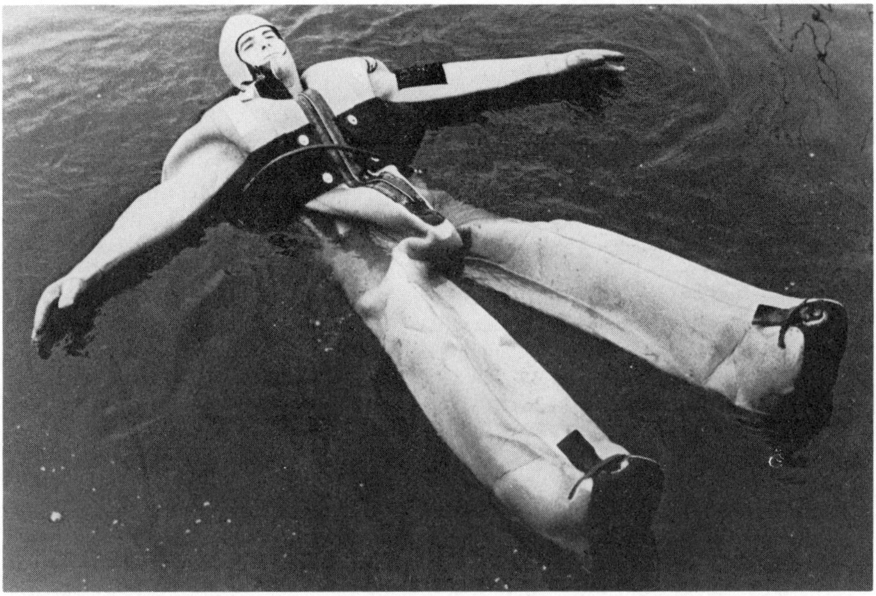

Figure 1-10. Example of a dry, foam survival suit for use during accidental immersion in cold water.

Acclimatization

There is no evidence that a training or habituation program of cold-water immersion can alter the physiology of human thermoregulation to an extent sufficient to reduce significantly the core cooling rate when humans are confronted with a severe thermal challenge (32). However, acclimatization can have important local effects on some areas of the body, such as the hands (33). Minor changes in metabolic rate and vasoconstriction of cold-acclimatized individuals are inconsequential in comparison to changes in subcutaneous fatness or the effect of wearing special insulating garments. This is not to say there is no value in such training. Indeed, there is good evidence that habituation or "familiarization" with cold-air or cold-water exposure leads to improved performance of mental tasks during cold stress (32). Familiarization with cold-water immersion could play a major role in the psychology of survival during cold-immersion accidents. Many sad stories of accidental immersion in cold water document the panic and irrational behavior experienced by humans shocked for the first time by severe cold stress. These seem to be cases of "the physiology is still willing, but the psychology is not."

References

1. Cooper KE, Martin S, Riben P: Respiratory and other responses in subjects immersed in cold water, Jour Appl Physiol *40*:903-910, 1976.
2. Goode RC, Duffin J, Miller R, Romet TT, Chant W, Ackles K: Sudden cold water immersion. Resp Physiol *23*:301-310, 1975.
3. Keatinge WR, Evans M: The respiratory and cardiovascular response to immersion in cold and warm water. Q Jour Exp Physiol *46*:83-94, 1961.
4. Keatinge WR: Survival in Cold Water. Oxford, Blackwell Scientific Publishing, 1969.
5. McKay WR: Man in cold water: Heart rate and electrocardiographic responses. M.Sc. thesis, University of Victoria, Victoria, B.C., 1977.
6. Gale CC, Hayward JS, Green WL, Wu SY, Schiller H, Jackson I: Endocrine response to cold in man. Fed Proc *34*:301, 1975.
7. Johnson DG, Hayward JS, Jacobs TP, Collis ML, Eckerson JD, Williams RH: Plasma norepinephrine responses of man in cold water. Jour Appl Physiol: Respirat Environ Exercise Physiol *43*:216-220, 1977.
8. Cupples WA, Fox GR, Hayward JS: Effect of cold water immersion and its combination with alcohol intoxication on urine flow rate of man. Can Jour Physiol Pharmacol *58*:319-321, 1980.
9. DeForest RE, Beckman EL: Some contraindications to use of life jacket for survival. Arch Environ Health *4*:56-64, 1962.
10. Fitzgibbon T, Hayward JS: EEG and evoked potentials of conscious man during moderate hypothermia. EEG Clin Neurophysiol (submitted).
11. Bullard RW, Rapp GM: Problems of body heat loss in water immersion. Aerospace Med *41*:1269-1277, 1970.
12. Hayward JS, Eckerson JD, Collis ML: Thermal balance and survival time prediction of man in cold water. Can Jour Physiol Pharmacol *53*:21-32, 1975.
13. Witherspoon JM, Goldman RF, Breckenridge JR: Heat transfer coefficients of humans in cold water. Jour Physiol (Paris) *63*:459-462, 1971.
14. Hayward JS, Collis M, Eckerson JD: Thermographic evaluation of relative heat loss areas of man during cold water immersion. Aerospace Med *44*:708-711, 1973.
15. Hayward JS, Eckerson JD, Collis ML: Effect of behavioral variables on cooling rate of man in cold water. Jour Appl Physiol *38*:1073-1077, 1975.
16. Cannon P, Keatinge WR: The metabolic rate and heat loss of fat and thin men in heat balance in cold and warm water. Jour Physiol *154*:329-344, 1960.
17. Craig AB, Dvorak M: Thermal regulation during water immersion. Jour Appl Physiol *21*:1577-1585, 1966.
18. Hayward JS, Eckerson JD, Collis ML: Thermoregulatory heat production in man: Prediction equation based on skin and core temperatures. Jour Appl Physiol: Respirat Environ Exercise Physiol *42*:377-384, 1977.
19. Haight JSJ, Keatinge WR: Failure of thermoregulation in the cold during hypoglycaemia induced by exercise and ethanol. Jour Physiol *229*:87-97, 1973.
20. Carlson LD, Hsieh ACL, Fullington F, Elsner RW: Immersion in cold water and body tissue insulation. Aerospace Med *29*:145-152, 1958.
21. Keatinge WR: The effects of subcutaneous fat and of previous exposure to cold on the body temperature, peripheral blood flow and metabolic rate of men in cold water. Jour Physiol *153*:166-178, 1960.

22. Pugh LGCE, Edholm OG, Fox RH, Wolff HS, Hervey GR, Hammond WH, Tanner JM, Whitehouse RH: A physiological study of channel swimming. Clin Sci *19*:257-273, 1960.
23. Timbal J, Loncle M. Boutelier C: Mathematical model of man's tolerance to cold using morphological factors. Av Space Environ Med *47*:958-964, 1976.
24. Kreider MB: Death and survival during water immersion: Account of plane crashes near Cape Cod and Hamilton Bay. Aerospace Med *38*:1060-1062, 1967.
25. Sloan REG, Keatinge WR: Cooling rates of young people swimming in cold water. Jour Appl Physiol *35*:371-375, 1973.
26. Mitchell JW, Galvez TL, Hengle J, Myers GE, Siebecker KL: Thermal response of human legs during cooling. Jour Appl Physiol *29*:859-865, 1970.
27. Fox GR, Hayward JS, Hobson GN: Effect of alcohol on thermal balance of man in cold water. Can Jour Physiol Pharmacol *57*:860-865, 1979.
28. Martin S, Diewold RJ, Cooper DE: Alcohol, respiratory, skin and body temperature changes during cold water immersion. Jour Appl Physiol: Respirat Environ Exercise Physiol *43*:322-215, 1977.
29. Keatinge WR: The effect of work and clothing on the maintenance of the body temperature in water, Q Jour Exp physiol *46*:69-82, 1961.
30. Hayward JS, Eckerson JD, Collis ML: Man in Cold Water: Cooling Rate in Heavy Winter Clothing. Cleveland, U.S. Coast Guard, 1975 (reference No. 09-7025-75).
31. Hayward JS: Design Concepts of Survival Suits for Cold Water Immersion and Their Thermal Protection Performance. Canoga Park, Calif., SAFE Association, 1980.
32. Lapp MC, Gee GK: Human acclimatization to cold water immersion. Arch Environ Health *15*:568-579, 1967.
33. LeBlank J: Local adaptation to cold of Gaspé fishermen. Jour Appl Physiol *17*: 950-952, 1962.

CHAPTER TWO

Hypothermia and the Pediatric Patient

Richard S. K. Young, M.D., and Keith H. Marks, M.B.

This chapter addresses two separate clinical situations involving hypothermia and pediatric patients. The first section summarizes current knowledge about the neurological outcome of children who drown in cold water. In this setting, children suffer an acute cold injury with superimposed cerebral hypoxia and ischemia. In the second part of this chapter, the effects of hypothermia on the premature infant are discussed. Acute cold injury is much less common in this clinical situation. Instead, the primary danger to fragile neonates is the effect of chronic cold stress.

Neurological Outcome of Children Drowning in Cold Water

Morbidity and Mortality from Childhood Drowning Accidents

Before one can reach a valid conclusion about hypothermia's ameliorating effects on the anoxic injury sustained in drowning, one should review the neurological outcome of children who drown in "warm" water. Although drowning is one of three major causes of accidental death in children in the United States, there is still considerable disagreement about the morbidity and mortality associated with serious immersion accidents. Certain authors have maintained that the prognosis of children who drown is excellent (1, 2), while others draw a far more bleak picture (2, 3).

Much of the confusion about the prognosis of children who have suffered drowning accidents results from an inability to determine the degree of hypoxic injury sustained by the victim. The three studies that specifically examine the outcome of children with prolonged cardiac arrest (for whom cardiopulmonary resuscitation was required on arrival at the emergency room) conclude that these children invariably suffer neurological sequelae (3, 4, 5) (Figures 2-1, 2-2, and 2-3). Other factors that correlate positively with poor neurological outcome include need for mechanical ventilation, coma on admission (5), and initial blood pH less than 7.0. Since all of these factors may reflect cerebral hypoxia, it is likely that the final neurological outcome of drowning victims is closely related to the amount of brain injury incurred at the time of drowning.

Prognosis after Near-Drowning in Cold Water

Does drowning in cold water protect the child from the injurious effects of cerebral anoxia? Numerous anecdotal case reports and newspaper articles testify to the dramatic recovery of some children who had been submerged for as long as 40 minutes (6). Sekar and others (7) concluded that "undoubtedly, the outlook for neurologic recovery following prolonged submersion is favorably modified by the coexistence of hypothermia."

The conclusion of the single study by Kruus and associates (8)

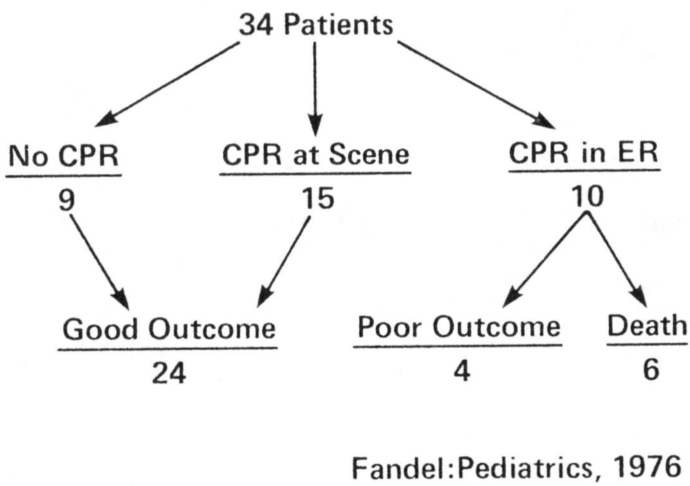

Figure 2-1. Neurological outcome of 72 patients according to whether cardiopulmonary resuscitation (CPR) was instituted. Note that patients requiring CPR on arrival at the emergency room (ER) either had a poor outcome or died.

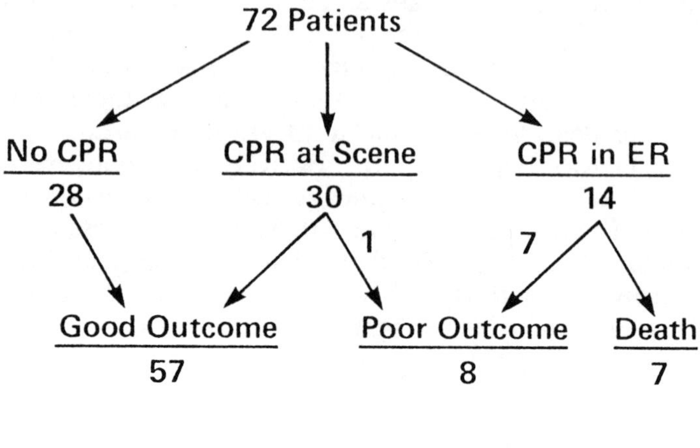

Figure 2-2. Neurological outcome of 34 patients as predicted by amount and length of CPR.

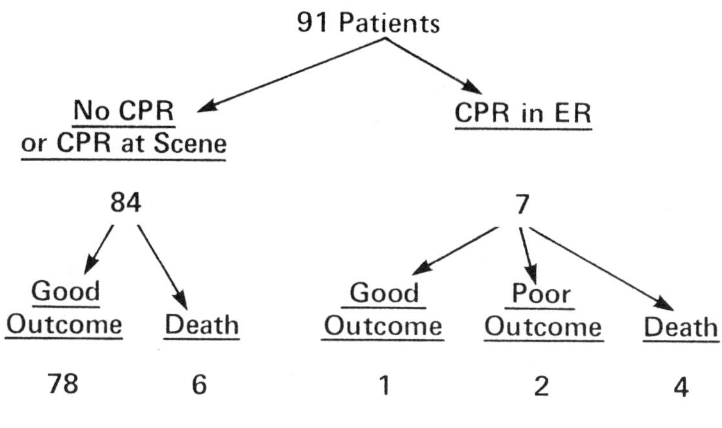

Figure 2-3. Neurological outcome of 91 patients in relation to amount and length of CPR. The majority of patients needing CPR in the emergency room either had poor neurological outcome or died.

evaluating the neurological outcome of a large group of children drowning in cold water is far less optimistic. Of the patients with an initial rectal temperature of less than 30°C, 70% had a poor neurological outcome as opposed to only 25% of patients with rectal temperatures of 35°C or more. Kruus and associates concluded that hypothermia, like a low arterial pH, is indicative of prolonged immersion and severe anoxia.

In our own experience with prolonged cold-water drowning accidents (Table 2-1), one of four patients made a slow but nearly complete recovery (6). The other three patients died 2 to 6 d after the immersion. All four showed cerebral edema, either clinically or at postmortem examination, suggesting that they had suffered severe cerebral anoxic injury.

Before attempting to reach a final conclusion about the possibly protective effects of hypothermia in the drowning victim, it would be worthwhile first to review the experimental literature.

Protective Effect of Hypothermia in Young Animals Subjected to Hypoxia

Both age and ambient temperature affect the amount of hypoxia an animal can tolerate. It was recognized more than a century ago that newborn and young animals could survive periods of hypoxia that were lethal to adults (9). This resistance to hypoxia is limited to the neonatal period, and an "adult pattern" of survival under hypoxic conditions may be attained as early as 2 wk after birth in dogs, cats, rabbits, rats, and guinea pigs.

Hypothermia may also protect the young animal from hypoxic injury. A beneficial effect of hypothermia has been shown in baby guinea pigs, kittens, puppies, baby rabbits, piglets, baby opossums, and baby hamsters subjected to asphyxia. Zakhary and associates demonstrated that hypothermia prolongs survival in puppies rendered hypoxic (Table 2-2).

Mohri and associates (11) noted that the combined protection afforded by age and hypothermia could modify neurological outcome. Puppies subjected to 50 min of cardiac arrest at temperatures of 14°C to 18°C appeared normal on recovery, but adult dogs treated in the same manner developed gait disturbances.

Whether hypothermia can protect the primate from hypoxic-ischemic injury is less certain. Early studies of fetal rhesus monkeys suggested that hypothermia has no beneficial effect on anoxic survival (12). More recent studies of juvenile rhesus monkeys have shown that they can tolerate periods of cardiac arrest as long as 75 min when cooled to temperatures of 16°C to 20°C (13). Nonetheless, 38% of the animals demonstrated transient incoordination, and 13% of the animals suffered occipital lobe infarction.

Table 2-1
Outcome of Near-Drowning Accidents in Children

Patient	Core Temperature (°C)	Age/Sex	Time Immersed	pH	Time to Establish Pulse	Clinical Course
1	27	7 yr/male	15 min	6.7	2.5 hr	Quadriplegic for 1 wk. Arms much weaker than legs. Followed commands at 3 wk. Spoke in short sentences at 6 wk. Almost completely recovered intellectual abilities by 8 mo. Complete motor recovery.
2	27	12 yr/ Male	10 min.	7.09	—	Mechanical ventilation insufficient. Worsening hypoxemia led to bowel infarction and death at 3 d. Cerebral edema on postmortem examination.
3	32	23 mo/ Male	20 min	6.63	1.5 hr	Seizures developed at 24 hr. Worsening hypoxemia led to hypotension and death at 3 d. Cerebral edema on postmortem examination.
4	25	23 mo/ Male	15 min	6.5	1.5 hr	Spontaneous respirations initially. Developed severe increased intracranial pressure. Died at 6 d.

Table 2-2
Effect of Temperature on Length of Survival in Newborn Dogs Rendered Hypoxic

Core Temperature	Length of Survival (Minutes)
Hyperthermia (42°C)	4.7
Normothermia (37°C)	15.0
Hypothermia (15°C)	30-60

Several recent studies suggest that pharmacological agents may increase survival time under hypoxic conditions. Ketosis induced by fasting or butanediol, hypoglycemia due to experimental diabetes, and physostigmine all increase the survival time of experimental animals under hyoxic conditions (9, 14). Isolating the mechanism whereby these metabolic variables may interact with hypothermia to prolong survival during hypoxic will require further study.

Cardiac Arrest and Hypothermia in Children Undergoing Open-Heart Surgery

Infants and children undergoing open-heart surgery under conditins of deep hypothermia and cardiac arrest are perhaps the best example of how the brain can tolerate complete anoxia when protected by hypothermia. In this highly controlled situation, the patient is rapidly cooled by both surface and internal means to 20°C (15), and cerebral metabolic demands are quickly minimized. Upon completion of the surgery, the hypoxic state is immediately reversed. Although early investigators (using somewhat lower temperatures of 14.5°C to 21.8°C) found that many patients died postoperatively and suffered severe brain damage to the basal ganglia and cerebellum (16, 17), more recent studies show that there is no significant difference between mean preoperative and postoperative intelligence quotients (18).

Summary

Although it is possible for children who drown in cold water to make a satisfactory recovery, a good outcome is by no means guaranteed. Children drowning in cold water differ in many respects from those who undergo cardiac arrest under deep hypothermia in an operating room. First, few drowning victims are cooled to the degree (20°C) obtained in an operating room. Second, the rate of cooling may be much slower than that accomplished in the operating room, with a resulting lag time between the cooling of the skin and the brain. Third, the hypoxic state during resuscitation may not be readily reversible because of pulmonary injury from aspiration, pneumonia, or respiratory distress syndrome.

Children who drown in cold water but suffer neurological sequelae probably do so because of one of the above factors. In addition, secondary brain injury may result from cerebral edema. Measures to combat cerebral edema may be ineffective when the edema is primarily cytotoxic rather than vasogenic in nature (19). It is therefore essential that the drowning victim receive vigorous resuscitation at the scene of the accident in order to reverse the hypoxic state as quickly as possible.

Thermoregulation in the Newborn

There is wide variation in the ability of the young of many mammalian species to maintain thermal stability. The young of the ungulates and some of the rodent species can be considered "precocious newborn" in that most of them maintain a very stable deep-body temperature over a wide range of ambient temperatures even within an hour or two of birth. In less-developed newborns such as rabbits, cats, dogs, and humans, thermal controlling mechanisms are at least partially functional at birth. Within narrow climatic limits they maintain normal body temperatures, but beyond the narrow limits they rapidly become grossly hypothermic or hyperthermic. Thermal control in these species develops rapidly during the following weeks of life. In the least-developed newborn such as marsupials, mice, squirrels, and hamsters, deep-body temperature remains close to environmental temperature and physiological responses to thermal conditions are barely, if at all, detectable. Thermal control develops during the subsequent weeks of life. The young of these species can be considered "immature newborn." All but the precocious newborn depend on maternal warmth, usually in the microclimate of a pouch or nest, for maintenance of body temperature compatible with essential activity.

Maintenance of normal body temperature within a fairly narrow range (35.5°C to 37.5°C rectal) is critical in the care of newborn infants. The advantages of good temperature control are well known: (1) improved survival, (2) increased rate of growth, (3) less apnea, (4) less fluid requirement, and (5) less susceptibility to hypoglycemia, acidosis, and hypoxia.

The newborn infant, especially the low-birth-weight infant, has the disadvantage of having a relatively large surface area, little subcutaneous fat, a thin epidermis, and increased skin water content and permeability, all of which all favor *heat loss*. Some degree of cold stress following delivery is almost inevitable, but, when the infant is lusty and the cold stress is short-lived and not excessively severe, the infant usually responds by increasing his or her metabolism and so suffers only a small drop in body temperature.

Hypothermia in the Newborn

Hypothermia is an abormally low temperature of less than 35.5°C skin temperature or less than 36.5°C rectal temperature or less than 35.9°C axillary temperature. The consequences of hypothermia in the newborn are well known and include the following: mortality is increased; metabolic rate and oxygen requirement are increased; growth may be impaired; and metabolic acidosis and hypoglycemia occur, as does an increased risk of kernicterus. In severe cases, neonatal cold injury may result (20, 21, 22, 23, 24).

Treatment of the Hypothermic Infant

The question of whether the hypothermic infant should be warmed slowly or rapidly is still controversial. Fast warming has been shown to increase oxygen consumption and possibly to cause apnea; however, rapid warming probably decreases the degree of metabolic acidosis and hypoglycemia.

Hypoglycemia, shock, acidosis, clotting disorders, and hypoxia in the hypothermic infant should be treated. And blood pressure, temperature, blood sugar, pH, and pO_2 should be monitored closely.

The metabolic response to cold is mediated via cutaneous thermal receptors and is seen when the average skin temperature is lowered to about 35°C to 36°C. the mechanisms responsible for increased heat production in response to cold are: (1) muscular activity and shivering during exposure to cold (in adults) and (2) nonshivering thermogenesis (in newborns).

Nonshivering Thermogenesis

Nonshivering thermogenesis is an increase in the rate of heat production during cold exposure due to processes that do not involve contraction of voluntary muscles. Lavoisier (in the 18th century) made the fundamental observation that energy (and thus heat) is produced in the body by the process of oxidation. All of the tissues in the body are capable of metabolizing or burning food materials with the release or production of heat within the body.

The control mechanisms that determine or limit the efficacy of nonshivering thermogenesis in the cold-stressed newborn infant are (1) the amount of brown adipose tissue present, (2) the sympathetic nervous system, (3) an adequate supply of glucose, and (4) a large supply of oxygen.

Newborn infants have a tissue called brown fat. It is located in the upper thorax, in the axillae, and beneath the skin in the upper part of the back. Brown fat differs from normal yellow fat in that its primary function is generating heat under cold stress. When an infant is cooled, the brown-fat deposits are stimulated by way of the autonomic nervous system to release and to burn stored fat. As this fat is combusted, the heat is transferred throughout the body via the blood stream. The influence of brown-fat metabolism on the infant's heat production can be observed by measuring skin temperature in various parts of the body. Under cold stress, the skin overlying the upper part of the back, or in the axillae, may be as much as 1°C to 1.5°C above the skin temperature of the lower back, abdomen, or extremities. This increased skin temperature reflects the heat being produced in the brown fat immediately beneath the skin of these areas.

A lusty full-term newborn can triple his or her heat production by nonshivering thermogenesis when subjected to a cold stress. This response is severely limited in the small, sick, asphyxiated premature infant.

Factors that may interfere with these control mechanisms and thereby reduce nonshivering thermogenesis are (1) sedation given to the mother immediately before delivery and (2) diseases or disorders of the central nervous system (e.g., meningomyelocele).

Shivering Thermogenesis

Shivering thermogenesis is the increased rate of heat production during cold exposure due to increased contractile activity of skeletal muscles not involving voluntary movements and external work. Just how much of a role shivering plays in neonatal thermogenesis is debatable. Small premature infants are capable of shivering, although it is usually not observable as gross movements of the extremities. The mechanisms affecting the conversion from nonshivering to shivering thermogenesis are not known.

Temperature of the Fetus

The temperature of the human fetus at term, measured in utero or immediately after delivery, is about 0.5°C higher than the maternal temperature. Heat is produced as a necessary consequence of fetal metabolic processes, but there is no means of heat loss via skin or lungs. The placenta acts as an efficient thermostatic organ of heat exchange. Cineradioangiography demonstrates that spinal arterioles, opening at the floor of the intervillous space, intermittently discharge "spurts" of maternal blood that enter the intervillous "lake." Into this lake project fetal cotyledons containing complex loops of anastomosing capillaries. This unique double circulation of blood has the capacity for dissipating all, or nearly all, of the heat from fetal metabolism. Some heat may be lost from fetal skin to amniotic fluid, but no experimental observations of this process have been made. A pregnant mother who develops a high fever compensates by increasing blood flow and increasing ventilation at expense of blood flow to the uterus and placenta. This reduces the heat-removal efficiency of the placenta and results in a high fever of the fetus.

Care in the Delivery Room

Most delivery rooms are air conditioned for the comfort of the mother and the medical personnel. Babies inevitably suffer cold stress at the time of delivery because of the large radiant, convective, and evaporative heat losses from their warm, wet skin. Under usual delivery-room conditions, an initial decrease in skin tempearature of 0.3°C per minute can be observed. Rectal temperature falls more slowly, but a total decrease of 2°C to 3°C is not unusual. In the smallest infants the fall is likely to be the greatest. Asphyxia, anesthesia, infection, and birth injury can all have an adverse effect on thermal stability.

It is impossible to prevent completely the losses of body heat that occur after birth, but measures can be taken to reduce the heat loss: (1) Drying the baby, particularly his or her head and face, which have a large surface area, is very effective. (2) A radiant heater used above the baby creates a suitable microclimate. (3) Wrapping the baby with a dry, warm blanket, an aluminum swaddler, or a transparent plastic bag works to reduce heat loss largely by minimizing evaporative loss. Procedures such as bathing and circumcision should *not* be performed in the delivery room.

Care in the Neonatal Intensive Care Unit

Normal skin temperature, as measured by a thermistor taped to the infant's anterior abdominal wall, is approximately 35.5°C to 36.5°C. The normal rectal temperature is 36.5°C to 37.5°C, and the axillary temperature is 35.9°C to 36.7°C.

Table 2-3
Neutral Thermal Environmental Temperatures

Age and Weight	Starting Temperature (°C)	Range of Temperature (°C)
0-6 hr		
Under 1200 gm	35.0	34.0-35.4
1200-1500 gm	34.1	33.9-34.4
1501-2500 gm	33.4	32.8-33.8
Over 2500 (and under 36 wk)	32.9	32.0-33.8
6-12 hr		
Under 1200 gm	35.0	34.0-35.4
1200-1500 gm	34.0	33.5-34.4
1501-2500 gm	33.1	32.2-33.8
Over 2500 (and under 36 wk)	32.8	31.4-33.8
12-24 hr		
Under 1200 gm	34.0	34.0-35.4
1200-1500 gm	33.8	33.3-34.3
1501-2500 gm	32.8	31.8-33.8
Over 2500 (and under 36 wk)	32.4	31.0-33.7
24-36 hr		
Under 1200 gm	34.0	34.0-35.0
1200-1500 gm	33.6	33.1-34.2
1501-2500 gm	32.6	31.6-33.6
Over 2500 (and under 36 wk)	32.1	30.7-33.5
36-48 hr		
Under 1200 gm	34.0	34.0-35.0
1200-1500 gm	33.5	33.0-34.1
1501-2500 gm	32.5	31.4-33.5
Over 2500 (and under 36 wk)	31.9	30.5-33.3
48-72 hr		
Under 1200 gm	34.0	34.0-35.0
1200-1500 gm	33.5	33.0-34.0
1500-2500 gm	32.3	31.2-33.4
Over 2500 (and under 36 wk)	31.7	30.1-33.2
72-96 hr		
Under 1200 gm	34.0	34.0-35.0
1200-1500 gm	33.5	33.0-34.0
1501-2500 gm	32.2	31.1-33.2
Over 2500 (and under 36 wk)	31.3	29.8-32.8
4-12 d		
Under 1500 gm	33.5	33.0-34.0
1501-2500 gm	32.1	31.0-33.2
Over 2500 (and under 36 wk)		
4-5 d	31.0	29.5-32.6
5-6 d	30.9	29.4-32.3
6-8 d	30.6	29.0-32.2
8-10 d	30.3	29.0-31.8
10-12 d	30.1	29.0-31.4

Table 2-3 — *Continued*

Age and Weight	Starting Temperature (°C)	Range of Temperature (°C)
12-14 d		
Under 1500 gm	33.5	32.6-34.0
1501-2500 gm	32.1	31.0-33.2
Over 2500 (and under 36 wk)		
2-3 wk		
Under 1500 gm	33.1	32.2-34.0
1501-2500 gm	31.7	30.5-33.0
3-4 wk		
Under 1500 gm	32.6	31.6-33.6
1501-2500 gm	31.4	30.0-32.7
4-5 wk		
Under 1500 gm	32.0	31.2-33.0
1501-2500 gm	30.9	29.5-32.2
5-6 wk		
Under 1500 gm	31.4	30.6-32.3
1501-2500 gm	30.4	29.0-31.8

Source: Adapted from Scopes and Ahmed (23). In the original setting, the walls of the incubator were 1° to 2° warmer than the ambient air temperatures.
Note: Generally speaking, the smaller infants in each weight group require a temperature in the higher portion of the temperature range. Within each time range, the younger the infant, the higher the temperature required.

After delivery, the aim should be to provide a thermal environment in which metabolic heat production is minimal. This is the range of ambient temperature within which the infant's oxygen consumption (an indirect measurement of heat production) and thermoregulatory water loss are at a minimum and normal body temperature is maintained. However, the thermal neutral zone of the naked infant is fairly narrow and cannot be measured routinely. These measurements have been made on infants of varying gestational ages under optimal conditions, and the results serve only as a general guide for setting the neutral temperature inside the incubator. Thus, at best, the suggested temperature range for the thermal neutral zone for infants in the nursery is only an approximate prediction of the thermal neutral conditions most likely to maintain normal body temperature at minimal metabolic cost to the infant. (See Table 2-3.)

Incubators: The temperature of the incubator should not be set according to the neutral thermal environment. The incubator temperature should be recorded simultaneously with the infant's axillary or skin temperature, because an infant may be showing indirect evidence of fever if his or her temperature remains the same when the incubator's temperature drops.

During phototherapy for infants in incubators, the skin temperature should be maintained at 36.5°C by using a servo-controlled incubator. When servo-control is used, the skin probe must be kept dry and securely taped to the skin on the upright side of the infant. The probe should be protected from the light by an aluminum patch. Servo-controlled incubators generally should *not* be used in routine care because they probably do not provide a thermoneutral environment. The temperature of the room and the location of the incubator should be considered.

Radiant Warmers: The use of radiant warmers provides maximum access to the sick infant and is ideal for exchange transfusions, sepsis workups, and other minor surgical procedures. A servo-control probe must be used when the infant is nursed under the radiant warmer, and it should be set to maintain abdominal skin temperature at 36.5°C. The infant must not be completely covered with sterile drapes because this would keep the heat radiating to the infant. Insensible water losses are increased, sometimes dramatically, in a patient under radiant warmers, and increased fluid requirements should be met.

Plastic Heat Shields and Plastic Bubble Blankets: These may be used to cover the infant in order to reduce heat loss and insensible water loss. The covering alters physical conditions and creates a microclimate around the baby that reduces heat loss by radiation. A Thermoguard plastic bubble bag may be useful during transport.

Clothes: Increased thermal insulation through the use of clothing and blankets widens the range of thermal control and widens but lowers the range of thermal neutrality. It lowers the ambient temperature at which an infant is at risk of hyperthermia and reduces the capacity of the infant to lose extra heat. It improves weight gain in premature infants in incubators probably by reducing heat loss. And it may have a positive effect on parent-infant bonding.

Clinical Guidelines and Suggestions: (a) The incubator should be kept away from cold walls, windows, and other objects. (b) For small infants, a plexiglass shield should be used, or a thermal blanket of bubble plastic should be used when there is a problem in keeping the temperature up. (c) The infant should never be placed on a cold, wet surface. (d) The infant and incubator should be kept away from air currents (e.g., air conditioners, windows, and oxygen lines). (e) Only warm, humidified oxygen should be given directly to an infant. (f)

The infant should be kept dry, especially in delivery room. (g) Adequate humidity (approximately 50%) should be provided in the incubator. (h) A radiant warmer should be used in the delivery room and when the infant is being handled. (i) The infant should not be left in the delivery room any longer than necessary. (j) When the infant is transported, adequate thermal control should be provided. (k) A cold infant should not be rewarmed too rapidly because apnea could result.

Other Clinical "Pearls": (a) A newborn infant's water requirement may increase significantly when he or she is kept under a radiant warmer. (b) A high or low temperature may indicate sepsis, asphyxia, intracranial hemorrhage, or meningitis. (c) When servo-control is used, temperature as a clinical sign is lost. Therefore, a record of incubator temperature should be maintained. (d) A full-term newborn in normal room temperature (25°C to 27°C) should not require an incubator. If he or she does, something is wrong. (e) Maternal Valium, Demerol, and Reserpine may decrease the metabolic response to cold stress in the newborn. (f) Even in a normal thermal environment, a cold-air current (e.g., oxygen) applied to a small area of the infant's body (e.g., face) causes cold stress and triggers increased oxygen consumption and metabolic rate.

References

1. Pearn JH, Bart RD, Yamaoka R: Neurologic sequelae after childhood near-drowning: A total population study from Hawaii. Pediatrics *64*:187-191, 1979.
2. Pearn J: Neurological and psychometric studies in children surviving freshwater immersion accidents. Lancet *1*:7, 1977.
3. Fandel I, Bancalari E: Near-drowning in children: Clinical aspects. Pediatrics *58*:573-579, 1976.
4. Peterson B: Morbidity of childhood near drowning. Pediatrics *59*:364-370, 1977.
5. Modell JH, Graves SA, Ketover A: Clinical course of 91 consecutive near-drowning victims. Chest *70*:231, 1976.
6. Young RSK, Zalneraitis EL, Dooling EC: Neurologic outcome in cold water near drowning. Jour Am Med Assn *244*:1233-1235, 1980.
7. Sekar TS, MacDonnell KF, Namsirikul, et al.: Survival after prolonged submersion in cold water without neurologic sequelae. Arch Intern Med *140*:775-779, 1980.
8. Kruus S, Bergstom L, Suutarinen T, et al.: Prognosis of near-drowned children. Acta Paediatr Scand *68*:315-322, 1979.
9. Scremin A, Scremin OU, Brechner T: Survival under hypoxia: Age dependence and effect of cholinergic drugs. Stroke *11*:548-552, 1980.
10. Zakhary R, Miller JA, Miller FS: Hypothermia, asphyxia, and brain carbohydrates in newborn puppies. Biol Neonate *11*:36-49, 1967.
11. Mohri H, Barnes R, Wintersheld LD, Dillard DH, Merendino KA: Challenge of prolonged suspended animation: A method of surface induced hypothermia. Annals Surg *168*:779, 1968.

12. Daniel SS, Dawes GS, James, et al.: Hypothermia and the resuscitation of the asphyxiated fetal rhesus monkeys. Jour Pediatr *68*:45-53, 1966.
13. Kopf GS, Mirvis DM, Myers RE: Central nervous systemic tolerance to cardiac arrest during profound hypothermia. Jour Surg Res *18*: 29-34, 1975.
14. Kirsch JR, D'Alecy LG, Mongroo JB: Butanediol induced ketosis increases tolerance to hypoxia in the mouse. Stroke *11*:506-512, 1980.
15. Mori A, Muaoka R, Yokota Y, et al.: Deep hypothermia combined with cardiopulmonary bypass for cardiac surgery in neonates and infants. Jour Cardiovasc Thorac Surg *64*:422-429, 1972.
16. Bjork V, Hultquist G: Contraindications to profound hypothermia in open heart surgery. Jour Thorac Cardiovasc Surg *44*:1-14, 1962.
17. Brumberg JA, Doty DB, Reilley EL: Choreoathetosis in infants following cardiac surgery with deep hypothermia and cardiac arrest. Jour Pediatr *84*:232-235, 1974.
18. Stevenson JG, Stone EF, Dillard DH, et al.: Intellectual development of children subjected to prolonged circulatory arrest during hypothermic open heart surgery in infancy. Circulation *50*(suppl 2):54-59, 1974.
19. Gudeman SK, Miller JD, Becker DP: Failure of high dose steroid therapy to influence intracranial pressure in patients with severe head injury. Jour Neurosurg *51*:301-306, 1979.
20. Hey EN, Katz G: The optimum thermal environment for naked babies. Arch Dis Child *45*:328-334, 1970.
21. Hull D: Temperature regulation and disturbance in the newborn infant. Clin Endo Metab *5*:39-54, 1976.
22. Klaus MH, Fanaroff AA, Martin RJ: The physical environment. *In*: Klaus MH, Fanaroff AA (eds.), Care of the High-Risk Neonate, pp. 94-112. Philadelphia, W. B. Saunders, 1979.
23. Scopes J, Ahmed I: Range of critical temperatures in sick and premature newborn babies. Arch Dis Child *41*:417-419, 1966.
24. Sinclair JC: Metabolic rate and temperature control. *In*: Smith CA, Nelson NM (eds.), The Physiology of the Newborn Infant, pp. 354-415. Springfield, Ill., Charles C. Thomas, 1974.

CHAPTER THREE

Thermoregulation and Hypothermia in the Elderly

K. E. Cooper, M.B., B.S., M.A., D.Sc., and A. V. Ferguson, B.Sc., Ph.D.

The assessment of thermoregulatory function and risk of hypothermia in the elderly still suffers from a lack of precise information concerning the conditions of temperature measurement and the impact of ill-defined pathological conditions. Close examinations of the brains of elderly persons almost always reveal multiple small scars probably caused by minute vascular occlusions, which did not result in obvious alterations in body function. Such minute infarcts, if they occurred in specific hypothalamic loci, could be expected to alter thermo-regulatory function. Similarly, slow, progressive degenerative changes occurring with advancing years, such as a reduction in the total number of nerve fibers in nerve trunks, might well lead to modified temperature regulation, but they would not be classified as known disease. It may be of value, however, to classify some of the known conditions that can predispose the elderly to hypothermia or produce apparent modifications in their temperature regulation, especially in response to cold exposure:

1. Changes in perception of environmental temperature, for example, without obvious disease or as a result of neurological disease (e.g., stroke).
2. Changes in the ability to generate heat in the cold, for example, minute but unrecognized brain lesions, immobilization (e.g., severe arthritis, stroke), myxoedema or panhypopituitarism, coma (diabetes, hypoglycemia, cerebral vascular accident, use of alcohol, use of street drugs, trauma), or subclinical malnutrition (?).
3. Failure of behavioral responses to cold, for example, senility,

mild confusion, or Alzheimer's disease.

4. Effects of prescription drugs, for example, drugs used to treat high blood pressure (e.g., aldomet, sympathetic transmitter modifiers), drugs used to alter mood (e.g., imipramine) or unrecognized myxoedema psychosis treated with clorpromazine, or tranquilizers and barbiturates.
5. Simple exposure (e.g., falling into cold water, being caught in an automobile in a blizzard) as could happen at any age.
6. Severe autonomic dysfunction that prevents control of blood vessels in the skin, for example, Shy-Drager syndrome, intermediolateral column degeneration, or hypothalamic tumors.

Factors of Importance in Studies of Hypothermia

If the disease processes that are more common in old age and the use of mood-altering or antihypertensive drugs lead to significant alterations in body temperature and hypothermia, then a random study of a very large sample of the human population over 65 years of age might be expected to reveal a bimodal distribution in body temperature. It might also be found that there is a shift of the mean or a wider spread about the mean in the body-temperature distribution curve of the elderly as compared with that of young adults. Some limited studies of this type have been done, but the problem in comparing such data lies in the differences in the circumstances of recording.

The environmental temperatures vary widely among studies. The method of assessing body temperature also varies. The "stress" of being studied may itself alter the subject's body temperature, and there are ethical problems that preclude the performance of many potentially useful experiments. It is difficult to find reliable data for the quantitative assessment of skin-blood flow in response to standardized perturbations of core temperature in young adults, and it is even more so in the elderly.

The methods available for measuring body temperature in a mass survey are limited. Oral temperature is simple to take, and its measurement is not unpleasant. It can, however, be markedly affected by mouth breathing or ingesting warm or cold foods and drinks. Tympanic temperature is also a valid index of core temperature, but its measurement requires sophisticated equipment and can be unpleasant. Rectal temperature would probably be the most reliable for a mass study, but its measurement would be unacceptable to many volunteers. The temperature of freshly voided urine has been used (1,2) on the basis that urine is secreted by the kidneys at core temperature and retained in the body core until voided. Some inconvenience accompanies the measurement of urine temperature, however, and minor inaccuracies can occur, especially in women. In addition, any recent rapid alteration in body temperature is unlikely to be recorded. However, the method has had successful use in surveys, and combined with a second method it can be valuable. Esophageal temperature, though a valid index of core temperature, could not be easily measured in a mass survey.

Results of Surveys of Body Temperature in the Elderly

What then have surveys of body temperature in the elderly revealed? No evidence for alterations in body temperature related to age was found by Finch and Hayflick (3). On the other hand, Fox and associates (4) found unusually low body temperatures in 10% of the elderly people they studied. An interesting study was made of body temperatures in the elderly population of an Orkney island (5). In this study, a wide range of body temperatures was found and the distribution appeared to be bimodal, although the numbers were perhaps too small to be certain. The two apparent temperature peaks were close to 35.8°C and 36.5°C. Others found low body temperatures in 17% of the random population over 69 years old studied in London (6).

Disparities among many studies, though in part related to the method of temperature measurement, can also be traced to two other factors, namely, the inclusion or exclusion of patients with disease or on medication and the environmental conditions under which the measurements were made. In most North American studies, the environmental temperatures were greater than 15°C, but in the Orkney study the external temperature was 3.7°C to 5°C and the houses were poorly insulated and very badly heated. What is still needed, then, is a large study in which the volunteers are placed for at least 12-hr periods in at least three different environmental temperatures before body temperatures are measured.

The thermosensory problems of the aged have been studied. The afferent information used by the thermoregulatory system consists of the thermoreceptors and their input to the central nervous system. It would appear that there are two different groups of warm and cold receptors: those in the skin and viscera carry information about the temperature in these regions, and those in the spinal cord and hypothalamus carry information on the thermal state of the central nervous system. The importance of this part of the system cannot be overstated, for without the ability to differentiate between warm and cold at these levels our thermoregulatory systems, both physiological and behavioral, would cease to function. Thus, it is of interest that clinical studies have been carried out that show a reduced ability of aged subjects to discriminate temperature. In 1955 Horvath and associates (7) exposed eight nude patients from 52 to 76 years of age to a cool 10°C environment and compared this group to a similarly exposed group of young patients. These workers found several changes in thermoregulatory responses between the two age-groups; but, most relevant to this part of the discussion, they found that, though the younger subjects all complained of discomfort in the cold, the older group of patients did not despite observed falls in their colonic temperatures. This study strongly suggests a decreased ability to feel the cold in the older group of patients. In a similar study, Watts (8) showed that the most elderly subjects (74 to 86 yr old) responded to the experience of cold discomfort with appropriate voluntary thermoregulatory behavior. However, the thermal preference data suggested that some of the subjects first experienced a feeling of cold at unusually low environmental temperatures. Another study centered on an investigation of elderly subjects who had already been treated for at least one incidence of hypothermia (2). One of the tests carried out on these patients assessed their ability to discriminate between two different temperatures. It was demonstrated that 20 young subjects could perceive mean-temperature differences of 0.8°C ± 0.2°C while elderly subjects could discriminate only between a mean-temperature difference of 2.3°C ± 0.5°C. A word of caution should precede an assessment of the significance of these thermal preference data. In a general survey of thermal preference in the aged (2) carried out on more than 1,000 subjects, the vast majority of the subjects stated that they were warm (as opposed to comfortable or cool). The same patients were then asked whether they would prefer to be warmer, cooler, or the same; the majority replied warmer. This series of replies appears somewhat paradoxical. Perhaps the elderly subjects were simply confused about the thermal environment. However, the weight of evidence suggests that the aged have a lowered ability to sense the cold. Such a disability, obviously puts them at great risk of developing hypothermia.

The need for further work in this area cannot be overestimated. Thermal preference data from human subjects merely suggest a deficit in the afferent part of the thermoregulatory system. A most productive avenue of research could be the study of the neurophysiological and functional characteristics of temperature-sensitive neurons in several species and in young and old groups of animals. In addition, changes in the physical characteristics of skin leading to differences in the skin's thermal conductance during old age can lead to nerve-ending temperatures not experienced in youth.

Thermoregulatory Mechanisms Involved in Animal Studies

The ability of the body to maintain its temperature during cold exposure depends in large measure in increasing the body's heat production and reducing the skin's thermal conductance by vasoconstriction. Again, under some circumstances, changes in these functions occur in the elderly.

There is no direct evidence suggesting changes in thermoregulatory control related directly to alterations in central-nervous-system function in aged humans. The reason for this deficit in our knowledge lies in the inaccessibility of this part of the temperature-regulating system to experimental study. In addition, many of the changes in the effector mechanisms of the thermoregulatory system that occur with increasing age may simply be a reflection of altered central-nervous-system control.

Age-related changes are known to occur within the central nervous system, as shown by several recent animal studies. Despite the fact that none of these studies has related such changes to temperature regulation, some of the work that may ultimately be shown to be relevant to this system is reviewed here.

Acetylcholine and noradrenaline are both neurotransmitters known to be intimately involved in the control of body temperature in the rabbit. Frolkis (9) demonstrated that the older rabbit (42 to 54 mo) is more sensitive to the intracerebroventricular application of these substances than the young animal. He showed that the threshold dose of these substances required to produce electroencephalographic changes in the hypothalamus is considerably lower in older animals. This evidence suggests a hypersensitivity of the brain to these substances that fits in well with evidence showing that their concentrations are reduced in the brains of old animals (10, 11).

It appears that further information on the central-nervous-system mechanisms involved in impaired thermoregulatory control in the aged might be obtained through a series of animal studies comparing the effects of various putative neurotransmitters. By microinjecting them into the hypothalamus, one causes temperature changes, and these temperature changes may differ according to the age of the animal.

Efferent Systems

Efferent systems have been investigated in several clinical studies. The more extensive knowledge of changes in the efferent system is due mainly to the relative ease with which it can be investigated.

Shivering

Shivering is the process by which voluntary muscular activity results in an increase in heat production at the expense of chemical energy. The process is usually initiated only when body temperature falls below normal, and it is mediated by the release of acetylcholine at the neuromuscular junction. Collins and associates (2) assessed the ability of 43 elderly subjects to shiver when placed in the cold. Only 4 of the subjects were observed to shiver. Although the short length of time these subjects spent in the cold (15 min) ruled out this test as a definitive test of their ability to shiver, a considerable number (15 of the subjects) admitted to feeling uncomfortable and cold. In another study, 8 elderly subjects who had survived hypothermia and 3 elderly controls who had no such history were compared (12). The controls were observed to shiver vigorously when exposed to cold-air flow, while the survivors of hypothermia showed no definite evidence of shivering. Similarly, Horvarth and associates (7) showed that only 1 of 8 subjects over 52 yr old was seen to shiver when placed naked in a 10°C environment and then only began 31 min after being placed in the cold. In contrast, a young control group (22 to 27 yr old) of subjects exposed to the same conditions all began to shiver from 2.7 to 23.2 min after being placed in the cold room. The performance of the old group also differed in that no tremors were observed, while tremors were always noted in the control subjects before they began to shiver.

The evidence so far presented shows a clear reduction in shivering in old subjects, as compared to young, when they are exposed to the cold. It seems that such a deficit may be related to the body's failure to activate this mechanism since the aged subject still has the muscles used in shivering. It is also of particular interest that MacMillan's team (1) was able to divide the elderly population into two groups: those who had previously developed hypothermia and who lacked the shivering response and those who had no such history and who shivered vigorously. This finding suggests that there may be a specific portion of the elderly population that is particularly susceptible to hypothermia.

Metabolic Rate

Metabolic rate is a measure of heat production derived from shivering and nonshivering thermogenesis. Without an active defense of the body's temperature, the metabolic rate of the whole human has a temperature Q_{10} of 2.3 (13). The basal metabolic rate is known to be reduced in the aged. Several studies have examined the changes in oxygen consumption (a quantitative measure of metabolic rate) that occur in aged subjects when they are exposed to the cold. Since the majority of the old subjects do not shiver, any consistent increase in metabolic rate is presumably due to the stimulation of nonshivering thermogenesis. In their study of survivors of accidental hypothermia, MacMillan and associates (12) found no consistent changes in oxygen consumption in elderly patients in the cold who had a previous history of hypothermia. In subjects with no such background, they found an average increase in oxygen consumption of 67%. Horvath and associates (7) in their comparison of old and young subjects in the cold also found no significant increases in oxygen consumption in the old subjects, though the young group did increase their metabolic rate in the cold. These data suggest a deficit in nonshivering as well as shivering thermogenesis in the elderly population. The evidence at this point is not conclusive because the observed differences between the old and young groups could simply be a reflection of the former group's inability to shiver. If the normal subjects could be shown to be utilizing both shivering and nonshivering thermogenesis during cold exposure, it could then be concluded that the aged group had deficits in both systems. Such evidence could readily be obtained by treating the young group of subjects with the beta-adrenergic blocking agent propranolol during cold exposure. This would block activation of nonshivering thermogenesis, which is mediated by the beta-adrenergic receptor. If metabolic rate were increased to a lesser extent following this treatment, one could conclude that both systems were utilized during cold exposure and thus that both showed deficits in the aged.

Peripheral Vasomotor Tone

Peripheral vasomotor tone is a vital mechanism in the control of normal body temperature. Vasodilatation and vasoconstriction of peripheral blood vessels allow humans to regulate heat loss very precisely. Collins and associates (2) in their assessment of thermoregulatory function in the aged classified subjects into three different groups according to changes in peripheral vasomotor tone observed during exposure to cold and warm environments: normal—vasoconstriction on cooling and vasodilatation on warming; abnormal—no vasoconstriction on cooling and vasodilatation on warming; and abnormal—no vasoconstriction on cooling and no vasodilatation on warming. Similarly, MacMillan and associates (12) found that elderly subjects with no history of hypothermia vasoconstricted in the cold while elderly subjects who had suffered from hypothermia showed no vasoconstriction in seven cases out of eight. Also of interest is evidence demonstrating that reflex vasodilatation in the hand is abnomal in the aged. This can normally be induced in healthy people by heating the cutaneous receptors of the trunk (14). Such vasodilatation is inhibited when the central temperature is below 36.5°C (15). However, in two aged survivors of hypothermia, vasodilatation in the hand occurred at abnormally low central temperatures, namely, 33.9°C and 35.8°C (16).

Wagner and associates (17) found that resting temperature tends to be inversely related to age and that, when exposed to cold, boys raised their rectal temperatures whereas men 46 to 67 yr old lowered their core temperatures. The fall in the older men appeared to be due to higher peripheral blood flow and a smaller and delayed metabolic response.

These studies have shown quite clear differences in the vasomotor responses of aged subjects during thermal challenge. Such changes could be due to alteration of the sensitivity of peripheral blood vessels to vasoconstrictor or vasodilator substances with increasing age, as has recently been demonstrated in animal studies (18). Alternatively, it could be due to a decreased sensitivity of the sympathetic nervous system to changes in temperature.

Additional quantitative information is still needed in order to detect the earlier and more subtle changes in vasomotor responses in the elderly that may predispose them to hypothermia. Measurements of vasomotor behavior could be developed further from the techniques of Cooper, Cranston, and Snell (19), Cooper (13), Fox, Hackett, and Turk (20), and Savard and associates (21).

Another area of concern is related to the intake of prescription drugs. Some drugs are known to lower body temperature by disrupting the processes of heat conservation and heat production. Chlorpromazine is one such drug, and devastating hypothermia resulting from its use in myxoedema psychosis is not unknown. It is more likely to lower temperature in the aged rabbit than in the young one (22). Barbiturates are always capable of disrupting thermoregulation and may predispose their users to hypothermia.

An interesting study by Chandramohan, Hariharasubramanian, and Johnson (23) demonstrated the hypothermic potential of alpha-methyldopa (Aldomet), particularly in elderly patients with cerebral vascular impairment or markedly reduced dietary tryptophan intake. Mood elevators may lead to hypothermia. Impramine hydrochloride, used as an antidepressant, is one of these (24). It is clear that we are only at the threshold of understanding the potential hypothermic hazard of many drugs in common use in the treatment of old people.

There seems no doubt that the incidence of hypothermia in the elderly does vary from country to country, from very high in Great Britain to almost nonexistent in Scandinavia (25). Nevertheless, it does occur in the United States of America, as Rango (26) has shown. Deaths from "excessive cold," in his report, are particularly frequent at ages 45 to 84 yr, with a peak in the 60-to-80 age range. Over the years 1970 to 1977, the hypothermia death rate in the over-65-yr-old age-group has been consistently more than four times that in the under-65-yr-old group, and it has tended to increase in the older patients. Increases in energy and food costs may well put many more Americans on fixed retirement incomes at risk of hypothermia in the coming years. A careful program of education about the possibility of hypothermia in the elderly, with emphasis on simple techniques of keeping warm, is needed, as is a new study of the thermoregulatory deficits that occur during cold exposure in the elderly.

It would not be proper to leave the subject of hypothermia in old people without mentioning briefly some of the problems in its management as well as some widely held myths. The chances of underlying disease are high in the elderly hypothermic patient. In some cases the authors have observed, rapid rewarming through hot peritoneal dialysis was successful. Other cases (for example, hypothermia in association with myxoedema) require slow rewarming in a room only slightly warmer than the patient's body temperature and the very cautious use of tri-iodothyronine to raise the metabolic rate. Bleeding from intraabdominal aneurysms, myocardial infarcts, severe infection, and even a ruptured appendix with peritonitis have also been observed in elderly hypothermic patients. In such cases, it may be advisable to rewarm the patients less vigorously. However, no method has as yet yielded a very high rate of recovery for hypothermia patients with serious underlying diseases.

Some experimental work has been done in the authors' laboratory in which young volunteers have been cooled to core temperatures of 35.5°C to 36°C. Subsequently, they have then been rewarmed passively in a hot tub, with a radiant heat cradle, and by exercise on a bicycle (21). In these cases, hand-blood flow and in the case of radiant heating forearm-blood flow do not return to measurable levels until the core temperature is close to the precooling level, usually about 36.5°C. This finding is in agreement with those of Cooper and associates (19) and MacMillan and associates (12). Preliminary though as yet unproven results indicate that the increase in blood flow in the heated skin is also similarly delayed. If this is so, then warnings about the dangers of peripheral vasodilatation will have to be reconsidered. But in the elderly the return of blood flow can occur at unusually low core temperatures (16); thus, surface rewarming techniques still rest on flimsy foundations.

References

1. Barwood A: Royal Air Force Institute of Aviation Medicon, personal communcation, 1949.
2. Collins KJ, Dore C, Exton-Smith AN, Fox RH, McDonald IC, Woodward PM; Accidental hypothermia and impaired temperature homeostasis in the elderly. Brit Med Jour *1*:353-356, 1977.
3. Schock NW: Systems integration. *In:* Finch CE, Hayflick L (eds.), Handbook of the Biology of Aging, pp. 159-188. New York, Van Nostrand.
4. Fox RH, MacGibbon R, Davies L, Woodward PM: Problem of the old and the cold. Brit Med Jour *1*:21-24, 1973.
5. Collacott RA: Screening for hypothermia in Orkney. Jour Roy Coll Gen Pract *25*: 647-651, 1975.
6. Eddy TP, Payne PR, Salvosac C, Wheeler EF: Body temperatures in the elderly. Lancet *2*:1088, 1970.
7. Horvath SM, Radcliffe CE, Hatt PK, Spurr GB: Metabolic responses of old people to a cold environment. Jour Appl Physiol *8*:145-148, 1955.
8. Watts AJ: Hypothermia in the aged: A study of the role of cold sensitivity. Environ Res 5:119-126, 1972.
9. Frolkis VV: The hypothalamic mechanisms of aging. *In*: Everitt AV, Burgess JA (eds.), Hypothalamus, Pituitary and Aging, pp. 614-633. Springfield, Ill, Charles C. Thomas.
10. Estes KS, Simpkins JW: Age related alterations in catecholamine concentrations in discrete preoptic area and hypothalamic regions in the male rat. Brain Res *194*:556-560, 1980.
11. Finch CE: Neuroendocrine mechanisms and aging. Fred Proc *38*:178-183, 1979.
12. MacMillan AL, Corbett JL, Johnson RH, Smith AC, Spalding JMK, Wollner L: Temperature regulation in survivors of accidental hypothermia of the elderly. Lancet *2*:165-169, 1967.
13. Cooper KE: Quantitative observations in disordered temperature regulation. *In*: The Scientific Basis of Medicine Annual Reviews, pp. 239-256. London, Athlone Press, 1965.
14. Kerslake DMcK, Cooper KE: Vasodilatation in the hand in response to heating the skin elsewhere. Clin Sci *9*:31-47, 1950.

15. Cooper KE, Johnson RH, Spalding JMK: The effects of central body and trunk skin temperatures on reflex vasodilatation in the hand. Jour Physiol (London) *174*:46-54, 1964.
16. Johnson RH, Park DM: Intermittent hypothermia. Jour Neurol Neurosurg Psychia *36*:411-416, 1973.
17. Wagner JA, Robinson S, Marino RP: Age and temperature regulation of humans in neutral and cold environments. Jour Appl Physiol *37*:562-565, 1974.
18. Fleisch JH: Age related changes in the sensitivity of blood vessels to drugs. Pharmacol Ther *8*:477-487, 1980.
19. Cooper KE, Cranston WI, Snell ES: Simple apparatus for examining thermoregulatory mechanisms in man. Jour Physiol (London) *171* (24P), 1964.
20. Fox RH, Hackett AJ, Turk J: Mobile equipment for studying body temperature regulation in man. Jour Physiol (London) *194* (55P), 1968.
21. Savard G: Personal communication, 1981.
22. Lipton JM, Whisenant JD, Gean JT: Hypothermia produced by peripheral and central injections of chlorpromazine in aged rabbits. Brain Res Bull *4*:631-635, 1979.
23. Chandramohan M, Hariharasubramanian N, Johnson, ES: Hypothermia in alphamethyldopa treatment. Indian Jour Physiol Pharmacol *20*(4):216-220, 1976.
24. McGrath MD, Paley RG: Hypothermia induced in a myxoedematous patient by imipramine hydrochloride. Brit Med Jour *2*:1364, 1960.
25. Hirvonen J: Accidental hypothermia. *In*: Lomax P, Schönbaum E (eds.), Body Temperature, Regulation, Drug Effects and Therapeutic Implications, p. 566. New York and Basel, Marcel Dekker.
26. Range N: Old and cold: Hypothermia in the elderly. A presentation to the President's Symposium on Energy and the Aged at the Gerontological Society Annual Meeting and to the United States Senate Special Committee on Aging, 1979.

CHAPTER FOUR

The Development and Rectification of Hiker's Hypothermia

W. C. Kaufman, Ph.D.

In studies of the effectiveness of cold-weather clothing and sleeping bags, the author and his associates have gathered data from human subjects and observed responses that raise questions concerning instructions for survival in the out-of-doors. The experiments use both physiological and physical methods to provide information that suggests shortcomings in the advice regularly given to the recreational outdoorsman.

One can only be impressed by the aura of irrefutability granted the basic rules for activity in the outdoors, which have approached the status of dogma. One's perception of thermal comfort does not always indicate one's physiological status. Perception provides an obvious awareness, but physiological changes may remain unperceived—or at least unperceived until marked changes have taken place. One may feel comfortably warm at the same time one's core temperature is decreasing markedly. Another contributor to this dogma is the advice of "authorities," who are authorities in that they have successfully lived in the outdoors for extended periods. These people are rarely the ones caught in emergencies, for they have learned to anticipate and prevent such occurrences. A consideration of physical and physiological principles suggests that their advice for handling emergencies may not always be fundamentally sound.

Hiker's hypothermia is perhaps less spectacular than immersion hypothermia in that the environment heat sink at first glance seems less severe. On the other hand, treatment of the victim may be much more difficult in that air or surface rescue with appropriate rewarming

The author gratefully acknowledges the continued support of the Eddie Bauer Company, Redmond, Wash., and the contributions of many research assistants and long-suffering subjects.

apparatus is unlikely to be available. Thus, prevention is still the surest cure. When the condition does occur, treatment may be primitive at best.

Consider first the development of hiker's hypothermia. The heat-balance equation provides guidance:

$$H = M \pm H_d \pm H_c \pm H_r \pm H_e$$

Where M is the major source of heat. For our purposes, it may range from about 100 to 400 kcal per hour.

In the cold outdoors, H_r (radiation) can be another heat source when the sun is bright, but it seems that most instances of hypothermia occur with overcast, with rain, or during the night.

Convective transfer (H_c) may be overrated as a danger in the properly dressed individual, but wind associated with wetness and the resulting evaporative loss is likely to be the most effective and dangerous avenue of heat loss (1, 2).

Conductive transfer (H_d) from feet and hands can cause great pain, but as an avenue of heat loss it may be relatively minor since peripheral chilling stimulates protective vasoconstriction. This vasoconstrictive response is likely to be very important under extremely cold conditions, under which subjects with painfully cold hands and feet have been observed to tolerate hours of exposure with high core temperatures and no shivering. Conversely, overprotection of hands and feet has produced uncontrolled shivering with warm hands and feet and a steadily falling core temperature.

Evaporative heat transfer (H_e) in the cold can always be considered negative and should under any circumstances be prevented.

Associated with these physical factors in heat transfer are anthropomorphic factors. The slender, slight, or ectomorphic individual endowed with a smaller thermal mass and a greater surface-to-mass ratio suffers more rapid heat loss (3, 4). Such an individual may also be somewhat less tolerant to the stress of vigorous exercise. In the author's experiments, slender females always lose heat at the greatest rate.

The physiological aspects of the development of hypothermia can also be considered. Little can be done to control metabolic heat production since it is a direct product of the energy expended. Metabolic heat production can be the source of a great deal of heat, and it can be managed to the advantage of the individual.

Protective vasoconstriction occurs when the proper chilling stimuli are allowed to be detected. On the other hand, heat-dissipating vasodilatation occurs when the individual allows himself or herself to become overheated.

In addition to vasodilatation, sweating begins. In the heavily clothed individual, sweating may have little effect in dissipating heat, but it does wet the clothing.

Vasodilatation due to a requirement for heat dissipation conflicts with the metabolic requirements of working muscles and may contribute to fatigue. It certainly contributes to cardiac stress.

Development of Hypothermia

Now let us construct a model of the candidate for hiker's hypothermia. The weather is threatening or darkness is coming on, and so it is necessary for the hiker to hurry. Improper management of energy expenditure and clothing leads to sweating and fatigue. Dehydration may accompany this condition. Competitiveness may keep the hiker from admitting to his or her condition, and he or she may reach a rather severe state of exhaustion and wetness before calling for a rest stop.

The individual's peripheral circulation has dilated, and he or she sits or lies on a cold surface of relatively high thermal conductivity. Heat is lost rapidly by this avenue. Sweating may cease, but the wet clothing continues to dry, chilling the vasodilated vessels of the skin. An oxygen debt may cause continued high levels of ventilation with accompanying evaporative heat loss (cold air, even when saturated, is relatively dry and, when breathed, readily accepts water vapor). Even the controversial declines reported in sublingual (pharyngeal, palatine) temperature (5, 6) may contribute markedly to the debilitated condition of an overheated, fatigued, wet, vasodilated individual with a physiology adjusted for maximum heat loss. In some animals pharyngeal hat loss is very effective (7).

Paradoxically, it appears that the prevention of overheating is likely to be a major factor in the prevention of hypothermia. The prevention of overheating requires the proper management of energy expenditure, clothing, and evaporation.

If rain has fallen or accidental wetting in snow or water has occured (and this may be coupled with a wind), evaporative heat loss may be greatly accelerated. Marked evaporative losses result from accidental wetting. Proper handling of evaporation is likely to lie, not in removing damp clothing, since the hiker may not have additional clothing that is dry, but rather in recognizing that wetness is uncomfortable but properly managed not overly dangerous. The warming of one kilogram of water from 4°C (the coldest that fluid water is likely to be) to 34°C (the skin temperature of the normally sweating individual) requires only 30 kcal. This is a miniscule expenditure of energy compared to the energy dissipated in the evaporation (drying) of one kilogram of water, 580 kcal. The rate of heat dissipation under these conditions, coupled with a wind, as Pugh has reported, can be startling—and lethal (1, 2).

Rectification of Hypothermia

The recognition of these physical and physiological factors in heat transfer and thermal homeostatic mechanisms should enable the knowledgeable outdoorsman to combat successfully any of the usually encountered cold stresses. This knowledge should also modify some of the commonly held ideas about combating cold.

When an individual hikes alone, the prevention of hypothermia is essential. Like hypoxia, hypothermia appears to be associated with factors that prevent the stricken individual from recognizing the affliction.

What can be done, rationally and practically, when a member of a group shows signs of stress in the cold—fatigue, perspiration, and sometimes mental or emotional change? First of all, further energy expenditure and heat loss must be avoided. The victim should sit or lie down to rest, and conductive heat loss should be reduced as much as possible. This means sitting or lying on relatively nonconductive surfaces—branches, leaves, or dirt rather than rock, snow, or ice—with extra clothing, sleeping bags, or packs between the victim's body and the surface (Figure 4-1).

The victim should wear a raincoat or a poncho, something to prevent evaporation if sweat or rain has wetted his or her clothing. Additional clothing, even if it is wet, reduces convective heat loss (Figure 4-2).

These actions should alleviate the most obvious factors in conductive and evaporative heat loss. There is a less obvious but very effective avenue of evaporative heat loss—obligatory respiratory evaporation, which under normal conditions may account for 10% of resting heat production (8). In the cold even saturated atmospheric air is very dry relative to air at the temperature of the body's core, the temperature to which respired air is warmed. This air when inspired is again saturated and accounts for significant heat dissipation.

The recognition of this fact suggests an additional method of heat conservation. When respiratory losses can be reduced, significant heat conservation can be established at a time when what appear to be insignificant amounts of heat can be terribly important. The best course

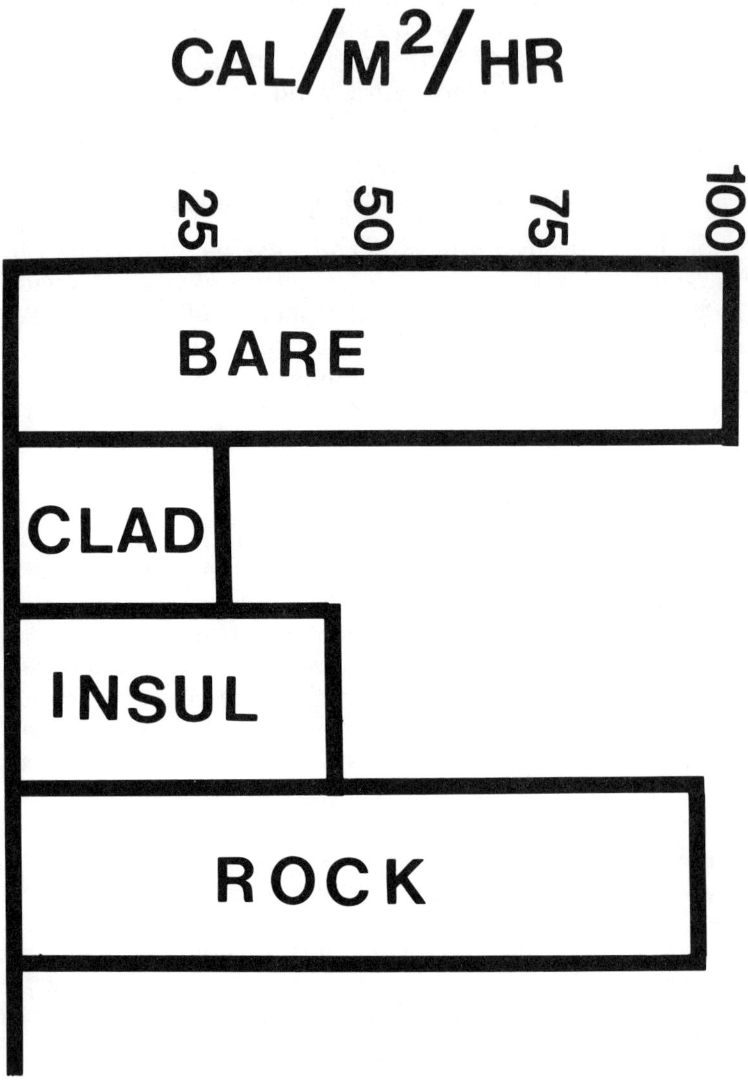

Figure 4-1. Conductive heat loss. Bare: a physical model is suspended in the air; clad: the model is protected by approximately 3 cm of thermal insulating material; insul: the model is dressed the same as in "clad" but now is in contact with approximately 6 cm of thermal insulating material; increased heat transfer is due mainly to compression of primary insulating material; rock: model is dressed the same as in "clad" but has been placed in direct contact with the rock surface that underlaid the insulating material in "insul." The experiment demonstrates the effectiveness of clothing in convective heat transfer and how conductive heat transfer can be minimized or increased.

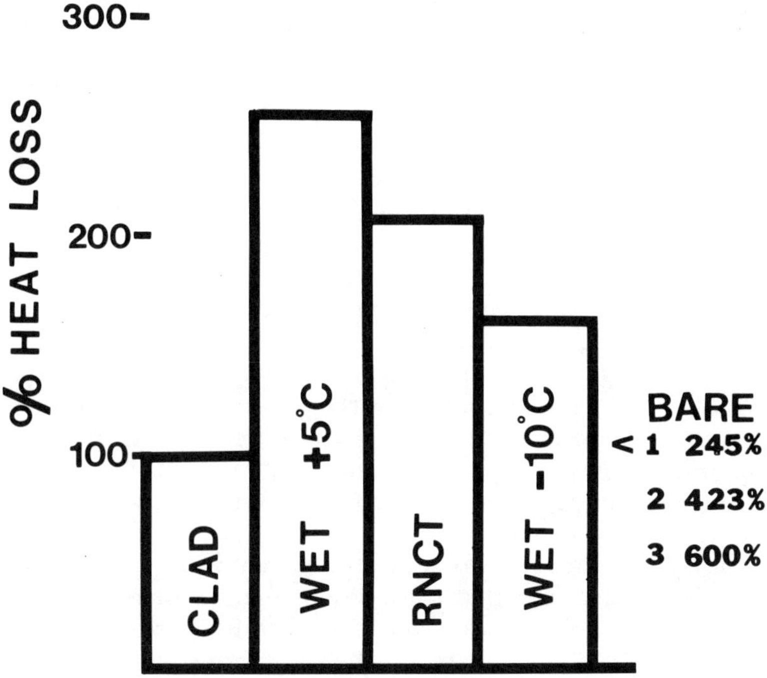

Figure 4-2. Evaporative heat loss. Clad: a physical model is protected by approximately 3 cm of thermal insulating material, and the wind is calm (0.5 m/sec); Wet + 5°C: the model is dressed as in "clad," but the insulating material is soaked with water; Rnct: as in "wet + 5°C," but there is a polyethylene "raincoat" over the insulating material; Wet −10°C: as in "wet + 5°C" but at −10°C, evaporative heat loss is impeded by film of ice. The experiment demonstrates the effectiveness of evaporation as an avenue of heat loss and how heat loss can be reduced by an impermeable garment or in freezing temperatures, where ice performs a similar function. Bare: heat loss from the unclad model as compared to "clad."

<1 air motion less than 1 mph (0.46 m/sec)
2 air motion 2 mph (0.90 m/sec)
3 air motion 3 mph (1.35 m/sec)

The method is a modification of that described by Siple and Passel (13).

clearly then is to cover the head, mouth, and nose with a cap and scarf to impede heat loss by making a crude heat exchanger and humidifier.

These suggestions, based on fundamental concepts, may seem paradoxical. They conflict with the commonly held ideas of correction, getting dry. Drying certainly helps and is desirable if it can be accomplished by changing to dry clothing. But on the trail this action may lead to additional rapid heat loss that may exceed the advantages obtained.

Preventing evaporation is likely to produce the discomfort associated with damp or wet clothing and may appear to conflict with the physiological mechanisms established by an organism that has been overproducing heat. The fact may be that, without the continued high level of metabolic heat production that put these responses into action, the heat loss that can occur from respiratory evaporation and rapid evaporation of sweat or rain from clothing may drop core temperature excessively when the individual has established the physiological heat-dissipation responses. Heat dissipation can reach levels that may be dangerous. In the fatigued individual, this condition may be difficult if not impossible to overcome, and the predisposition to, or even establishment of, the clinical hypothermic state may occur.

Two major physiological fundamentals should be considered: establishing or reestablishing heat-conservation responses and increasing metabolic heat production.

In the management of homeostatic mechanisms preventing hypothermia, it is important that the body recognize the requirement for heat conservation. This may require mild chilling at the beginning of the hike. The body must perceive the stimuli in order to activate the negative-feedback control loop. Overdressing of hands and feet may prevent this necessary perception. The author's experiments with winter ensembles produced two responses, one with high core temperatures and cool or even cold hands and feet and another with falling core temperatures and shivering with warm hands and feet. This finding led to a recommendation for distribution of thermal insulation over the body that placed the smallest amount over hands and feet and the greatest amount over the torso (9). Such clothing allowed the establishment of physiological conservation mechanisms and supported the usual skin-temperature gradients that are greatest over head and torso and fall peripherally to the lowest level at hands and feet. The results may be uncomfortable, but they are effective in heat conservation.

Where metabolic heat production is a factor, the matter is more complex, and it may be difficult to increase heat production in the fatigued individual. It is especially difficult in the victim approaching or entering clinical hypothermia.

The only mechanism for increased metabolism is external work (exercise). Modest exercise (for example, strolling) easily doubles or even triples heat production. Arithmetic indicates the theoretical effectiveness. For a 70-kg individual, when heat loss can be entirely prevented, basal heat production (70 kcal per hour) increases mean body temperature 1°C in 1 hr. Modest to moderate exercise doubles or triples that increase. Even in an individual in thermal balance, prevention of respiratory losses begins to increase body temperature; at rest by 0.1°C per hour, at moderate exercise by 0.2°C to 0.3°C per hour. When further heat loss is prevented and the sort of cardiovascular heat conservation mechanism that the diving response is thought to produce is involved, the reestablishment of normal temperature within the critical viscera, the heart and the brain, should be possible and the progress toward severe or dangerous levels of hypothermia arrested or reversed.

Exercise is not recommended for the severely hypothermic. But, in the absence of other means of rewarming, it seems a reasonable alternative to further heat loss and a decrease in core temperature (10).

In experiments with mildly hypothermic individuals, exercise levels of which the deteriorating victim is capable, when strongly encouraged and supported by a companion, produced changes in core temperatures (rectal, sublingual, and esophageal) comparable to those produced by inhalation rewarming (Figure 4-3).

Two controversial points deserve examination. The first is the afterdrop. The research of Golden and Hervey (11) done on live and dead pigs strongly supports the contention that afterdrop is a physical phenomenon modified only slightly by circulation. The author and his colleagues at the University of Wisconsin have performed experiments with chilled and rewarmed inanimate, fluid-filled spheres that produced afterdrops remarkably similar to those observed in mildly hypothermic subjects.

It appears that at least a major factor in afterdrop is physical, the result of the complex processes of heat transfer from warmer regions (core) to still colder regions (intermediate thermal masses) while the surface is being rewarmed and peripheral thermal masses are gaining and losing heat, depending on the direction of temperature gradients (Figure 4-4). Certainly, the magnitude and duration of the afterdrop are modified by rewarming methods, and the smaller and shorter afterdrop is associated with the most rapid (most effective?) method of rewarming.

Afterdrop can certainly be important when generally accepted concerns for changes in myocardial excitability are considered. In the severely hypothermic individual, it can be presumed that the minimization of afterdrop and the reversal of the direction of temperature change in the viscera are very important.

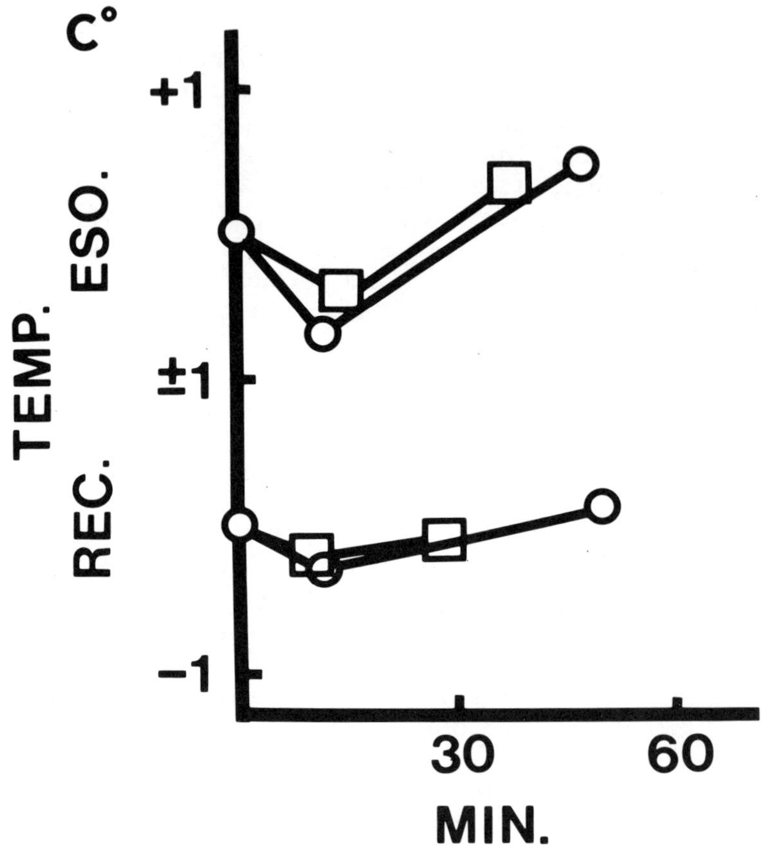

Figure 4-3. Afterdrop with inhalation and exercise rewarming. ESO.: esophegeal temperature, REC.: rectal temperature, squares: rewarming by inhalation of warmed, humidified oxygen, and circles: rewarming by mild exericse. These data are the mean values from experiments on four mildly hypothermic subjects. Responses of both esophageal and rectal temperatures are remarkably similar for both inhalation and exercise rewarming.

In one often recommended method of rewarming, body-to-body warming, afterdrop is likely to be affected by physiological response. An examination of fundamentals seems to recommend against the method. Even in the warmest torso, skin temperature is unlikely to be much above 33°C. Perhaps 33°C is not sufficient to produce vasodilatation in the skin vessels of the hypothermic individual, but there is evidence that it may be perceived as "warm" and so reduce stimuli

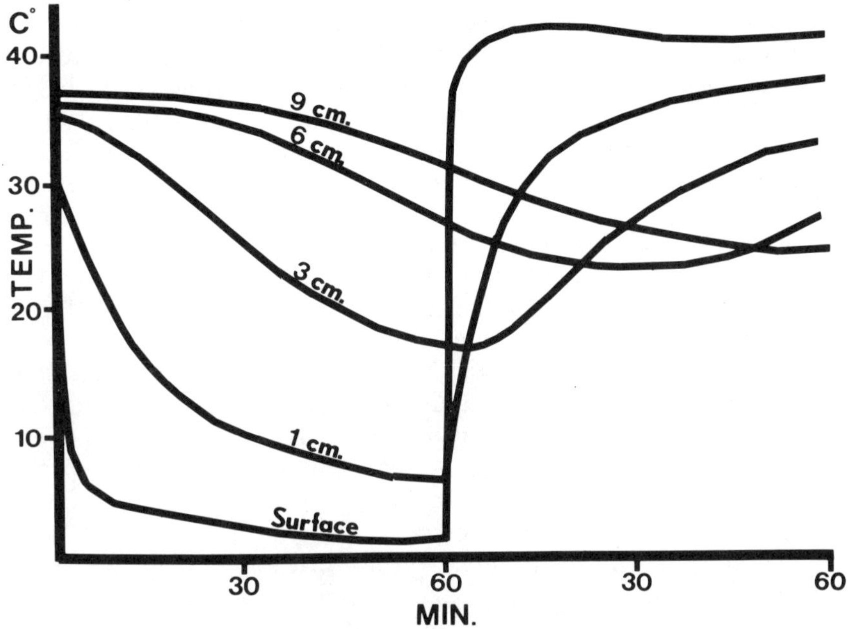

Figure 4-4. Temperatures within 3-kg fluid-filled spheres during chilling and rewarming by immersion. Numerals indicate depth of thermistor in sphere; 10 cm was approximately at center. In this inanimate object, time and magnitude of afterdrop are directly related to depth of the probe.

for heat conservation. It is also a temperature far below that which is normal for the core, and it is to be avoided, if possible. Blood perfusing a region of such a temperature is likely to cool the critical core regions further.

In general, it appears that surface rewarming, unless it can be done by hot bath, is to be avoided. What method does this leave for the isolated hiker? Any rewarming of the surface is likely to be counterproductive. The authors have observed research assistants who have entered a cold room repeatedly for short periods of time suddenly seized by uncontrolled shivering. Apparently, each short exposure to cold chilled the body while their return to a warm environment and the perception of warmth prevented the homeostatic heat conservation responses until the core had cooled enough to trigger shivering.

More than a decade ago, Dr. Arthur C. Brown of the University of Oregon Health Science Center in Portland discussed with me immersion studies in which he was able to manipulate water temperature in such a way that a steadily falling core temperature could be established. Each time shivering was stimulated, a slight increase of water temperature stopped the shivering and chilling could be continued. This process could be repeated until the core was cold enough to result in uncontrollable and continuous shivering. Apparently, the slight increase in surface temperature prevented the shivering response even though the heat balance of the body required it. Harnett and associates (12) also have discussed this response.

Experiences and experiments such as these suggest that surface heating is to be avoided, and they raise questions concerning the effectiveness of warming a hypothermic individual by an outdoor fire, where his or her perception of radiant heating may reduce or eliminate the effectiveness of heat-production and heat-conservation stimuli.

It is possible that huddling or bundling may prove beneficial, especially if several bodies participate. It seems likely that two or three unaffected bodies would increase thermal insulation surrounding an affected individual and might increase the thermal mass with a concurrent reduction in surface area so that heat losses might be reduced and metabolic heat sufficiently conserved to reverse a hypothermic trend. It seems unlikely that a single body applied to a hypothermic one could produce real results, and the work of Harnett and associates (12) supports this contention.

Consideration of fundamental concepts of physics and physiology provides knowledge that indicates basic inadequacies in traditionally held rewarming theories. The recreational outdoorsman, armed with a modicum of knowledge of physical and physiological principles and common sense, may experience discomfort but should not experience real difficulty. There are unsophisticated but theoretically sound methods of combating and correcting hypothermia in the victim to whom mechanical rewarming devices are unavailable.

For the isolated hypothermic hiker, peripheral heating is not likely to produce desirable results, but metabolic heat production can be sufficient to rewarm the stricken individual internally if accompanied by physiological heat-conservation responses and prevention of respiratory heat losses.

References

1. Pugh LGCE: Accidental hypothermia in walkers, climbers and campers: Report to the Medical Commission on Accident Prevention. Brit Med Jour *1*:123-129, 1966.
2. Pugh LGCE: Cold stress and muscular exercise with special references to accidental hypothermia. Brit Med Jour *2*:333-337, 1967.

3. Kollas J. Buskirk ER: Body cooling patterns in men who vary in body composition and size (abstr). Fed Proc *27*:699, 1968.
4. Pittman JD, Kaufman WC, Harris CE: Physiologic evaluation of sea survival equipment. Aerospace Med *40*:378-381, 1969.
5. Kaufman WC, Nichols T, Coffman R: Subnormal temperatures in men exercising in the cold (abstr). Fed Proc *35*:560, 1976.
6. Williams H, Arnold HD: The effects of violent and prolonged muscular exercise upon the heart. Phila Med Jour *2*:1233-1239, 1899.
7. Taylor CR, Lyman CP: Heat storage in running antelopes: Independence of brain and body temperatures. Amer Jour Physiol *222*:114-117, 1972.
8. Brebbia DR, Goldman RF, Buskirk ER: Water vapor loss from the respiratory tract during outdoor exercise in the cold. Jour Appl Physiol *11*:219-222, 1957.
9. Kaufman WC: Cold-weather clothing for comfort or heat conservation. Phys & Sports Med *10*:71-75, 1982.
10. Ames A, Goldthwaite DA, Griffith RS, Nexcht MB: An Evaluation of Methods of Re-warming Men. Washington, D.C., Environmental Protective Series, Reprint No. 134, Office of the Quartermaster General of the Army, August 31, 1948.
11. Golden FStC, Hervey GR: The mechanism of the afterdrop following immersion hypothermia in pigs. Jour Physiol *272*:26-27, 1977.
12. Harnett RM, O'Brien EM, Sias FR, Pruitt JR: Initial treatment of profound accidental hypothermia. Av Space Environ Med *51*:680-687, 1980.
13. Siple PA, Passel CF: Measurements of dry atmospheric cooling in subfreezing temperatures. Proc Amer Phil Soc *89*:177-199, 1945.

PART II. The Physiology of Hypothermia

CHAPTER FIVE

Cerebral Circulation during Hypothermia

Milton J. Hernández, Ph.D.

Although the control of cerebral circulation in both health and disease has received considerable attention over the past two decades, the mechanisms that govern cerebral blood flow (CBF) during hypothermia remain poorly understood. In this chapter, the following aspects of cerebral circulation are reviewed: anatomy and hemodynamics, CBF during early life, and, finally, effects of hypothermia on CBF.

Anatomy and Hemodynamics

The human brain receives approximately 15% of the total cardiac output, or 50 ml. per minute per 100 gm of brain tissue. Blood is delivered to the brain by two pairs of arteries, the internal carotids and the vertebrals. The internal carotid arteries deliver approximately 65% of the blood destined for the brain, and the vertebrals account for the remainder. These four arteries enter the skull and coalesce at the base of the brain to form a polygon-shaped anastomoses known as the circle of Willis. This structure was named after the English anatomist Thomas Willis, who described it in his *Cerebri Anatome* (1). The circle of Willis is a functional anastomoses capable in most cases of redirecting the blood supply to compensate for deficiencies in the normal patterns of blood flow to specific areas of the brain. For example, the decrease in blood flow to a region that might be expected from chronic or acute occlusion of one of the four main channels to the brain can be minimized by an increase in flow through the other three arteries. This potential redistribution in flow is important in clinical conditions.

The brain, cerebellum, and medulla are supplied by a series of paired arteries that arise from either the circle of Willis or the vertebral-basilar system. After delivering oxygen and other nutrients to the brain, the venous blood flows out through a series of veins and sinuses that drain primarily into the internal jugular veins.

Cerebral Vascular Physiology

According to Poisseulle's law, blood flow through any particular organ is proportional to the pressure that drives it and inversely proportional to the resistance it meets. The driving pressure is determined by the efficiency with which the heart pumps blood and the resistance by the cross-sectional diameter of the vessels that deliver blood.

One of the peculiarities of the cerebral vascular bed is that a great part of the resistance to flow is mediated in the large arteries, both in and around the circle of Willis, as well as in the larger cerebral arteries (2). In other organs, most of the resistance occurs in the small distal arterioles and relatively little occurs in the larger arteries. In the brain, though the small vessels do contribute significantly to cerebral vascular resistance (CVR), their share is only about 50% of total CVR, with the other 50% coming from the larger vessels.

There are a number of physiological characteristics of the cerebral circulation in both humans and experimental animals that have been the subject of extensive reviews in the recent literature (3, 4, 5). They include the autoregulation of CBF, the response of CBF to increased arterial CO_2 tension, the coupling of CBF and cerebral metabolism, and the responses of CBF to hypoxia.

CBF Autoregulation

CBF autoregulation can be defined as constancy in the amount of blood delivered to the brain despite wide variations in mean arterial blood pressure (MABP) (3, 6). In humans and experimental animals, CBF is maintained at a relatively constant level in the MABP range from approximately 70 to 160 torr. Once the lower limits of autoregulation are exceeded, cerebral ischemia ensues, and, depending on its duration, neurological deficits may arise. On the hypertensive end of the pressure axis, the reverse occurs; when MABP is too great, CBF "breaks through." This "breakthrough" of autoregulation is also believed to entail neurological consequences (7).

In terms of CVR, the "typical" cerebral vessel must adjust its diameter during autoregulation of CBF. During hypotension, the vessels must dilate to compensate for the decrease in driving pressure;

during elevations in MABP, they must constrict if they are to maintain CBF.

Autoregulation of CBF probably results from a combination of myogenic, neurogenic, and metabolic factors. The initial, virtually instantaneous adjustments in CVR required during autoregulation result from the inherent myogenic properties of the smooth-muscle wall of the cerebral arteries but are modified both by the sympathetic nerves as well as by cerebral metabolism.

One theory advanced to explain how autoregulation occurs is based on the fact that under aerobic or anaerobic conditions the brain produces either carbon dioxide or lactic acid (8). Both of these metabolites generate H^+, which when present around cerebral vessels elicits vasodilatation. Another substance that may be implicated in the metabolic control of CBF is adenosine (9). According to that theory, brief periods of lowered cerebral perfusion delay the washout of metabolically produced substances in any given segment of the brain's microcirculation. The slight, localized accumulation of carbon dioxide brings about the opening of the vessels in question. This theory, though attractive, is probably incomplete, for it presupposes that CVR is mediated exclusively in the very small parenchymal vessels.

Clinically, the presence or absence of autoregulation is an indication of whether or not the cerebral vasculature is normal (10). In cases of severe head trauma, for example, CBF autoregulation is abolished (11). Dysautoregulation of varying degrees has also been noted in other pathological conditions (7, 10). Measurements of CBF during various manipulations of MABP are utilized to test autoregulation under clinical conditions. Head tilts and various vasoactive drugs can be used to induce the desired levels of hypo- or hypertension under these conditions. With the advent of a relatively noninvasive technique (the ^{133}Xenon-inhalation technique), measurements of CBF have been greatly facilitated.

CBF Responses to Increased Arterial CO_2 Tension

Carbon dioxide is a powerful cerebral vasodilator in adult experimental animals and in humans, and the responses of the cerebral vasculature to changes in arterial pCO_2 have been well documented (6, 12). CBF responds linearly to CO_2 between the approximate arterial pCO_2 levels of 20 to 80 torr. This response is characteristic of various species, including humans. CBF is altered from 1.5 to 3 ml per minute per 100 gm per torr change in arterial pCO_2. A flattening of the CBF-CO_2 response slope (i.e., "CO_2 reactivity") is, like the absence of autoregulation, an indicator of abnormal status in the cerebral vasculature.

Coupling of CBF and Cerebral Metabolism

The level of blood flow to the brain is dictated by the organ's metabolic needs (3). The higher the cerebral metabolism, the higher the CBF, and vice versa. The mediator of these increases is thought to be H^+ evolved from CO_2 or lactate, but recent studies suggest that adenosine may be involved as well (9). Thus, when large increases in cerebral metabolic rates occur, such as during rapid eye movement (REM) sleep (13) or an epileptic seizure (14), CBF increases accordingly. Recent advances in the measurement of regional CBF have shown quite elegantly that squeezing a rubber ball (15) or performing other higher cortical functions (16) elicits increases in CBF in the appropriate areas of the brain.

Responses of CBF to Hypoxia

In humans and experimental animals, CBF is unaffected by alterations in the O_2 tension of arterial blood as long as it is higher than approximately 50 torr (3). Levels of arterial hypoxia below 50 torr pO_2 trigger compensatory increases in CBF (8). The mechanism that initiates this vasodilitation is unclear, and it is only in cases of profound hypoxia that anaerobic production of lactate increases to levels sufficient to elicit an increase in CBF. Prolonged periods of cerebral hypoxia, as in cases of ischemia, may result in serious neurological damage.

Cerebral Circulation During Early Life

Although the factors that regulate the adult cerebral circulation have been studied in detail, the regulation of CBF during the newborn period has received scant attention in the past. From experiments conducted on rats (17, 18), dogs (19, 20, 21, 22, 23), nonhuman primates (24), and humans (25, 26), it appears that CBF is considerably lower in the newborn than in the adult. In addition, several studies indicate that cerebral vascular responses to hypercarbia are less developed in neonates than in adults (20, 27). However, few conclusions can be drawn from the literature available because of the variety of species employed, the wide range of physiological conditions under study, and, possibly, the methodological limitations of the techniques employed to measure CBF.

It should be noted that, despite this seeming paucity of information on the responses of the neonatal cerebral circulation and metabolism to stressful conditions, a number of recent studies point to a notable resistance of the developing brain to several of the insults so common in early life, including hypoxia, ischemia, hypoglycemia, and asphyxia.

Hypoxia

Preliminary studies of CBF in the author's laboratory have shown that CBF does not increase with hypoxia in the newborn dog until the arterial pO_2 decreases to a level below approximately 35 torr (28). This limit is lower than that of the adult, in whom decreases in arterial pO_2 below approximately 50 torr produce increments in CBF (3).

Ischemia

The author and his colleagues (22) have recently shown that the phenomenon of CBF autoregulation is present in the newborn dog. Decreases in MABP to approximately 30 torr resulted in no changes in CBF. Thus, the newborn dog's brain appears to be well protected from ischemia during hypotension, down to very low levels of MABP. More recent unpublished results from a study employing an autoradiographic technique suggest that the limit for autoregulation, on a regional basis, may actually be lower than the author and his colleagues previously reported (22).

Hypoglycemia

The author and his colleagues (29) also recently reported that both CBF and cerebral metabolic rate for oxygen ($CMRO_2$) are undisturbed during profound hypoglycemia in the newborn dog. At very low arterial blood glucose concentrations, CBF and $CMRO_2$ were not significantly changed from control levels. Therefore, the newborn dog's brain appears to be extremely tolerant of hypoglycemia.

Asphyxia

Clinical observations in the past have pointed to the newborn's remarkable tolerance of asphyxia (profound hypoxia combined with hypercarbia). In newborn dogs, the author and his colleagues (21) found that a profound redistribution of regional cerebral blood flow (rCBF) occurs during asphyxia, such that blood flow to the forebrain decreases and blood flow to the hindbrain increases. They believe that these changes may serve to preserve vital cardiovascular centers in the brain stem during asphyxia and that this results in the newborn's known resistance to this insult.

Effects of Hypothermia on CBF

Very little information is available on the cerebral circulation and oxidative metabolism during hypothermia. The few studies conducted to date indicate only that CBF and $CMRO_2$ decrease with body temperature. Absent from the literature are studies on the effects of hypothermia on autoregulation, CO_2 responses, and responses to hypoxia. This is especially true of studies on newborns. The physiological mechanisms that dictate either survival or nonsurvival after hypothermic stress are poorly understood.

Ehrmantraut, Ticktin, and Fazekas (30) studied the effects of marked hypothermia on CBF and $CMRO_2$ in two adult males. In the first case, at 30°C, CBF was 31 ml per minute per 100 gm, and $CMRO_2$ was 1.6 ml O_2 per minute per 100 gm. Upon the victim's rewarming to 37.8°C, both CBF and $CMRO_2$ returned to almost normal levels. In the second case, a more severe degree of hypothermia was present, with a core temperature of 23°C, CBF was 31 ml per minute per 100 gm, $CMRO_2$ equaled 1.5 ml O_2 per minute per 100 gm. Again, when the victim was rewarmed, both values returned to normal levels. It should be noted that neither patient was severely hypotensive during either hypothermia or normothermia and so dysautoregulation was not the cause of their lowered CBF. Rather, in light of what is now known of the delicate coupling of CBF and cerebral metabolism (3), it is likely that CBF was decreased to match the lowered metabolic rate imposed by hypothermia. Similar results were reported by Stone, Donnelly, and Frobese (31) in humans and by Rosomoff and Holaday (32) in dogs. However, the arterial-inflow technique employed by Rosomoff and Holaday is known to seriously misrepresent true CBF values. Interestingly, Rosomoff and Holaday (32) noted that MABP decreased in their experiments when body temperature was lowered to approximately 30°C. If MABP dropped at the rate of 5 torr per 1°C as they suggested, then their hypothermic dogs' MABP (not reported) might be below the lower limits of the autoregulation plateau.

More recently, Kawashima and associates (33) measured CBF in hypothermic dogs by using the radioactive microsphere technique. They also reported that hypothermia (23.9°C) decreased CBF from

53 to 14 ml per minute per 100 gm with no major reductionism in MABP. Anzai and associates (34) also utilized this technique to measure CBF in more discrete regions of the brain than those described by Kawashima and associates (33). A remarkably uniform decrease in regional CBF was noted throughout the brain; it ranged from 62% in the brain stem to 82% in the posterior lobe. MABP during hypothermia was also lowered but was still within the autoregulatory range. In another recent study, Steen, Milde, and Michenfelder (35) studied the effects of prolonged hypothermia and rewarming on CBF, $CMRO_2$ and levels of energy-yielding metabolites. In dogs rendered hypothermic for 24 hr, CBF was 20 ml per minute per 100 gm, $CMRO_2$ equaled 2.0 ml O_2 per minute per 100 gm, and ATP and phosphocreative levels were normal. Upon the dogs' rewarming to 37°C, $CMRO_2$ increased to 3.4 ml O_2 per minute per 100 gm, but CBF equaled only 30 ml per minute per 100 gm, a value approximately 30% to 40% of normal levels. Interestingly, ATP and phosphocreative levels were also lower than control values upon the dogs' rewarming.

Obviously more research needs to be done in studying the interaction between hypothermia and CBF, since many hypothermia victims are also victims of drowning.

References

1. Willis T: Cerebri Anatome. London, 1664.
2. Stromberg DD, Fox JR: Pressures in the pial arterial microcirculation of the cat during changes in systemic arterial blood pressure. Circ Res *31*:229-239, 1972.
3. Lassen NA: Control of cerebral circulation in health and disease. Circ Res *24*:749-760, 1974.
4. Kuschinsky W, Wahl M: Local chemical and neurogenic regulation of cerebral vascular resistance. Physiol Rev *58*:656-689, 1978.
5. Purves MJ: The Physiology of the Cerebral Circulation. Cambridge University Press, Cambridge, 1972.
6. Hernández MJ, Brennan RW, Bowman GS: Cerebral blood flow autoregulation in the rat. Stroke *9*:150-155, 1978.
7. Strandgaard L, Olesen J, Skinhoj E, Lassen NA: Autoregulation of brain circulation in severe arterial hypertension. Brit Med Jour *1*:507-510, 1973.
8. Siesjö BK: Brain Energy Metabolism. Wiley, Winchester, 1978.
9. Rubio R, Berne RM, Bockman EL, Curnish, RR: Relationship between adenosine concentration and oxygen supply in rat brain. Amer Jour Physiol *228*:1896-1902, 1975.
10. Agnoli A, et al.: Studies during drug-induced hypertension in normal subjects and in patients with cerebral vascular diseases. Cir Res *38*:800-812, 1968.
11. Fog M: Autoregulation of cerebral blood flow and its abolition by local hypoxia and/or trauma. Scand Jour Lab Clin Invest Suppl *102*:VB, 1968.
12. Reivich M: Arterial pCO_2 and cerebral hemodynamics. Amer Jour Physiol *206*:25-35, 1964.

13. Townsend RE, Prinz PN, Obrist WD: Human cerebral blood flow during sleep and waking. Jour Appl Physiol *35*:620-625, 1973.
14. Meldrum BS, Nilsson B: Cerebral blood flow and metabolic rate early and late in prolonged epileptic seizures induced in rates by bicuculline. Brain *99*:523-542, 1976.
15. Olesen J: Contralateral focal increase of regional cerebral blood flow in man during arm work. Brain *94*:635-646, 1971.
16. Ingvar DH: Patterns of brain activity revealed by measurements of regional cerebral blood flow. See Brain Work, Ingvar DH and Lassen NA (eds.), pp. 397-413. Copenhagen, Munksgard, 1975.
17. Barker JN: Fetal and neonatal cerebral blood flow. Amer Jour Physiol *210*:897-902, 1966.
18. Moore TJ, et al.: Brain glucose metabolism in the newborn rat. Amer Jour Physiol *221*: 1746-1753, 1971.
19. Gregoire NM, Gjedde A, Plum F, Duffy TE: Cerebral blood flow and cerebral metabolic rates for oxygen, glucose, and ketone bodies in new born dogs. Jour Neurochem *30*:63-69, 1978.
20. Hernández MJ, Brennan RW, Vannucci RC, Bowman GS: Cerebral blood flow and oxygen consumption in the newborn dog. Amer Jour Physiol *234*:R209-R215, 1978.
21. Hernández MJ, Hawkins RA, Brennan RW: Regional cerebral blood flow during neonatal asphyxia. *In:* Cerebral Metabolism and Neural Function, pp. 196-201. Baltimore, Williams & Wilkins, 1980.
22. Hernández, MJ, Brennan RW, Bowman GS: Autoregulation of cerebral blood flow in the newborn dog. Brain Res *184*:199-202, 1980.
23. Kennedy C, Grave GD, Jehle JW, Sokoloff L: Changes in blood flow in the component structures of the dog brain during postnatal maturation. Jour Neurochem *19*:2423-2433, 1972.
24. Behrman RE, Lees MJ: Organ blood flows of the fetal, newborn and adult rhesus monkey: A comparative study. Biol Neonate *18*:330-340, 1971.
25. Garfunkel JM, Baird HW, Ziegler J: The relationship of oxygen consumption to cerebral functional activity. Jour Pediatr *44*:64-72, 1954.
26. Lou HC, Lassen NA, Friis-Hansen B: Impaired autoregulation of cerebral blood flow in the distressed newborn infant. Jour Pediatr *94*:118-121, 1979.
27. Reivich M, Braun A, Shapiro H, Rawson J, Sano N: Reactivity of cerebral vessels to CO_2 in the newborn rhesus monkey. Europ Neurol *6*:132-136, 1971.
28. Casciotti MS, Hernández MJ, Vannucci RC, Bowman GS, Brennan RW: Cerebral blood flow and oxidative metabolism in the hypoxic newborn dog. Physiologist *22*:18, 1979.
29. Hernández MJ, Vannucci RC, Salcedo A, Brennan RW: Cerebral blood flow and metabolism during hypoglycemia in newborn dogs. Jour Neurochem *35*:622-628, 1980.
30. Ehrmantraut WR, Ticktin HE, Fazekas JF: Cerebral hemodynamics and metabolism in accidental hypothermia. Arch Intern Med *99*:57-59, 1957.
31. Stone HH, Donnelly C, Frobese AS: The effect of lowered body temperature on the cerebral hemodynamics and metabolism of man. Surg Gynecol Obstet *103*:313-317, 1956.
32. Rosomoff HL, Holaday DA: Cerebral blood flow and cerebral oxygen consumption during hypothermia. Amer Jour Physiol *179*:85-88, 1954.
33. Kawashima Y, et al.: Changes in distribution of cardiac output by surface-induced deep hypothermia in dogs. Jour Appl Physiol *40*:876-882, 1976.
34. Anzi T, Turner MD, Gibson WH, Neeley WA: Blood flow distribution in dogs during hypothermia and posthypothermia. Amer Jour Physiol *234*:H706-H710, 1978.
35. Steen PA, Milde JH, Michenfelder JD: The detrimental effects of prolonged hypothermia and rewarming in the dog. Anesthesiology *52*:224-230, 1980.

CHAPTER SIX

Hypothermia: A Timing Disorder of Circadian Thermoregulatory Rhythms?

Martin C. Moore-Ede, M.D., Ph.D.

Hypothermia is a significant cause of morbidity and mortality, especially among the elderly (1). The chronic exposure of individuals to reduced environmental temperatures in which they develop hypothermia is a public health and socioeconomic problem of enormous proportions. It can be addressed only through a concerted, multifaceted effort. Since science is "the art of the soluble" (2), we should focus our attention on problems that have the highest probability of yielding to experimental investigation. One such area of profitable inquiry appears to be the identification of those factors that may predispose an individual to hypothermia when he or she is faced with reductions in ambient temperature.

Thermoregulation in humans is normally very efficient, maintaining core body temperature within a few tenths of a degree in the face of a wide range of environmental temperatures. Body temperature, however, is not regulated at a constant level over the day but rather oscillates with a prominent circadian (about 24-hr) rhythm. This diurnal variation was first recognized by Hunter in 1778 (3). Using one of the first thermometers, he showed that body temperature in humans falls to a minimum during sleep and rises to a maximum during daytime activity. Since Hunter's time, the endogenous nature of circadian temperature rhythms has become well established (4, 5).

This chapter presents evidence to show that a disorder of the circadian timing system may predispose an individual to hypothermia. More specifically, the failure to thermoregulate against falling ambient temperature may be caused by dissociation of the circadian timing of

Supported by NSF grant PCM-76-19943, NIH grants NS-13921 and GN-22083, NASA grant NSG-9054, and NIH Research Career Development Award NS-00247-01.

heat-production and heat-loss mechanisms. It is also argued that, since elderly people appear to be more susceptible to circadian dissociation, this mechanism may contribute to hypothermia in older subjects. To provide a theoretical basis for this discussion, the organization of the circadian timing system and the regulation of body-temperature rhythms are reviewed first.

The Circadian Timing System

Most physiological and behavioral variables show prominent circadian rhythms, each with its own characteristic phase relationship to environmental time cues. These circadian rhythms are endogenously generated within the organism, and they persist when the animal is placed in a constant aperiodic environment. Under such conditions, circadian rhythms show a free-running period usually close to but significantly different from 24 hr. Circadian rhythms can only be synchronized to a 24-hr period by specific environmental periodicities, the most important of which are the light-dark cycle and the timing of food intake. Over the past 25 yr, the properties of free-running circadian systems and the mechanisms of entrainment have been extensively documented (6).

Circadian rhythms in physiological and behavioral variables are generated by an internal system of oscillators that are coupled together by periodic neural and endocrine mechanisms (7). There is evidence that the internal synchronization between circadian oscillators in humans is maintained by two central pacemakers with different endogenous periods. One of these regulates the timing of the sleep-wake cycle and a number of associated rhythms (e.g., plasma growth hormone, urinary calcium excretion), and the other regulates the timing of the core-body-temperature rhythm (as well as other rhythms such as plasma cortisol and REM sleep) (8, 9). Occasionally when a person is deprived of environmental time cues, these two pacemakers can become "internally desynchronized" so that the sleep-wake cycle free runs with a different periodicity from the core-body-temperature rhythm (10). In such a desynchronized subject, the sleep-wake cycle might show a 33-hr period at the same time as the body-temperature rhythm continues to display a period of 25 hr.

These two central pacemakers are located in separate anatomical sites. The suprachiasmatic nuclei (SCN) of the hypothalamus appear to be the pacemaker controlling the sleep-wake cycle and related rhythms. When these nuclei are destroyed in lesioning experiments, sleep and wakefulness become randomly distributed throughout day and night instead of being consolidated to one part of the day (11, 12). However, Fuller and associates (13) recently showed that the core-body-temperature rhythm persists after the SCN are destroyed; this indicates that the pacemaker driving core temperature is located outside the SCN.

Circadian Thermoregulatory Rhythms

In humans, the circadian rhythm of core body temperature shows a 1°C change over the course of each cycle. A typical record from a subject living a regular 24-hr day is shown in Figure 6-1. Core body temperature starts to rise each morning before the subject awakes and before the lights come on. It then rapidly rises to a plateau level after the subject's waking and is maintained at that level throughout the day. In the evening, body temperature falls again to reach a minimum between 4 and 5 A.M.

Both heat-loss and heat-production mechanisms contribute to the generation of the circadian rhythm of core body temperature. The

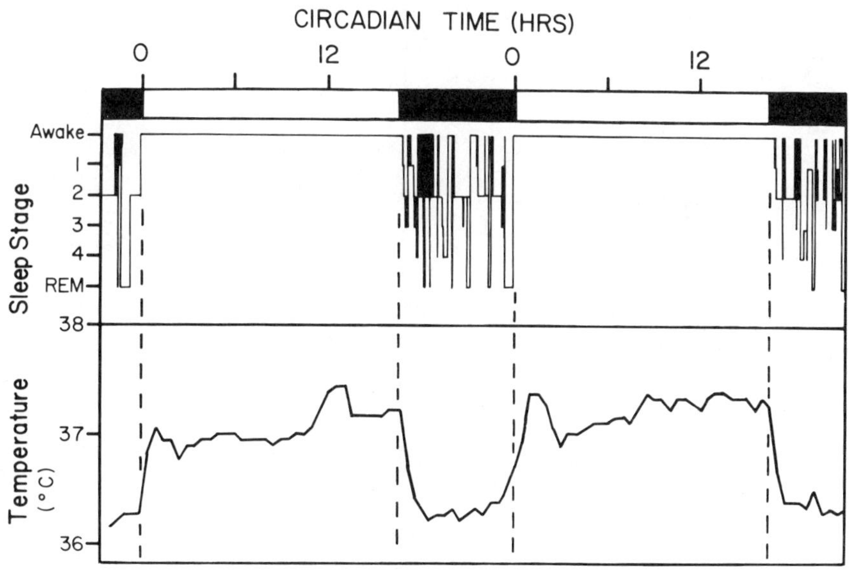

Figure 6-1. Circadian sleep-wake cycle (upper panel) and body-temperature rhythms (lower panel) of normal human subject recorded over a 48-hr period of observation. Lights on from 7 A.M. (circadian time 0) to 11 P.M. (circadian time 16) each day are indicated by the white bar above the figure; the black bar indicates the hours of darkness.

rhythmic fall in body temperature in each cycle is in part caused by increases in skin blood flow and therefore increased loss of heat by the body (14, 15, 16, 17, 18). Similarly, a rhythm in metabolism or heat production has been shown to be present in several species of mammals (15, 19, 20). In addition, behavioral changes at certain phases of the cycle may contribute to the control of the body temperature rhythm (21, 22, 23).

The interaction of heat loss and heat production in generating the circadian rhythm of body temperature is illustrated by data from squirrel monkeys (*Saimiri sciureus*) in Figure 6-2. The fall in body

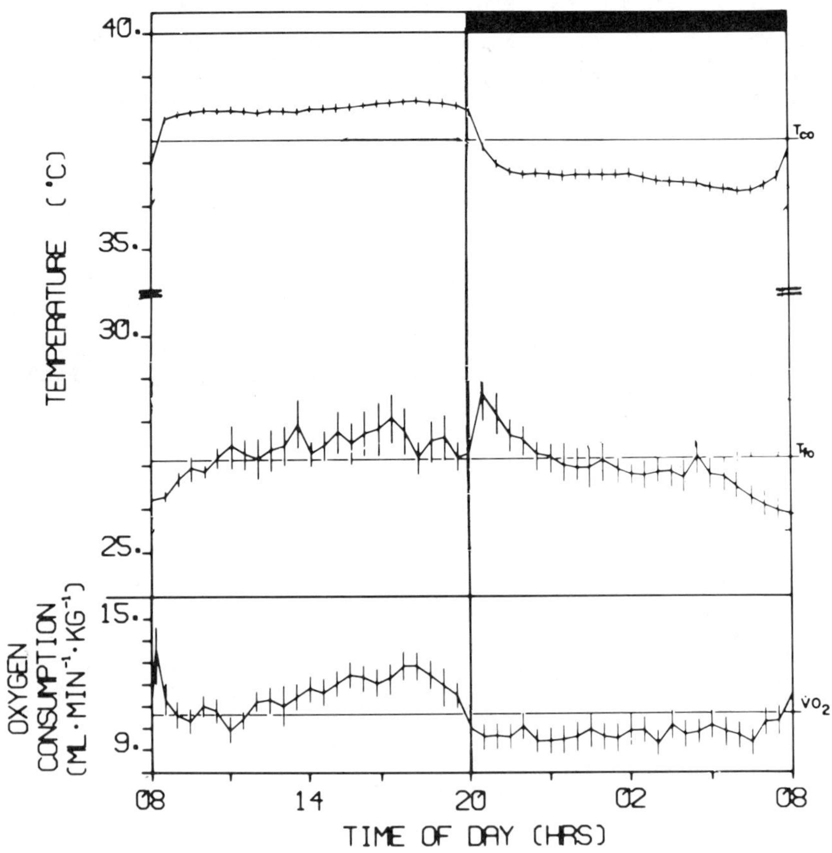

Figure 6-2. Circadian rhythms of core body temperature (upper panel), foot skin temperature (middle panel), and oxygen consumption (lower panel), from four squirrel monkeys (*Saimiri sciureus*) (mean ± SEM) entrained to an LD 12:12 light-dark cycle with lights on from 8 to 20 hr each day.

temperature at the end of the subjective day can be seen to be a combination of a fall in heat production (indicated by a decrease in oxygen consumption) starting before the onset of darkness and a rapid rise in heat loss (indicated by the increase in foot skin temperature) immediately after the onset of darkness. Similarly, the morning increase in core body temperature in anticipation of light is achieved by a sharp rise in oxygen consumption (and heat production) while skin temperature (and heat loss) falls. The skin temperature then stays low until daytime elevated body temperatures have been achieved.

There is evidence that heat production and vasomotor heat loss may be timed by separate pacemakers within the circadian system. In humans who have become internally desynchronized so that their sleep-wake cycle and core-body-temperature rhythms free run with different periods, the skin-temperature rhythm (and therefore a major component of thermoregulatory heat loss) is coupled with the sleep-wake cycle and shows a period independent from the core-body-temperature rhythm (9, 24). A similar dissociation between skin-temperature and core-body-temperature rhythms has also been observed in the squirrel monkey (15).

Impaired Thermoregulation in the Absence of Circadian Cues

Does temporal dissociation between heat-loss and heat-production mechanisms impair thermoregulation? The answer to that question came serendipitously. While studying the body-temperature rhythms of squirrel monkeys in a temperature-controlled chamber in the absence of environmental time cues, the author and his colleagues noticed one night that the body temperature of a monkey had fallen precipitously. On checking the temperature record from the chamber, it became apparent that the thermostat had failed overnight and that the ambient temperature had fallen from 28°C to 20°C. When they (25) reproduced this drop in ambient temperature they found that the monkeys maintained in light-dark cycles thermoregulated perfectly (Figure 6-3) so that this body temperature changed by no more than 0.1°C to 0.2°C. However, if the monkeys were maintained without a light-dark cycle in constant illumination, the same 8°C drop in ambient temperature resulted in significant falls in core body temperature of up to 2°C. The responses did not depend on the time of day that ambient temperature was reduced. Subsequent studies have shown that in a 24-hr light-dark cycle, an 8°C fall in ambient temperature does not cause a fall in core body temperature at any phase of day or night. However, falls in core temperature can be induced at all phases

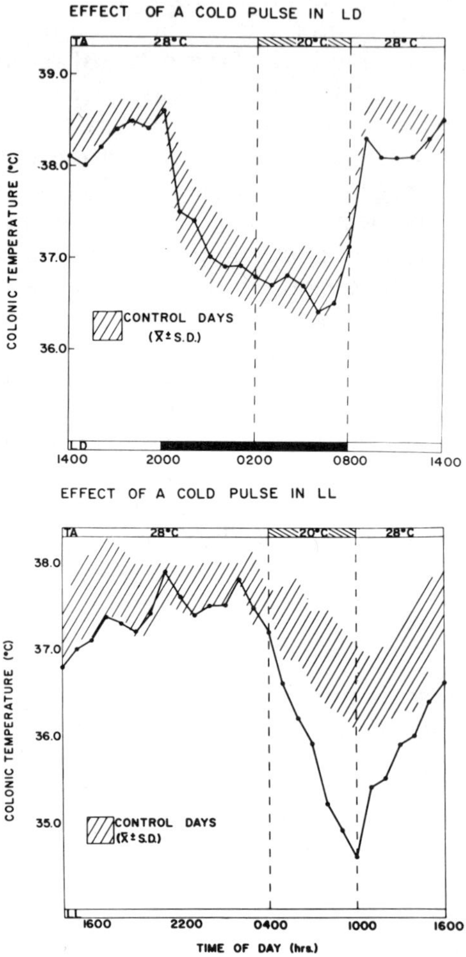

Figure 6-3. Effect of a 6-hr cold exposure on core (colonic) body temperature in a squirrel monkey (*Saimiri sciureus*) entrained to an LD 12:12 cycle (upper panel) and free running in constant illumination (LL) (lower panel). At the top of each graph, the ambient temperature (T_A) is indicated on the day the cold pulse was applied; the lighting conditions are indicated at the bottom of each panel (the black bar indicates darkness). The shading represents the mean ± SD of colonic temperature from the previous 3 d, and the solid line is the colonic temperature on the day the cold pulse was given. The data are normalized so that each cycle (24 hr in upper panel; 25 hr in lower panel was set equal to 360° of circadian phase angle. (From Fuller, Sulzman, and Moore-Ede [25], reprinted with permission from *Science 199*: 794-796, 1978.)

of the temperature rhythm in animals free running in constant light. This impairment of thermoregulation in constant environments has recently been confirmed in rodents by Satinoff (26) and also by Holley and Ninget (27).

In order to determine whether the failures to thermoregulate were related to the constant illumination per se, the author and his colleagues (28) also studied the response to drops in ambient temperature in squirrel monkeys mantained in constant illumination but synchronized to a 24-hr period by the application of restricted feeding schedules. They had previously shown that food was an effective time cue in synchronizing circadian rhythms in the squirrel monkey, just like the light-dark cycle, and that consistent phase relationships among the various rhythms within the animal could be maintained by the provision of periodic feeding (29). In food-synchronized animals, drops in ambient temperature did not cause any fall in core body temperature (Figure 6-4), this implied that it was the dissociation of the circadian system in constant environments, rather than the provision of constant light per se, that contributed to the failure of thermoregulation.

To test this hypothesis, the author and his colleagues used a technique by which circadian internal desyncrhonization could be reliably induced in squirrel monkeys. They had previously demonstrated that cortisol is an important mediator of temporal information within the circadian system (30). Through the preparation of adrenalectomized monkeys with chronically implanted catheters, it was possible to regulate artificially the plasma-cortisol rhythm through the provision of intravenous infusions of cortisol. The monkeys were studied in an isolation chamber with the infusion catheter led outside the chamber so that the animals were unaware of the timing of steroid administration. By placing the animals in constant illumination so that their circadian rhythms free ran with an endogenous 25-hr period and at the same time providing cortisol infusions with a 24-hr periodicity, the investigators were able to induce internal desynchronization. The rhythms that were synchronized by cortisol were entrained to a 24-hr period, whereas the other rhythms in the animal free ran with their normal endogenous 25-hr periodicity.

In these internally desynchronized animals, consistent large falls in body temperature were obtained whenever ambient temperature was reduced (29). An example is shown in Figure 6-5. This finding could not be explained by the fact that these animals were adrenalectomized, since no falls in core body temperature were observed in adrenalectomized animals synchronized by a light-dark cycle.

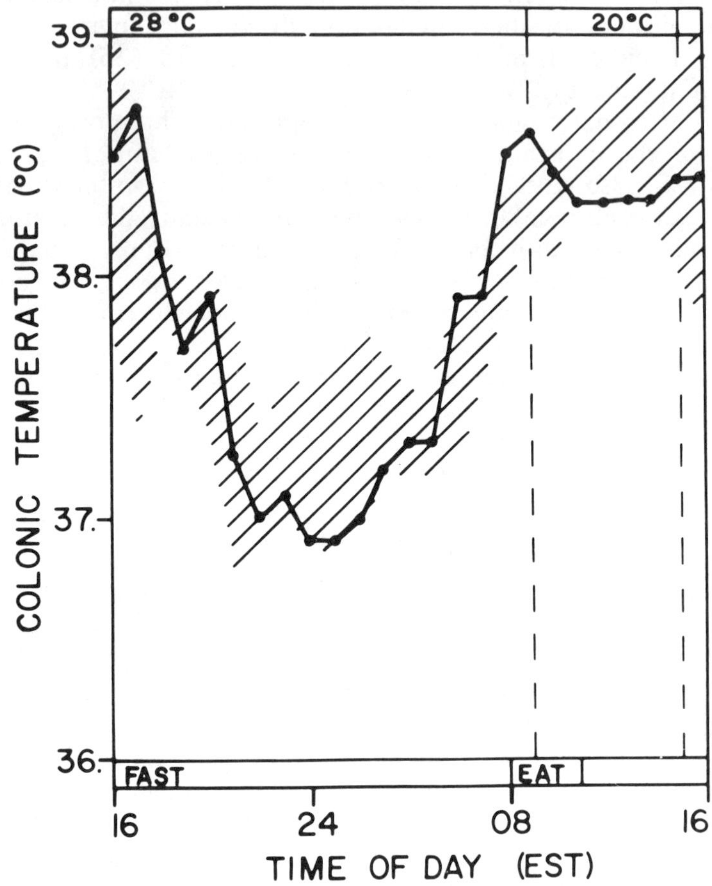

Figure 6-4. Effect of a 6-hr cold exposure on core body temperature in a squirrel monkey (*Saimiri sciureus*) maintained in constant illumination but provided with a restricted 24-hr feeding schedule (EAT indicates daily mealtime) that entrained its circadian system. The axes and data presentation are as described for Figure 6-3, except that time of day is plotted on the abscissa. (From Fuller, Sulzman, and Moore-Ede [28], reprinted with the permission of Pergamon Press, Inc.)

Circadian Dissociation and Hypothermia

Dissociation between the heat-production and the heat-loss mechanisms involved in thermoregulation thus appears to result in a reduced ability to regulate against drops in ambient temperature. This suggests that precise internal temporal relationships are required between

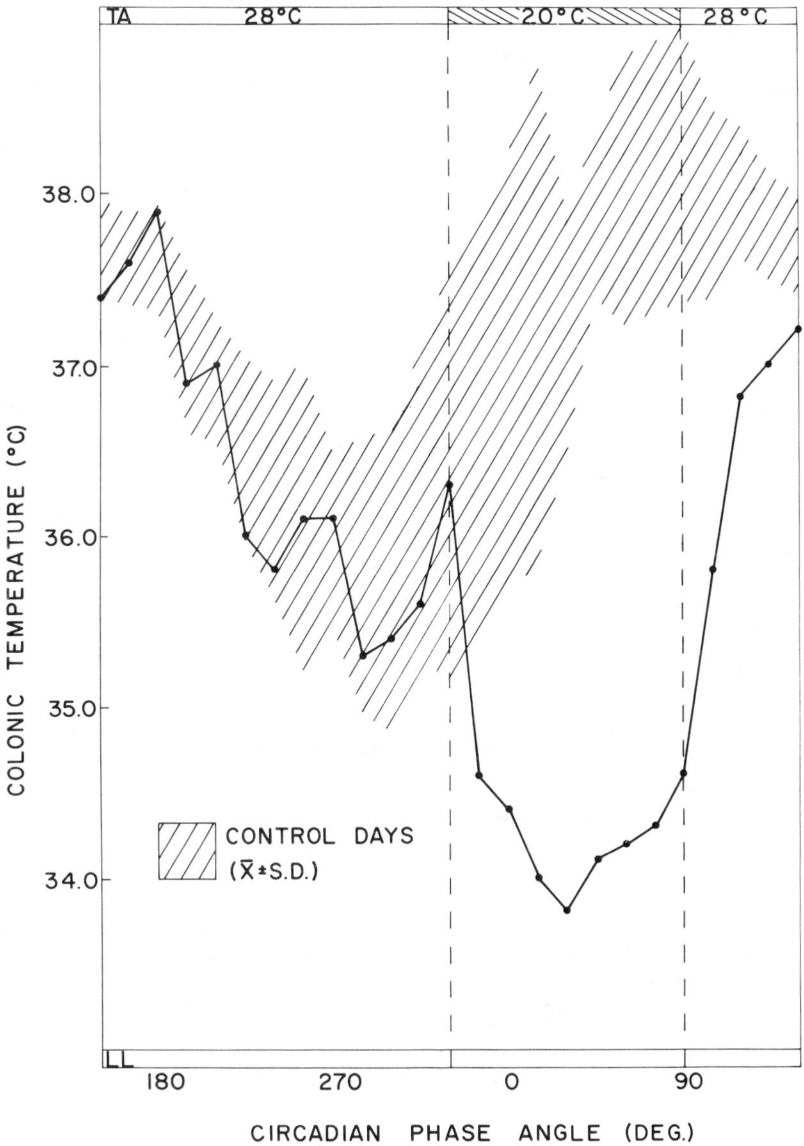

Figure 6-5. Effect of a 6-hr cold exposure in a squirrel monkey (*Saimiri sciureus*) internally desynchronized by periodic cortisol administration as described in the text. Axes and data presentation are as in Figure 6-3. (From Fuller, Sulzman, and Moore-Ede [28], reprinted with permission of Pergamon Press, Inc.)

heat-production and heat-loss mechanisms in order to achieve stable homeostasis.

What relevance does this impairment of thermoregulation have for the clinical syndrome of hypothermia? One observation that suggests a correlation is that elderly subjects are particularly prone to hypothermia. With increasing age, the circadian system begins to dissociate (31) and internal desynchronization has been reported to be more frequent (8). Thus, in the very population that is most susceptible to hypothermia there is also an increased incidence of circadian dissociation. Clearly, much work needs to be done in order to confirm the theory that such failures in thermoregulation occur in humans, but these studies offer a testable hypothesis that seems well worth exploring.

This is not the first report of failures in physiological function when organisms are deprived of circadian time cues. In constant light, tomato plants fail to thrive (32) and fruit flies show a significant reduction in their life span (33). The provision of a light-dark cycle with a period close to 24 hr corrects both of these conditions. Humans are confronted with aperiodic environments in intensive care wards (with constant levels of lighting and noise), in polar environments (during midwinter and midsummer), and even in the 24-hr activity of cities. The full importance of the loss of these periodic cues is not fully understood.

A number of clinical conditions caused by disorders of the circadian timing system are now coming to light. These include failures to entrain to environmental light-dark cycles (34, 35, 36, 37), phase disorders in which the sleep-wake cycle and other rhythms are entrained at inappropriate phase relationships to the light-dark cycle (38), and amplitude disorders and arrhythmias in which disruption of the sleep-wake cycle occurs because of damage to the pacemaker (6). These observations reinforce the conclusion that clinical syndromes can as much involve the fourth dimension of medicine (that of time) as the three spatial dimensions.

References

1. Fox RH, Woodward PM, Exton-Smith AN, Green MF, Donnison DV, Wicks MH: Body temperatures in the elderly: A national study of physiological, social, and environmental conditions. Brit Med Jour *1*:200-206, 1973.
2. Medawar PB: The Art of the Soluble. London, Methuen, 1967.
3. Hunter J: Of the heat of animals and vegetables. Phil Trans Roy Soc Lond (Biol) *68*: 7-49, 1778.
4. Ogle JW: On the diurnal variations in the temperature of the human body in health. St George's Hosp Rep *1*:220-245, 1866.

5. Aschoff J: Circadian rhythm of activity and body temperature. *In*: Hardy JD, Gagge AP, Stolwijk JAJ (eds), Physiological and Behavioral Temperature Regulation, pp. 905-919. Springfield, Ill., Charles C. Thomas, 1970.
6. Moore-Ede MC, Sulzman FM, Fuller CA: The Clocks That Time Us: Anatomy and Physiology of the Mammalian Circadian Timing System. Cambridge, Mass., Harvard University Press, 1982.
7. Moore-Ede MC, Sulzman FM: Internal temporal order. *In*: Aschoff J (ed.), Handbook of Behavior Neurobiology, pp. 215-241. New York, Plenum Press, 1981.
8. Wever RA: The Circadian System of Man: Results of Experiments under Temporal Isolation. New York, Springer-Verlag, 1979.
9. Czeisler CA, Weitzman ED, Moore-Ede MC, Zimmerman JC, Knauer RS: Human sleep: Its duration and structure depend on its circadian phase. Science *210*:1264-1267, 1980.
10. Aschoff J, Gerecke U, Wever R: Desynchronization of human circadian rhythms. Japan Jour Physiol *17*:450-457, 1967.
11. Ibuka N, Kawamura H: Loss of circadian rhythm in sleep-wakefulness cycle in the rat by suprachiasmatic nucleus lesions. Brain Res *96*:76-81, 1975.
12. Rusak B, Zucker I: Neural regulation of circadian rhythms. Physiol Rev *59*:449-526, 1979.
13. Fuller CA, Lydic R, Sulzman FM, Albers HE, Tepper B, Moore-Ede MC: Circadian rhythm of body temperature persists after suprachiasmatic lesions in the squirrel monkey. Amer Jour Physiol *241*:R385-R391, 1981.
14. Aschoff J, Heise A: Thermal conductance in man: Its dependence on time of day and ambient temperature. *In*: Itoh S, Ogata K, Yoshimura H (eds.), Advances in Climatic Physiology, pp. 334-348. New York, Springer-Verlag, 1972.
15. Fuller CA, Sulzman FM, Moore-Ede MC: Circadian control of thermoregulation in the squirrel monkey (*Saimiri sciureus*). Amer Jour Physiol *236*:R153-R161, 1979.
16. Smith RE: Circadian variations in human thermoregulatory responses. Jour Appl Physiol *26*:554-559, 1969.
17. Bloch M: Rhythmic diurnal variation in limb blood flow in man. Nature *202*:398-399, 1964.
18. Gauthrie M: Circadian rhythm in the vasomotor oscillations of skin temperature in man. Int Jour Chronobiol *1*:103-139, 1973.
19. Aschoff J, Pohl H: Rhythmic variations in energy metabolism. Fed Proc *29*:1541-1552, 1970.
20. Kreider MB, Iampietro PF: Oxygen consumption and body temperature during sleep in cold environments. Jour Appl Physiol *14*:765-767, 1959.
21. Cabanac M, Hildebrandt G, Massonnet B, Strempel H: A study of the hypothermal cycle of behavioral temperature regulation in man. Jour Physiol (London) *257*:275-291, 1976.
22. Ingram DL, Walters DE, Legge KF: Vaiations in behavioral thermoregulation in the young pig over 24 hour periods. Physiol Behav *14*:689-695, 1975.
23. De Castro JM: Diurnal rhythms of behavioral effects on core temperature. Physiol Behav *21*:883-886, 1978.
24. Czeisler CA: Internal organization of temperature, sleep-wake, and neuroendocrine rhythms monitored in an environment free of time cues. Ph.D. thesis, Stanford University, Stanford, Calif., 1978.
25. Fuller CA, Sulzman FM, Moore-Ede MC: Thermoregulation is impaired in an environment without circadian time cues. Science *199*:794-796, 1978.
26. Satinoff E: Personal communication, 1981.
27. Holley D: Personal communication, 1982.
28. Fuller CA, Sulzman FM, Moore-Ede MC; Effective thermoregulation in primates

depends upon internal circadian synchronization. Comp Biochem Physiol (A) *63*:207-212, 1979.
29. Sulzman FM, Fuller CA, Moore-Ede MC: Comparison of synchronization of primate circadian rhythms by light and food. Amer Jour Physiol *234*:R130-R135, 1978.
30. Moore-Ede MC, Schmelzer WS, Kass DA, Herd JA: Cortisol mediated synchronization of circadian rhythm in urinary potassium excretion. Amer Jour Physiol *233*:R230-R238, 1977.
31. Sacher GA, Duffy PH: Age changes in rhythms of energy metabolism, activity, and body temperature in *Mus* and *Peromyscus*. *In*: Samis HV, Capobianco S (eds.), Aging and Biological Rhythms, pp. 105-124. New York and London, Plenum Press, 1978.
32. Hillman WS: Injury of tomato plants by continuous light and unfavorable photoperiodic cycles. Amer Jour Bot *43*:89-96, 1956.
33. Pittendrigh CS, Minis DH: Circadian systems: Longevity as a function of circadian resonance in *Drosophila melanogaster*. Proc Natl Acad Sci USA *69*:1537-1539, 1972.
34. Miles LEM, Raynal DM, Wilson MA: Blind man living in normal society has circadian rhythms of 24.9 hours. Science *198*:421-423, 1977.
35. Elliott AL, Mills JN, Waterhouse JM: A man with too long a day. Jour Physiol (London) *212*:30-33, 1971.
36. Kokkoris CP, Weitzman ED, Pollak CP, Spielman AJ, Czeisler CA, Bradlow H: Long-term ambulatory temperature monitoring in a subject with a hypernychthermal sleep-wake cycle disturbance. Sleep *1*:177-190, 1978.
37. Weber AL, Cary MS, Connor N, Keyes P: Human non-24-hour sleep-wake cycles in an everyday environment. Sleep *2*:347-354, 1980.
38. Czeisler CA, Richardson GS, Coleman RM, et al.: Chronotherapy: Resetting the circadian clocks of patients with delayed sleep phase insomnia. Sleep *4*:1-21, 1981.

CHAPTER SEVEN

Neuropharmacological Aspects of Thermoregulation

Peter Lomax, M.D., D.Sc.

Modern concepts of thermoregulation derive from the classic studies initiated some 40 yr ago by Ranson and his colleagues (1), although the theoretical considerations stem from the ideas developed by Liebermeister (2) on the basis of clinical observations during the second half of the 19th century. Over the past two decades, a great deal of attention has been directed toward the role of the several neurotransmitters in the central thermoregulatory pathways in maintaining thermal homeostasis. Recently, the list of putative central neurotransmitters has been expanded considerably with the identification of neural peptides in the central nervous system and the demonstration that many of these may have effects on body temperature either under thermoneutral conditions or during response to environmental thermal stress.

A large number of centrally active drugs has been shown to modify or disrupt thermoregulation in different species, and many can lead to clinically important disorders, not infrequently to a life-threatening degree. With increasing research into the mode of action of neuropharmacological agents, there is growing evidence that many exert their effects indirectly by a modification of transmitter release rather than by a direct action at neuronal receptor sites. Thus, the elucidation of the function of transmitters involved in the thermoregulatory pathways assumes added importance in explaining the pathogenesis of drug-induced disorders of thermoregulation and in developing rational stratagems for the therapeutic management of these syndromes.

The research discussed in this chapter was supported in part by ONR contract N00014-75-C-0506 and USPHS grant AAO 3513-03.

In this chapter, current concepts of central thermoregulation are discussed together with the neuronal pathways involved. On the basis of these considerations, thermoregulatory disorders resulting from the use of centrally active drugs that are of relevance to clinical practice are discussed. Finally, a common condition that appears to be the result of a specific thermoregulatory change—postmenopausal hot flushes—is described.

The Regulation of Body Temperature

As early as 1845, Bergmann (3) suggested that thermosensitive sites in the brain are responsible for regulating cutaneous heat loss. Evidence rapidly accrued to support this hypothesis, but it was not until 1938 that Magoun and associates (4) localized the major thermoregulatory centers to the rostral hypothalamus in the cat. Subsequent evidence has confirmed the preeminence of the preoptic and supraoptic nuclei of the hypothalamus in regulating body temperature in numerous species, including humans (Figure 7-1).

Inputs come to the rostral hypothalamus from thermosensors located throughout the body, and there is some debate as to which temperature the thermostats are "looking at." However, most of the evidence favors the transduced hypothalamic temperature as the regulated temperature. When an animal is subjected to thermal stress (e.g., entering a cold environment), appropriate thermoregulatory

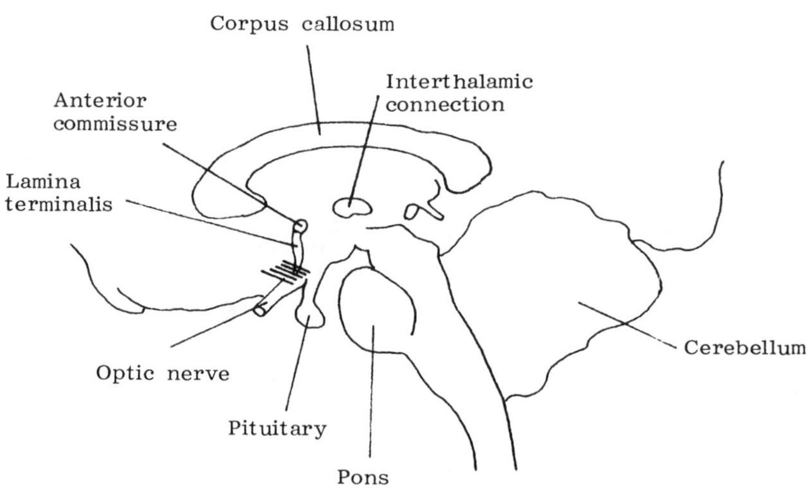

Figure 7-1. Midsagittal section of the human diencephalon. The cross-hatched area indicates the site of the rostral hypothalamic thermoregulatory centers.

adjustments take place that prevent any change in the core (i.e., hypothalamic) temperature from occurring. Various models have been proposed to explain this observation. There is increasing acceptance of the hypothesis that the thermoregulatory centers operate as a proportional controller in which the thermoregulatory responses are proportional to the offset between the actual temperature of the central neurons and the threshold temperature (the "set point") maintained by comparator neurons in the rostral hypothalamus. The set point varies according to input from peripheral sensors. When the hypothalamic temperature is above the set temperature, responses that increase heat loss are activated (cutaneous vasodilatation, sweating, behavioral responses); when the set temperature is higher, heat loss is decreased and/or heat production is increased (shivering, behavioral responses). Figure 7-2 illustrates the proportional controller system.

In several physiological and pathological states the resetting of the central thermostats is evident. Body temperature is lowered in many species during sleep, and vasodilatation and increased heat dissipation result; regulation continues normally at the lower level. Studies of temperature regulation during exercise indicate a downward adjustment of the set point that is mediated by input from the muscles; this change is reflected in the considerable increase in sweating seen

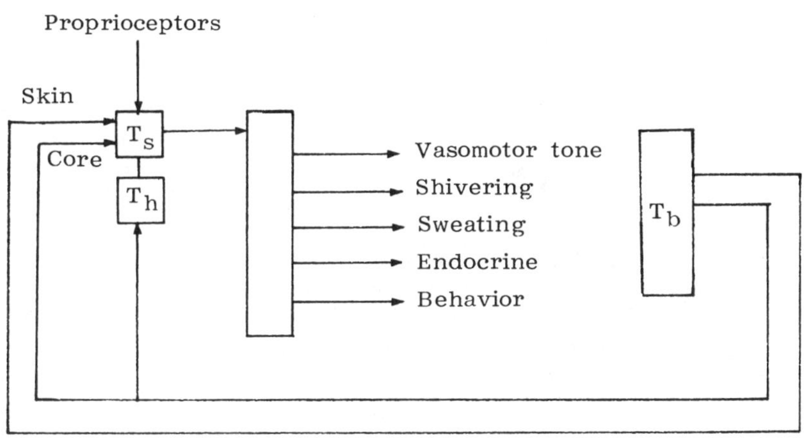

Figure 7-2. Schematic representation of the mammalian thermoregulatory system (T_s, set temperature; T_h, hypothalamic temperature; T_b, deep-body temperature). Thermal inputs from the body core and the body surface are integrated and determine the level of T_s. T_h is compared to T_s and, according to the direction and magnitude of the offset, the appropriate thermoregulatory effector systems are activated to prevent any change in T_b in the face of an internal or external thermal stress.

with the onset of exercise in humans. During the fever the set point is elevated due to the action of endotoxins on the rostral hypothalamic thermostats; body temperature is then regulated at this higher level. There is evidence to support the concept that the vasomotor events accompanying postmenopausal hot flushes may be the result of a sudden lowering of the set point caused by a hormonal imbalance (this topic is discussed later in the chapter).

Neurotransmitters in the Thermoregulatory Pathways

The effects of virtually every natural compound in the central nervous system on temperature regulation have been investigated. Only a limited number of these has yet been demonstrated to fulfill a neurotransmitter role. Recently, complex electrophysiological responses seen with some compounds have been characterized as modulatory, although there is no consensus on the definition of modulation (5). Such compounds do not appear to exhibit the properties of synaptic release and one-to-one cellular communication. From these studies has arisen the concept of neuromodulators exerting diffuse multicellular influences, although evidence of nonsynaptic release is lacking in the central nervous system. However, such a mechanism seems to underlie explanations of the effects of several of the compounds postulated to be of physiological importance in thermoregulation.

An abbreviated list of the transmitters that may be involved in the thermoregulatory pathways is provided in Table 7-1. These are compounds for which there is substantial evidence of effects on body temperature in different species. Some of these compounds cause thermoregulatory changes under normal thermoneutral conditions, and others have been implicated as modifying the responses to

Table 7-1
Putative Neurotransmitters in the Central Thermoregulatory Pathways

Monoamines	Acetylcholine	Norepinephrine	5-HT
	Dopamine		
Polyamines	Histamine	Spermine	Spermidine
Amino Acids	DOPA	GABA	Histidine
	5-HTP	Taurine	Tryptophan
Peptides	ACTH	Angiotension II	Bombesin
	Beta-endorphin	Enkephalins	LHRH
	MIF	Neurotensin	SRIF
	TRH	Vasopressin	
Others	Cyclic nucleotides		
	Prostaglandins		

environmental thermal stress or as participating in the thermoregulatory component of pathological conditions.

A detailed review of all the neurotransmitters is beyond the scope of this chapter and so only those that may be of clinical significance in drug-induced or other disorders of thermoregulation are discussed.

Acetylcholine

Almost 50 yr ago, Cushing (6) injected pilocarpine into the lateral cerebral ventricle of a patient and noted a fall in body temperature accompanied by vasodilatation and sweating. This was the first demonstration of cholinergic receptors in the human central nervous system and probably the first description of a specific neurotransmitter in the thermoregulatory pathways. Cholinergic systems in the central nervous system generally, and especially those involved in the control of body temperature, have been studied in detail over the past two decades. The role of acetylcholine in thermoregulation has been reviewed most recently by Crawshaw (7). Acetylcholine is involved at multiple synaptic junctions on the afferent and efferent thermoregulatory pathways in the brain. In the rostral hypothalamus, it leads to depolarization and a downward setting of the thermostats.

In individuals poisoned by cholinesterase inhibitors (which increase both peripheral and central cholinergic activity), disturbances of body temperature (to as low as 29.5°C in one case) or moderate to severe fever may occur. Ambient thermal conditions may be the major determinant of the direction and magnitude of the body-temperature change, although the relative contribution of peripheral (effector) thermoregulatory components is also an important factor.

Norepinephrine

Norepinephrine is involved at multiple sites in the thermoregulatory pathways. Activation of alpha-receptors in the preoptic centers appears to stabilize the neurons and cause a rise in body temperature. Noradrenergic synapses are also involved in the efferent heat-loss pathways, and their activation may cause a drop in core temperature. There remain, however, several apparent anomalies concerning the thermoregulatory effects of norepinephrine that need further investigation. (See Cox and Lomax [8].)

5-HT

As with norepinephrine, there appears to be considerable interspecies variation in the central effects of 5-HT on thermoregulation.

(See Cox and Lomax [8].) In primates, 5-HT and its precursor (5-HTP) lead to a rise in temperature when injected into the brain. Neurochemical maneuvers that deplete 5-HT levels in the brain reduce responses to cold challenge in the monkey. This finding has been interpreted to indicate 5-HT synapses in the afferent pathways from peripheral cold receptors.

Dopamine

Reports of the effects of dopamine and dopaminomimetics on body temperature have been fairly consistent. A fall in core temperature occurs in most species, including primates, following activation of central dopamine receptors. Dopamine acts directly or indirectly to lower the thermoregulatory set point and may exert a tonic influence to suppress the level.

Histamine

Both H_1- and H_2- histamine receptors have been identified in the central thermoregulatory pathways. Activation of the former, located in the rostral hypothalamic centers, leads to a downward setting of the thermostats. The H_2-receptors appear to be located in the efferent heat-loss pathways. Thus, histamine tends to reduce body temperature by two separate and distinct mechanisms. (For a review of the evidence, see Lomax and Green [9].)

Amino Acids

Several amino acids, mainly those that are precursors of the central nervous system neurotransmitters (Table 7-1), lead to changes in body temperature. Whether these effects reflect physiological mechanisms or pharmacological responses requires demonstration of synaptic release of amino acids. Although the evidence is evocative in the cases of GABA and taurine, final conclusions await further investigation.

Peptides

Since the initial report (10) that intracerebral injection of TRH produces autonomic responses and a fall in body temperature, the possible role of several polypeptides identified in the hypothalamus in thermoregulation has been investigated. (For a review of the evidence, see reference 11.) These studies were spurred on by the discovery of the enkephalins and endorphins and the search for the physiological significance of these molecules. Since the effects of the narcotic analgesics on body temperature became well established, it has been postulated that the opioid receptor may be involved in normal thermal homeostasis. In the case of the opioid peptides, the lack of significant thermoregulatory effects after the blockage of the opioid receptors by antagonists, such as naloxone, has tended not to support the initial suppositions. For the other peptides (Table 7-1) firm conclusions cannot yet be drawn. Certainly, the possibility of synaptic release exists, mainly in the case of the hypothalamico-hypophyseal-releasing hormones and ADH. Recently, it has been suggested that ADH may constitute an endogenous antipyretic (12). As with the amino acids, the evidence for peptidergic neurotransmission in the central thermoregulatory pathways is certainly less than complete, and the subject remains an active area of investigation.

Prostaglandins

Over the last few years, there has been considerable discussion as to whether the genesis of fever after bacterial infections involves the release of prostaglandins (of the E series) into the rostral hypothalamus. (See Milton [13].) The concept was particularly attractive because it formed a rational explanation for the action of acetylsalicylic acid and other inhibitors of prostaglandin synthetase in reducing fever. After initial reports that a rise in temperature is evoked in most species by central injection of PGE, many further studies appeared that were inconsistent with the hypothesis that the fatty acid mediates the response to bacterial pyrogen. The current status of the prostaglandin "enigma" has been summaried by Veale, Cooper, and Pittman (14).

Cyclic Nucleotides

Several of the neurotransmitters that may be involved in thermoregulation or fever stimulate the formation of cAMP or gGMP in neural tissue. Although intracerebral injection of these nucleotides may induce body-temperature changes, Milton and Danscombe (15), after extensive study of the subject, concluded "that the cyclic nucleotides . . . [do not] have a direct role in normal body temperature regulation . . . [nor is] cAMP . . . directly involved . . . in fever."

Centrally Active Compounds and Clinical Disorders of Thermoregulation

The considerable volume of research on the physiological and pharmacological aspects of thermoregulation during the past two decades has led to a growing understanding of the mechanisms underlying clinical disorders of body temperature, particularly the neural mechanisms involved. Much of this work is still incomplete, and this review can only briefly touch on some of the recognized syndromes, many of which are of current interest and ongoing investigation.

Antipyretics

The antipyretic drugs have been used empirically in the treatment of fever for more than a century, but it has only been within the last few years that more precise information on their mode of action has emerged. Although the antipyretics act at peripheral sites to reduce inflammation, their antipyretic effect appears to be due to interference with the action of endogenous pyrogen on the thermoregulatory centers. As noted above in the section on prostaglandins, this conclusion presupposes that the pyrogen increases at the rate of PG synthesis that mediates the rise in body temperature. In any event, there is little doubt that the antifebrile action of the antipyretics is mediated within the central nervous system. (For reviews, see Veale, Cooper, and Pittman [14] and Krupp and associates [16].)

Phenothiazines

The widespread use of phenothiazines in the treatment of psychiatric disorders renders them one of the most commonly prescribed group of drugs. Many of these compounds, especially in high doses, affect body temperature, and they have been used therapeutically because of this property. Soon after the synthesis of chlorpromazine, it was used in conjunction with general anesthetics to produce "artificial hibernation" (17) and small doses (5-10 mg per diem) have been used with body cooling to treat hyperpyrexia resulting from heat stroke, infection, cerebral trauma, or malignant disease.

In elderly patients in particular, life-threatening hyperthermia or hypothermia can take effect rapidly if phenothiazines, especially in high doses, are taken during exposure to extremes of environmental heat and humidity or cold. Myxedematous patients are particularly likely to become hypothermic under phenothiazine therapy (18).

With small doses of these compounds the major factor inducing the body-temperature changes appears to be the rapidly occurring vasodilatation in exposed skin areas and increased radiant heat exchange. Although the individual phenothiazines exhibit varying degrees of anticholinergic, antihistaminic, and antiadrenergic activity, there is no conclusive evidence to implicate any specific central site or mechanism of action to explain the body-temperature changes seen after low doses. However, it is possible that the adverse (toxic) thermoregulatory effects appearing with the high doses used in psychotherapy may reflect central nervous system responses.

Amphetamines

Moderate doses of amphetamines do not have any significant effect on body temperature in normal, healthy adults. Yet, hyperthermia is a prominent life-threatening consequence of amphetamine poisoning. Cases of heat stroke, circulatory collapse, and coma following ingestion of amphetamines were first reported over 20 yr ago, when there were cases of a similar syndrome in cyclists after extreme exertion and amphetamine use. The clinical literature has been reviewed by Sellers and associates (19).

After they are ingested, amphetamines readily enter the central nervous system, where they have direct noradrenergic and dopaminergic effects; they compete with sympathomimetic amines for neuronal uptake and indirectly release norepinephrine and dopamine, inhibit MAO, and sometimes accumulate as "false" neurotransmitters in nerve endings. Because of this multiplicity of actions, the effects of amphetamines on thermoregulation are complex and difficult to interpret in terms of basic physiological mehcanisms. In humans, the hyperthermic effect may be compounded by both central and peripheral actions: changes in set point, activation of heat-conservation pathways, thermogenesis in peripheral tissues, mobilization of free fatty acids, and direct effects on muscles increasing heat production.

Although the occurrence of amphetamine-associated hyperthermia is not common, the death rate approaches 65% when this complication accompanies acute intoxication. Abuse of the drug accounts for the majority of these cases. Whether legislation against the indiscriminant prescribing of these drugs, for which few if any clinical indications exist, will reduce the problem remains an unanswered question.

Ethanol

The most frequent predisposing factor in accidentla hypothermia in young people is drug abuse, and in a large number of such cases blood ethanol levels of 150 to 300 mg per deciliter are discovered at autopsy. The mechanism(s) by which ethanol affects thermoregulation are unclear. Peripheral vasodilatation and enhancement of heat loss in cold environments are frequently said to be a major factor, but experiments in laboratory animals and in humans have failed to demonstrate this contention. The state of intoxication is also considered to diminish the capacity of the victim to take suitable measures or precautions to combat the cold environment. However, the blood ethanol levels of victims are generally not great enough to make the victims unaware of the potential threat.

Recent animal studies suggest that ethanol may have a direct action on the thermoregulatory centers and cause a downward setting of the thermostats. The consequent activation of heat loss and/or inhibition of heat production in a cold environment leads to a rapid fall in core temperature such that doses of the drug that produce blood ethanol levels comparable to moderate intoxication in humans (about 150 mg per deciliter) prove to be rapidly fatal at an environmental temperature of 4°C. Under thermoneutral conditions (20°C), animals show complete recovery from similar doses. The evidence presently available suggests that a combination of factors—a downward setting of the thermostats and effects on peripheral heat production combined with the environmental cold stress—may lead to an irreversible thermal state in which the animal is unable to mobilize its thermal defenses (20).

Humans are increasingly being exposed to climatic extremes in polar-region development, military situations, space exploration, and broadening recreational activities. The problems associated with the concomitant use of drugs, including ethanol, require further study.

Thermoregulatory Disorders in the Menopause

Hot flushes are the most common and characteristic changes associated with the female climacteric. Until recent times, the underlying mechanisms of the syndrome have not received a great deal of attention, and the episodes have been vaguely attributed to a sudden and transient rise in sympathetic drive. Several factors have recently tended to focus attention on the condition: the increasing number of women in responsible professional positions for whom the attacks are more than an "inconvenience," the occurrence of severe flushes in younger patients undergoing oophorectomy, the growing reluctance of physicians to use estrogen therapy for prolonged control of the syndrome, and the need for alternative forms of treatment.

A major step in the study of postmenopausal hot flushes has been the objective measurement of attacks to replace the subjective assessments used previously (21). Thus, a detailed study was made of the pathophysiological changes in 275 episodes in which skin temperature (as an index of flushing), skin conductance (as an index of sweating), and deep-body temperature were monitored continuously (22). In addition, the subjects were able to signal the onset and end of each attack with an electronic marker. Figure 7-3 illustrates an actual record characteristic of a typical flush. It should be noted that the subject signaled the onset of the attack almost 1 min prior to any change in the measured parameters and indicated the termination at the time the skin temperature was highest. In the series, the mean duration of the subjective symptoms was 9.4 ± 0.46 min, whereas the measured responses returned to the normal level only after 40.9 ± 3.0 min. It is clear from these observations that the patients' subjective feelings are not the result of the flushing and sweating per se but derive from the central events that trigger the attacks. It can be noted from Figure 7-3 that the increased heat loss from cutaneous vasodilatation and sweating result in a fall in core temperature. Taken together, these observations suggest that the hot flush represents a coordinated thermoregulatory event that is triggered by a sudden downward setting of the central thermostats. This leads to increased heat loss

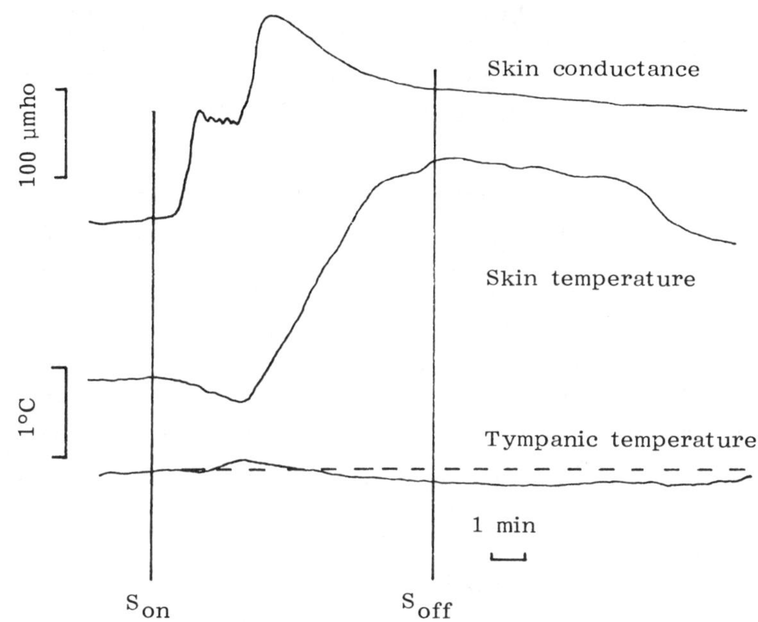

Figure 7-3. Recordings of skin conductance and skin and core (tympanic) temperature during a hot-flush episode in a postmenopausal subject. S_{on} and S_{off} are the signals made by the subject at the start and finish of the subjective symptoms of the flush. The recordings did not return to the baseline levels in this particular case because the next flush followed too quickly.

and a fall in deep-body temperature. The set point then readjusts to the normal level and the sequence of events is reversed. It can be postulated that it is the change in the set point that causes the subjective sensations.

Clearly, it is the failing ovarian function and decline in estrogen levels that precipitate the menopausal syndrome. Since the hot flushes seem to be triggered from the rostral hypothalamus, it is likely that altered neuroendocrine function in this region may underlie the disorder. The release from negative feedback of estrogen would be expected to increase the release of LHRH from neurosecretory cells in the hypothalamus; such cells are located in and around the preoptic/anterior hypothalamic nuclei that are the site of the major thermoregulatory centers. The onset of the flushes coincides with the low point in LH pulsatile release (23) at which time the LHRH release is maximal (24). These several findings suggest that the neuronal mechanisms regulating LHRH release, or LHRH itself, may be mediating the change in set point.

The concept of an integrated thermoregulatory disorder underlying the hot flush syndrome suggests a number of novel therapeutic approaches to the treatment of the disorder based on the considerable data, reviewed above, concerning modulation of the central thermostats and their responses to a variety of centrally active drugs.

Conclusion

The multitude of neurochemical and neuropharmacological influences on the central thermoregulatory pathways and centers is quite remarkable, and their complexity renders an exhaustive reivew almost beyond the scope of a single author. Certainly, many of the clinical disorders of thermoregulation should be amenable to a rational therapeutic approach once the underlying pathophysiological changes are understood. This end can only be attained with the continued advance of research in the field.

References

1. Ransom SW: Regulation of body temperature. *In*: Fulton JF, Ranson SW, Frantz AM (eds.), The Hypothalamus and Central Levels of Autonomic Function, pp. 342-399. Baltimore, Williams & Wilkins, 1940.
2. Liebermeister C: Handbuch der Pathologie und Therapie des Fiebers. Leipzig, Vogel, 1875.
3. Bergmann C: Nichtchemischer Beitrug zur Kritik der Lehre von Calor animalis. Arch Anat Physiol 1845, p. 300.

4. Magoun HW, Harrison F, Brobeck JR, Ranson SW: Activation of heat loss mechanism by local heating of the brain. Jour Neurophysiol *1*:101-114, 1938.
5. Dismukes RK; New concepts of molecular communication between neurons. Behav Brain Sci *2*:409-416, 1979.
6. Cushing H: The similarity in the response to posterior lobe extract (pituitrin) and to pilocarpine when injected into the cerebral ventricles. Proc Natl Acad Sci USA *17*: 171-177, 1931.
7. Crawshaw LI: Acetylcholine. *In*: Lomax P, Schönbaum E (eds.), Body Temperature, pp. 305-335. New York, Dekker, 1979.
8. Cox B, Lomax P: Pharmacologic control of temperature regulation. Ann Rev Pharmacol Toxicol *17*:341-353, 1977.
9. Lomax P, Green MD; Histamine. *In*: Lomax P, Schönbaum E (eds.), Body Temperature, pp. 289-304. New York, Dekker, 1979.
10. Metcalf G: TRH: A possible mediator of thermoregulation. Nature (London) *252*:310-311, 1974.
11. Symposium: The newer putative central neurotransmitters: Roles in thermoregulation. Fed Proc *40*:2735-2768, 1981.
12. Veale WL, Cooper KE: Arginine vasopressin and endogenous antipyresis: The evidence and significance. Fed Proc *40*:2750-2753, 1981.
13. Milton AS: Modern views on the pathogenesis of fever and the mode of action of antipyretic drugs. Jour Pharmaceut Pharmacol *28*:393-399, 1976.
14. Veale WL, Cooper KE, Pittman QJ: The role of prostaglandins in fever and temperature regulation. *In*: Ramwell P (ed.), Prostaglandins vol. 3, pp. 145-167. New York, Plenum, 1977.
15. Milton AS, Danscombe MJ: Cyclic nucleotides in thermoregulation and fever. *In*: Cooper KE, Lomax P, Schönbaum ED (eds.), Drugs, Biogenic Amines and Body Temperature, pp. 129-135. Basel, Karger, 1977.
16. Krupp PJ, Zeil R: Antipyretics. *In*: Lomax P, Schönbaum E (eds.), Body Temperature, pp. 383-401. New York, Dekker, 1979.
17. Laborit H-M: Clinical hypothermia. *In*: Lomax P, Schönbaum E (eds.), Body Temperature, pp. 595-611. New York, Dekker, 1979.
18. Borbély AA, Loepfe-Hinkkanen M; Phenothiazines. *In*: Lomax P, Schönbaum E (eds.), Body Temperature, pp. 403-426. New York, Dekker, 1979.
19. Sellers EM, Martin PR, Roy ML, Sellers EA: Amphetamines. *In*: Lomax P, Schönbaum E (eds.), Body Temperature, pp. 461-498. New York, Dekker, 1979.
20. Lomax P, Bajorek JG, Chesarek WA, Chaffee RRJ; Ethanol induced hypothermia in the rat. Pharmacology *21*:288-294, 1980.
21. Silverman RW, Bajorek JG, Lomax P, Tataryn IV: Monitoring the pathophysiological correlates of postmenopausal hot flushes. Maturitas *3*:39-46, 1981.
22. Tataryn IV, Lomax P, Bajorek JG, Chesarek W, Meldrum DR, Judd HL: Postmenopausal hot flushes: A disorder of thermoregulation. Maturitas *2*: 101-107, 1980.
23. Tataryn IV, Meldrum DR, Frumar AM, Lu KH, Judd HL, Bajorek JG, Chesarek W, Lomax P: The hormonal and thermoregulatory changes in postmenopausal hot flushes. *In*: Cox B, Lomax P, Milton AS, Schönbaum E (eds.), Thermoregulatory Mechanisms and Their Therapeutic Implications, pp. 202-207. Basel, Karger, 1980.
24. Ravnikar V, Elkind-Hirsch KE, Schiff I: The association between LHRH, LH and vasomotor flushes. Proc 62nd Ann Meeting Am Endocrinol Soc, abstract No. 310, p. 160, 1981.

CHAPTER EIGHT

Fluid Shifts in Hypothermia

Murray P. Hamlet, D.V.M.

Although changes in fluid balance in the human response to cold have been known for some time (1, 2), their impact on the management of hypothermic patients is not widely recognized. This chapter relates the physiological response to cold to a rational fluid-replacement regime for use in the resuscitation of hypothermia victims.

Field Experience or Predisposing Factors

Military after-action reports clearly define the progressive dehydration associated with increased work in the cold and the increased effort required to obtain water from snow or ice. The limited availability of liquid water, the lack of knowledge about water replacement, and the stress of forced activity place the soldier in jeopardy of dehydration during cold-weather exercises. Command emphasis on obtaining and drinking water is often lacking, and thirst alone does not override the aggravation of making liquid water from snow and ice. The thirst mechanism appears to be depressed in the cold, adding to the problem (3). Dehydration has a significant impact on temperature regulation. As blood viscosity increases, peripheral flow is impaired. Surface (shell) blood flow decreases, and the ability to move heat from the core to the shell diminishes. In a cold environment, peripheral cooling increases. For example, hand cooling increased 18% with a 4.2% body weight deficit (water) in a voluntary dehydration study (unpublished observation).

The views, opinions, and/or findings contained in this report are those of the author and do not purport to reflect the positions of the Department of the Army or the Deparment of Defense.

The clinical history of hypothermic patients is important in determining the duration of cold exposure and possibly their dehydration state. Civilians working in a cold environment dehydrate in the same way field soldiers do. Hikers, fishermen, and seamen may not have adequate water intake prior to or during their cold exposure. The elderly and infirm often have a low fluid intake. The diuresis induced by alcohol imbibition will contribute to the users' volume depletion.

Fluid-Loss Mechanisms

When humans are exposed to a cold environment, a number of physiological responses occur that tend to decrease effective circulating volume. There is an immediate peripheral vasoconstriction in the body's attempt to shut off peripheral heat loss. This peripheral constriction causes sequestration of plasma volume in peripheral vessels without trapping red cells (4). This process causes an increase in hematocrit, blood viscosity, and hemoglobin concentration (5, 6). This sequestered plasma water is readily available and rapidly mobilized during a rewarming procedure. Along with this sequestration, a recompartmentalization of water from vascular space to extracellular space occurs (7, 8). There is a loss of plasma volume, blood volume, or both (2). The mechanism for this movement is not clearly defined.

Water loss due to respiration, perspiration, and urination is significant in the cold. Respiratory loss is great as a result of the low relative humidity of cold, dry air. Exercise with its increased respiratory rate increases this loss. Perspiration continues in the cold but is not perceived as readily as it is in a warm environment. Clothing rapidly absorbs the moisture, and there is a more rapid loss through evaporation into the cold, dry air. The individual does not see water collecting on his or her skin or in his or her clothing and so does not realize that a significant loss is occurring. Water loss through sweating may be 1000 to 2000 ml per day. Respiratory loss may be as high as 300 to 500 ml per day (9).

Animal studies clearly define a recompartmentalization of the fluids during cooling (4). There are a progressive loss of circulating volume during cooling and a subsequent rise during rewarming. There is also an intracellular shift of water during hypothermia (8, 10). This shift is exemplified by the mild cellular edema observed in the brain and other organs during cooling and in postmortem examinations of hypothermic victims. The renal output continues during cooling and accounts for some of the vascular volume loss. These experiments were performed during short-term cooling episodes, and they give one indication by extrapolation of the fluid shifts during long-term cooling.

There is a well-defined increase in urinary output during cooling, termed cold diuresis (11). Cold diuresis differs from water diuresis in that cold diuresis involves an increase in total solute excretion (2, 12). There is an increase in chloride, sodium, and magnesium levels. Two mechanisms have been proposed for the diuresis. The first suggests that as peripheral constriction occurs there is a rise in circulating volume and arterial pressure. This rise is quickly controlled by an increased urine outflow (1, 13). The second proposed mechanism is that even in the face of decreased renal blood flow and glomerular filtration rate (14) there is an overriding decrease in tubular absorption and oxidative activity leading to increased urine production. This depressed oxidative tubular activity results in reduced sodium and water resorption (15). Because increased sodium, chloride, and magnesium excretion occur after artificial pitressin suppression of water loss, there appear to be two independent mechanisms for urinary output with cold exposure (2). Lennquist and associates (16) described the osmolar diuresis very well. Whatever the cause and process, the result is an initial diuresis during which significant water loss occurs. Combining the increased loss through diuresis, sweating and respiration with a reduced intake, and recompartmentalization of water, the result is the marked rise of hematocrit, increased plasma protein, and vascular volume depletion commonly observed in the hypothermia victim (17, 18, 19).

The longer the cooling, the greater the severity of the vascular volume decrement. Cold-water immersion without a survival suit generally produces no great fluid shifts because of the rapid rate of cooling. Land-based-accident victims, however, often take longer to cool, and there is more time for the combined effects of cold diuresis and recompartmentalization. Some water may be sequestered in the small vessels of the limbs as peripheral constriction occurs and circulation retreats toward the core. With peripheral constriction, interstitial loss, cold diuresis, change in circulation pattern from the shell to the core, and lack of water intake, the hypothermic victim ends up with a loss of circulating volume. Some of the volume loss is available in other compartments and will partially return on rewarming, but overall fluid balance is negative. Replacement therapy during rewarming must take into account this returning water so that vascular overload with subsequent pulmonary and cerebral edema can be avoided (20).

During replacement therapy, one should keep in mind that there is a significant amount of fluid available in the victim's body that will be rapidly mobilized during rewarming. (See Table 8-1). The water (plasma) in the stagnant peripheral bed will flow quickly and will be colder than the core and high in hydrogen ion and potassium. Recompartmentalized water will tend to return to its origin as the body's temperature rises. Intracellular water will move to the extracellular space, and extracellular water will then move to the vascular space as circulation increases.

As temperature rises, the central and peripheral vascular systems regain their tone and the vascular volume goes from very large and partially stagnant to one that is smaller with greater flow rates. The addition of fluids to the vascular space early in the therapy may tend to overload the patient as he or she is rewarmed and

Table 8-1
Fluid Replacement in the Treatment of Hypothermia

Type of Accident	Intravenous Replacement
Dry land:	
Slow cooling—elderly, drunks, injury or diseased states	Requires fluid replacement—continued and controlled central venous pressure monitoring
Rapid cooling—rain, wind, severe cold, infants	Requires modest intravenous replacement—depending on body size and rate of cooling
Warm-water immersion:	
Slow cooling—with personal flotation device (PFD), summer immersion, long duration	Volume is depleted—requires that central venous pressure is kept low early
Slow cooling and drowning—no PFD, summer submersion, and pool drowning	Requires monitoring and replacement as necessary—guarding against pulmonary and cerebral edema; freshwater drowning victims may be overloaded, saltwater drowning victims, depleted
Cold-water immersion:	
Rapid cooling—canoeing, falling out of boat with PFD	Vascular volume is near normal
Rapid cooling and drowning—no PFD, going through the ice, falling out of boat	Volume is near normal—requires ventilatory support and guarding against pulmonary and cerebral edema
Slow cooling—through the ice, hanging on the edge of ice, clothing floats, survival suit in the ocean	Small body: has near normal fluids, large body: longer duration requires fluid replacement
Slow cooling and drowning—survival suit but no PFD, hanging on edge of ice and then going under	Requires guarded intravenous support—mannitol to dry the lungs and brain in order to prevent cerebral and pulmonary edema

renal excretory function lags behind increasing volume. Animal studies define an initial loss of vascular volume but a partial return during rewarming without additional intravenous support (8). The addition of large volumes of water is not indicated, but decreasing blood viscosity early in therapy improves both cardiac output and arterial flow. Replacement therapy should be directed at partial replacement of circulating volume. Special attention to fluid type (glucose-ionic content), temperature, and rate of replacement are important factors to be considered when a very marginal cardiac function is being treated. Simple dilution decreases the viscosity, dilutes the potassium content, and increases cardiac output.

Warming the fluid adds some heat to the myocardium. Blood pressure rises but may be compromised by peripheral dilation as peripheral warming occurs. Rewarming without volume replacement is catastrophic because of this peripheral vasodilatation and loss of circulating volume. "Rewarming shock" is the term applied to this phenomenon, which is generally associated with peripheral warming techniques rather than core rewarming procedures. Attempts at peripheral field rewarming for the severely hypothermic (comatose) person without volume replacement are ill advised. Slower rates of replacement for the elderly may be indicated.

The fluid replacement therapy of drowning victims is different than that of other hypothermia victims (21, 22). Victims of rapid submersion in cold water in which drowning and hypothermia occur concomitantly generally have normal electrolytes and require minimal volume replacement. Freshwater-submersion victims usually have higher than normal arterial pressure and volume because of the rapid osmotic absorption of water across the alveolus. Hemodilution occurs, and care should be taken to avoid adding to the rapidly developing pulmonary edema through the administration of intravenous fluids to the already-expanded vascular volume. In cases of long-term cold-water immersion, such as those occurring in victims wearing survival suits, intravenous fluids are indicated since the victims are volume depleted. If drowning occurs at the end of the immersion accident, however, volume expansion may be contraindicated in the face of the victim's severe pulmonary and cerebral edema (23). The hypothermia is not the victim's major problem, and it protects them against the hypoxemia of drowning.

References

1. Burton AC, EDholm OG: Man in a Cold Environment. London, Edward Arnold Ltd., 1955.

2. Bass DE, Henschel A: Responses of body fluid compartments to heat and cold. Physiol Rev *36*:128-144, 1956.
3. U.S. Navy. Cold Weather Medicine. Bethesda, Md., National Naval Medical Center, 1978.
4. D'Amato HE, Hegnauer AH: Blood volume in hypothermic dog. Amer Jour Physiol *173*:100-102, 1953.
5. Keatinge WR: Survival in Cold Water. Oxford, Blackwell Press, 1969.
6. Hervey GR: Physiological changes encountered in hypothermia. Proc Roy Soc Med *66*: 1053-1058, 1973.
7. Harari H, Regnier B, Rapid M, Lemaire F, Legall JR: Haemodynamic study of prolonged deep accidental hypothermia. Europ Jour Intensive Care Med *1*:65-70, 1975.
8. Popovic V, Popovic P: Hypothermia in biology and medicine. New York, Grune and Stratton, 1974.
9. Vogt Lorentzen F: Cold: Physiology, Protection and Survival. AGARD Report No. 194, Advisory Group for Aerospace Research Development, NATO. London, Technical Editing and Reproduction Ltd., 1974.
10. Barbour HG, McKay EA, Griffith WP: Water shifts in deep hypothermia. Amer Jour Physiol *140*:9-19, 1944.
11. Little DM: Hypothermia. Anesthesiology *20*:842-877, 1959.
12. Adolph EF, Molnar GW: Exchange of heat and tolerance to cold in men exposed to outdoor weather. Amer Jour Physiol *146*:507-537, 1946.
13. Coniam SW: Accidental hypothermia. Aesthesia *34*:250-256, 1979.
14. Tansey WA: Medical Aspects of Cold Water Immersion. Report No. 763, U.S. Naval Submarine Medical Center. Groton, Conn., Naval Submarine Research Laboratory NTIS Document AD-775-687, 1973.
15. Segar WE, Ripley PA, Barila TG: Urinary composition during hypothermia. Amer Jour Physiol *185*:528-532, 1956.
16. Lennquist MD, Granberg PO, Bertil W: Fluid balance and physical work capacity in humans exposed to cold. Arch Environ Health *29*:241-249, 1974.
17. Kanter GS: Bicarbonate excretion during hypothermia. Can Jour Biochem Physiol *41*: 91-96, 1963.
18. Andrews, CI, Orkin LR: Environmental cold in man. Anesthesiology *25*:549-559, 1964.
19. Reuler JB: Hypothermia: Pathophysiology, clinical settings, and management. Ann Intern Med *89*:519-527, 1978.
20. Harnett RM, Silas FR, Pruitt JR: Resuscitation from Hypothermia. A Literature Review. Clemson, S.C., Clemson University, College of Engineering, 1979.
21. Jeffords DL: The Pathophysiological Difference between Salt and Fresh Water Drowning: Fact or Fallacy. Groton, Conn., U.S. Naval Submarine Medical Center, 1973.
22. Modell JH, Graves SH, Ketover A: Clinical course of 91 consecutive near-drowning victims. Chest *70*:231-238, 1976.
23. Conn AW: Near-drowning and hypothermia. Can Med Assoc Jour *120*:397-400, 1979.

CHAPTER NINE

The Relationship of Glucose Metabolism to Hypothermia

Milton Mager, Ph.D.,
and Ralph Francesconi, Ph.D.

One of the distinguishing characteristics of mammals is their ability to maintain a relatively constant body temperature despite large variations in environmental temperature. Clearly, the development of homeothermy in the higher animals necessitates complex mechanisms for heat production and heat loss as well a finely controlled balance between heat production and heat loss. Although heat loss varies widely in response to fluctuating ambient temperature, heat production responds adaptively and actively to retain homeothermy, especially under extremely cold environmental conditions (1).

How is the heat produced to maintain the constancy of body temperature in homeotherms? Girardier (2) referred to two types of heat production, which he called minimal and thermoregulatory. He further subdivided minimal heat production into essential energesis and obligate heat. Essential energesis is that energy expended and heat

The views, opinions, and/or findings contained in this report are those of the authors and should not be construed as an official Department of the Army position, policy, or decision, unless so designated by other official documentation. In conducting the research described in this report, the investigators adhered to the "Guide for Laboratory Animal Facilities and Care," as promulgated by the Committee on the guide for Laboratory Animal Facilities and Care of the Institute of Laboratory Animal Resources, National Academy of Sciences, National Research Council. Human subjects participated in these studies after giving their free and informed voluntary consent. Investigators adhered to AR 70-25 and USAMRDC regulation 70-25 of use of volunteers in research. The authors wish to express their deep gratitude to Ms. Cynthia Bishop and Ms. Sandra Beach for their excellent secretarial assistance. We wish also to thank our collaborators, Dr. N. Freinkel, Dr. S. Robinson, and Dr. T. Shirashi, as well as the technical personnel and test subjects for their outstanding contributions.

produced in anabolic and catabolic reactions that maintain cell structural integrity, that energy expended and heat produced to maintain solute and ion concentrations at appropriate concentrations at the cellular level, and that energy expended and heat produced in discharging the specialized function of the cell (e.g., impulse transmission, endocrine secretion, etc.) Obligate heat is that portion of the total body heat generated by continuous cellular metabolism. In fact, among higher organisms it has been demonstrated that the development of homeothermy is concomitant with a marked rise in general metabolic rate. The calorigenic action of the thyroid hormones, for example, can be thought of as acting at the level of basal obligate heat production.

Girardier (2) also referred to regulatory heat as the supplemental heat produced that permits homeotherms to survive under the wide range of temperatures noted in Figures 9-1 and 9-2. Regulatory heat is largely associated with increased muscular activity (shivering thermogenesis); increased metabolic activity of brown-fat tissue (nonshivering thermogenesis); and increased oxidative activity of additional organ systems, most notably the liver and the kidneys.

Regulatory heat production is, of course, maximal at colder ambient temperatures and decreases as ambient temperature increases.

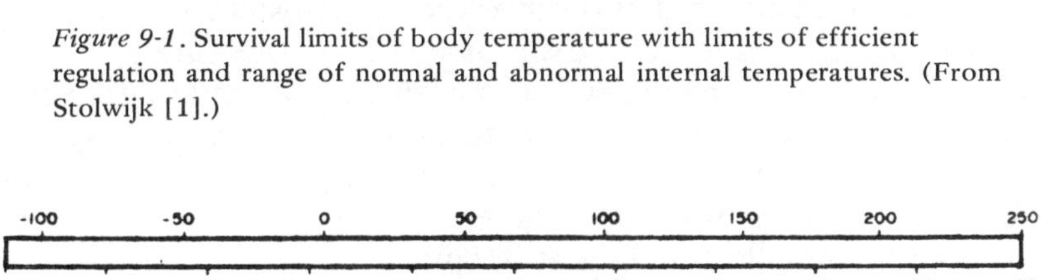

Figure 9-1. Survival limits of body temperature with limits of efficient regulation and range of normal and abnormal internal temperatures. (From Stolwijk [1].)

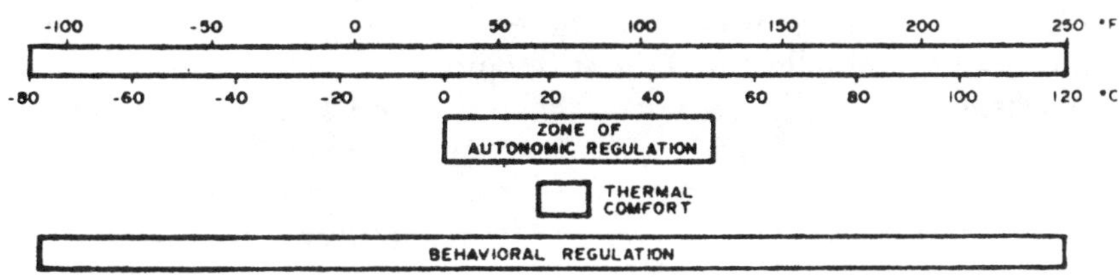

Figure 9-2. Environmental temperature ranges for thermal comfort and limits of autonomic regulation and behavior regulation. (From Stolwijk [1].)

Table 9-1
Heat Production-Homeotherm, Basal State

1. Total Heat Production = (Minimal & Regulatory) Heat Production
2. Minimal = Essential Energesis + Obligate Heat
   a. *Essential:* Anabolic and catabolic reactions, active transport of solutes, nerve impulse transmission, pulmonary and renal function, etc., all produce heat.
   b. *Obligate* heat is produced by normal metabolic processes under continuous stimulation. Not centrally controlled, but probably by thyroid hormone.
3. *Regulatory*—Continuous CNS Regulation. Effectors:
   a. Skeletal muscle (shivering thermogenesis)
   b. Brown fat (nonshivering thermogenesis)
   c. Liver (oxidative activity)

Obligate heat production is effective in regulating temperature around the neutral zone (or the zone of thermal comfort in Stolwijk's ([1]) version), while essential energesis continues to be constant independent of ambient temperature. This entire classification is outlined in Table 9-1.

Neuroendocrine Role in Thermogenesis

The catecholamines, norepinephrine, and epinephrine, have been shown to participate in the response to cold exposure in the following ways: cardiovascular adjustments resulting in, for example, peripheral vasoconstriction, redistribution of blood flow to various organs, or increased cardiac output; incremented shivering thermogenesis during acute or chronic cold exposure and nonshivering thermogenesis in animals acclimatized to cold; and mobilization and increased oxidative metabolism of lipid and carbohydrate substrates. Usually, this catecholaminergic response can be assessed by measuring the levels of epinephrine, norepinephrine, normetanephrine, and metanephrine in the urine of mammals exposed to cold. In his review, Gale (3) summarized results that demonstrated that the exposure of baboons to 6°C for 10 wk resulted in a threefold increase in urinary norepinephrine and a smaller increment in epinephrine; there also occurred a 50% rise in adrenal hydroxycorticosteroid output, evidently all three increments associated with a 20%-to-30% increase in overall resting O_2 consumption. In humans, the exposure of lightly clad males to an ambient temperature of 14°C to 15°C resulted in a more rapid turnover of iodine-131-labeled thyroxin, a decrement in plasma-protein-bound iodine, increased removal of inorganic iodide, and heightened thyroidal uptake of iodine-131 concomitant with a 20%-to-25%

increase in basal metabolic rate. However, it has recently been suggested that increased food intake and fecal bulk, rather than tissue utilization, may result in increased thyroid excretion. In animals that acclimatize to cold, evidence seems to indicate a synergism between thyroid hormones and catecholamines in stimulating brown adipose tissue in order to increase mobilization and oxidation of lipids for heat generation.

In recent studies, chemical ganglionic and adrenergic blockade has been used to investigate further the mechanisms of increased heat production. Gale (3) summarized data demonstrating that infusion of trimethaphan comphorsulfonate, a ganglionic blocker, caused a decline in plasma FFA and glucose, no effects on metabolic rate, and reduced FFA turnover, all of which contributed to a 1.7°C decrease in rectal temperature. When the infusion was terminated or exogenous catecholamines were administered, heat production quickly increased and rectal temperature rose 1.5°C to 2°C after 60 min. These experiments strongly suggested the involvement of catecholamines in the mechanism of the thermogenic response to cold stress.

In large mammals, such as goats and baboons, administration of the alpha-adrenergic blockers phenoxybenzamine or phentolamine did not prevent the increased metabolic response ordinarily occurring as a result of artificial cooling of the preoptic area of the anterior hypothalamus. Propanolol, a beta-adrenergic blocker, likewise failed to attenuate this thermogenic effect. By contrast, beta-adrenergic blockade of nonshivering thermogenesis in rodents indicates a catecholaminergic mechanism, particularly in neonatal and cold-acclimatized animals. It is possible that catecholamine-stimulated heat production is most effective during acute cold exposure among most mammals and in stimulating brown-fat lipolysis and thermogenesis in chronic cold exposure among animals manifesting adequate brown-fat mass.

Thus, it is apparent that during cold exposure peripheral stores of carbohydrate and lipid are being mobilized and combusted in order to maintain body temperature. Therefore, any reductions in the hormones controlling this metabolic process or in the responsivity to hormone stimulation will lead to decrements in available substrate and to a generalized hypothermia.

Thermoregulation and Aging

When groups of young (4-to-6 wk-old) and old (1-yr-old) mice were exposed to acute cold (0°C) stress, the average rectal temperature of the old animals fell by 3°C and that of the young mice remained essentially unchanged (4). The young animals increased their O_2 consumption by 82%, and the mature mice did so by 57%, but only the young mice demonstrated deceased concentrations of hepatic glycogen. Since increases in thermogenic capacity during cold exposure depend on sufficient supplies of metabolic substrate, it is reasonable to conclude that the attenuated thermogenesis is due to a reduced rate of hepatic oxidation of glycogen (glucose) reserves.

Additionally, it had been demonstrated that the glycogenolytic response to catecholamines decreases progressively with advancing age. Therefore, the decrement in rectal temperature can be explained directly from a decreased rate of carbohydrate catabolism pursuant to reduced catecholaminergic response.

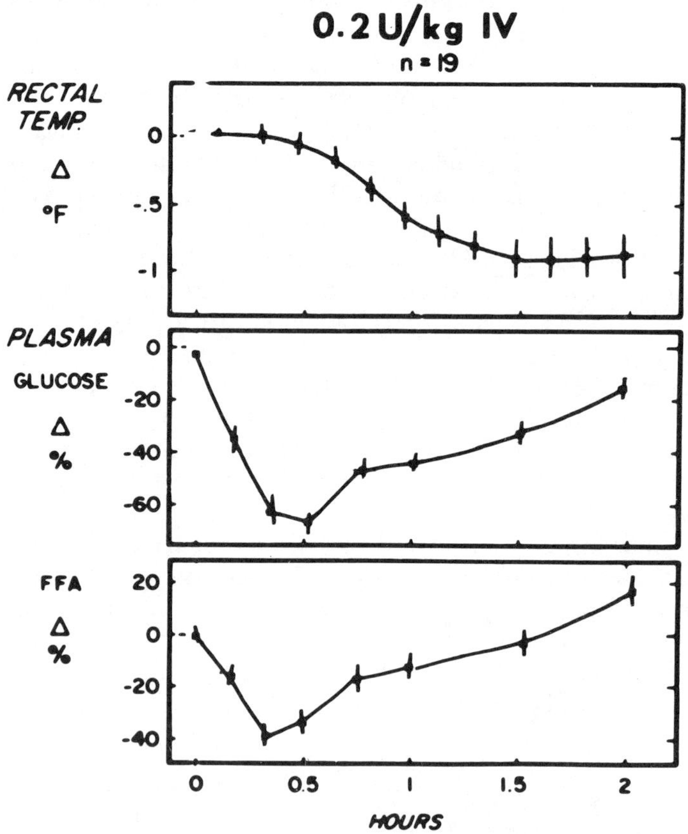

Figure 9-3. Effect of intravenous insulin (0.2 u/kg) on rectal temperature, plasma glucose, and free fatty acids in normal young males.

Hypothermia of Hypoglycemia

Hypothermia during insulin shock treatment was noted almost 40 yr ago (5) and was subsequently attributed to the hypoglycemic effect of insulin (6). In fact, the inability to thermoregulate under conditions of insulin shock has been used as a clinical sign of hypoglycemia (7, 8). Two-deoxy-D-glucose (2-DG) administered to humans also elicits a marked hypothermic effect (9), but the metabolic response is quite different from that of insulin. Two-DG blocks intracellular glucose utilization by competitive inhibition of phosphohexose isomerase, an enzyme essential in the metabolism of glucose. The resultant intracellular glucopenia triggers a sympathicoadrenomedullary response and results in a marked rise in levels of plasma glucose and free fatty acids (10).

Figure 9-3 is a composite graph of a typical metabolic and thermic response to intravenous insulin (0.2 U per kilogram) in young males. Nadir levels of plasma glucose are reached by 30 min and are essentially back to normal 2 hr after the injection; however, core temperature is still depressed at the end of this observation period. After 2-DG infusions (50 mg per kilogram), rectal temperature (T_{re}) fell 1.1°C in 2 to 2.5 hr and remained below basal levels for 6 hr (11). Since plasma glucose and insulin and urinary catecholamines increased, it can be concluded that the observed hypothermia with 2-DG is triggered by intracellular glucopenia. Subsequent studies in mice indicated that deprivation of glucose centrally is the major determinant in hypothermia of hypoglycemia.

The mechanism for the observed reduction in body temperature associated with the administration of insulin and 2-DG is not clearly defined. Molnar and Read (12) implicated decreased heat production, and Thompson and associates (13) reported increased heat loss as the cause of decrease in T_{re}. However, Mager and his associates have consistently noted a decrease in O_2 consumption with the administration of both insulin and 2-DG to animals (14, 15, 16) and have concluded that glucopenia in the central nervous system affects centers controlling heat production in the periphery. The resultant hypothermia is accompanied by a decreased peripheral utilization of metabolic substrates. Figures 9-4 and 9-5 depict these data for the T_{re} and O_2-consumption changes of mice administered insulin and 2-DG. In other experiments, it was noted that propanolol, a beta-blocker, exacerbates the decreased T_{re} produced by intracranial 2-DG, insulin, or norepinephrine (Figure 9-6); however, results of experiments with phentolamine (an alpha-blocker) indicated that 2–DG and insulin

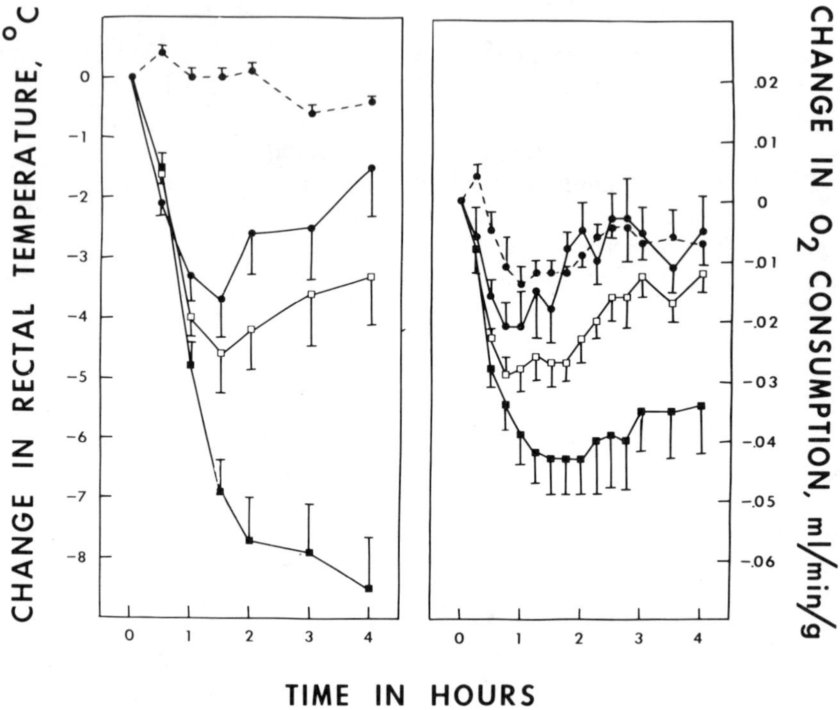

Figure 9-4. Effect of intravenous injection of insulin on body temperature and oxygen consumption responses in mice. Each point represents the mean difference and standard error from control values of 35 to 40 animals for temperature-dose response curves. Five different groups of 4 mice each were used at each dose level for the assessment of oxygen consumption. Closed circles and broken line denote data from saline controls. Closed circles and solid line represent data from mice receiving 0.05 unit insulin, and open squares represent data from mice receiving 0.07 unit insulin. Mice represented as the closed square were administered 0.1 unit insulin. (From Mager, Robinson, and Freinkel [14].)

may not be eliciting release of endogenous norepinephrine. The more pronounced fall in T_{re} accompanying propanolol injection may be reflecting a compromise in the counterregulatory recall of fuels from the periphery (17).

Thermoregulation, Caloric Restriction, and Cold

In separate studies designed to investigate the ability of young, healthy males to thermoregulate under conditions of restricted caloric intake

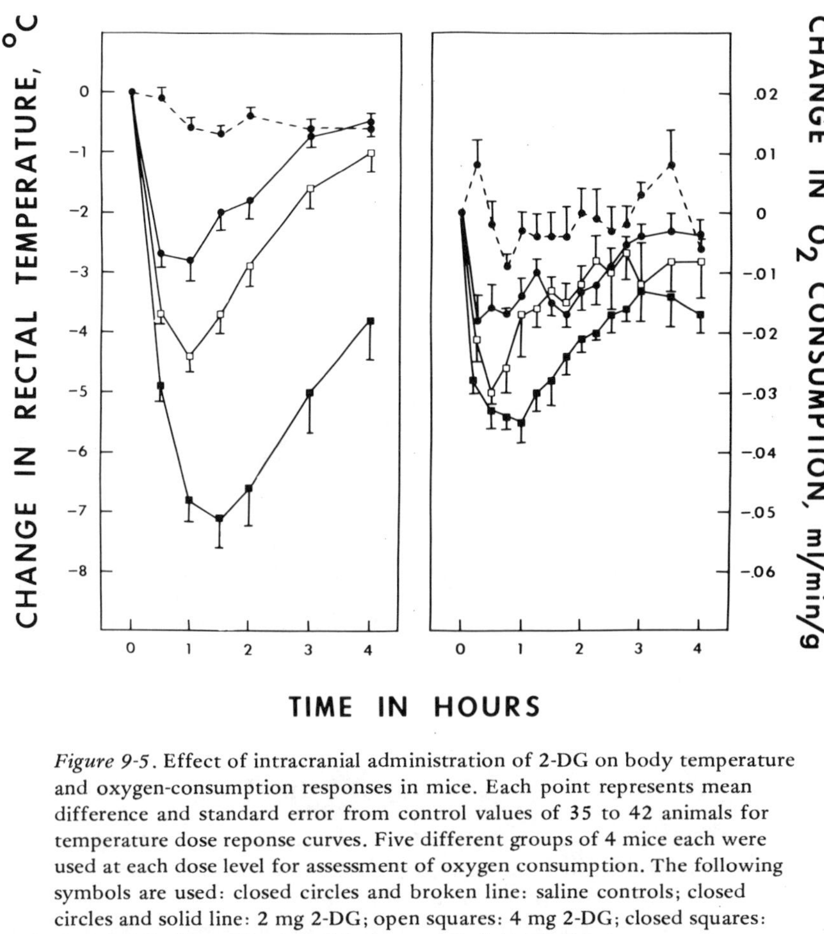

Figure 9-5. Effect of intracranial administration of 2-DG on body temperature and oxygen-consumption responses in mice. Each point represents mean difference and standard error from control values of 35 to 42 animals for temperature dose reponse curves. Five different groups of 4 mice each were used at each dose level for assessment of oxygen consumption. The following symbols are used: closed circles and broken line: saline controls; closed circles and solid line: 2 mg 2-DG; open squares: 4 mg 2-DG; closed squares: 8 mg 2-DG. (From Mager, Robinson, and Freinkel [14].)

and cold, no problem was encountered in maintaining normal T_{re} and in mobilizing and utilizing peripheral metabolic substrates (18). Thus, young males exposed to 60°F and consuming no calories for 14 d were able to maintain their normal core temperatures and circulatory plasma glucose at approximately 80% of control levels. Additionally, the metabolic mixture that is being oxidized for total heat production under these conditions of cold and starvation is the same caloric density (4.06 kcal per gram) as humans use under fasting conditions in a thermoneutral environment.

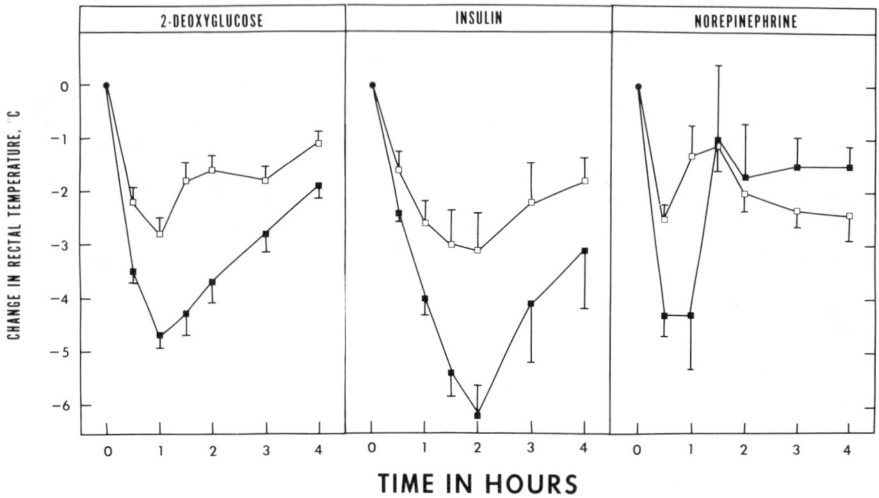

Figure 9-6. Effect of intracranial injection of propranolol (5 μg) on temperature response of mice to intracranial administration of 4 mg of 2-DG ($n = 20$), 0.05 unit of insulin ($n = 8$), and 10 μg of norepinephrine ($n = 8$). Each point represents mean difference and standard error from control values. Open squares represent hypothermic agents alone; closed squares are the same agents in combination with propranolol. (From Mager, Robinson, and Freinkel [14].)

Thermoregulatory Effects of 5-thio-D-glucose

With the observation that analogues of D-glucose can competitively inhibit glucose oxidation, the authors have used additional metabolic inhibitors to elucidate further the relationship between glucose metabolism and body temperature. Thus, since it had been demonstrated (19) that phosphorylated intermediates of the glucose analogues competitively inhibit the reactions of the glycolytic cycle, the authors (20) hypothesized that such metabolic inhibition would subsequently affect core temperature and, further, that magnitude of the effects might depend on the site of administration, dosage, and ambient temperature.

In a series of experiments, adult male mice (Swiss-Webster) were injected intracerebrovntricularly or intraperitoneally with appropriate concentrations of the glucose analogue, 5-thio-D-glucose (5-TG). Two environmental temperatures, 4°C and 22°C, were selected; 4°C is well below the thermoneutral environment for mice, and 22°C may be in the lower thermoneutral range. Where appropriate, blood was collected by cardiac puncture and plasma was separated, frozen, and subsequently analyzed for glucose levels.

Figures 9-7 and 9-8 demonstrate the T_{re} response to several concentrations of 5-TG when injection is made intracerebroventricularly. Figure 9-8 indicates that by 15 min after the administration of 37.5 μg of 5-TG at 4°C, a significant dose-dependent hypothermic response occurred. At the highest dosage (100 μg), the hypothermic response was so profound that three of the animals succumbed by 120 min with an average T_{re} below 20°C. At 22°C ambient temperature, analogous but more moderate hypothermia was effected; T_{re} ordinarily returned to normal levels by 120 min at this temperature.

When the 5-TG was given by intraperitoneal injection as demonstrated in Figures 9-9 and 9-10, generally hypothermic responses were elicited. Again, at the colder environmental temperature, the highest

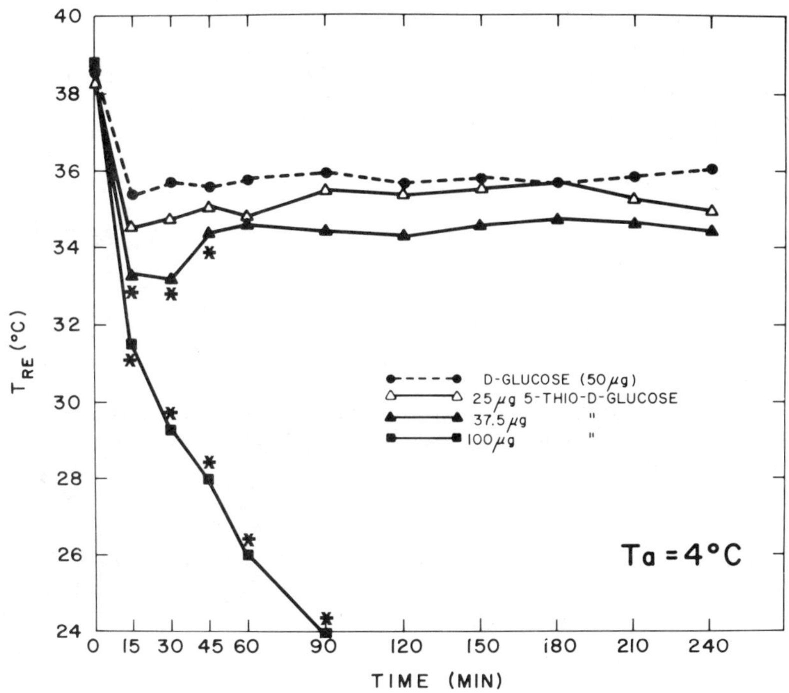

Figure 9-7. Effects of intracerebroventricular administration of 5-TG on the T_{re} of mice at an ambient temperature of 4°C. (From Francesconi and Mager [20].)

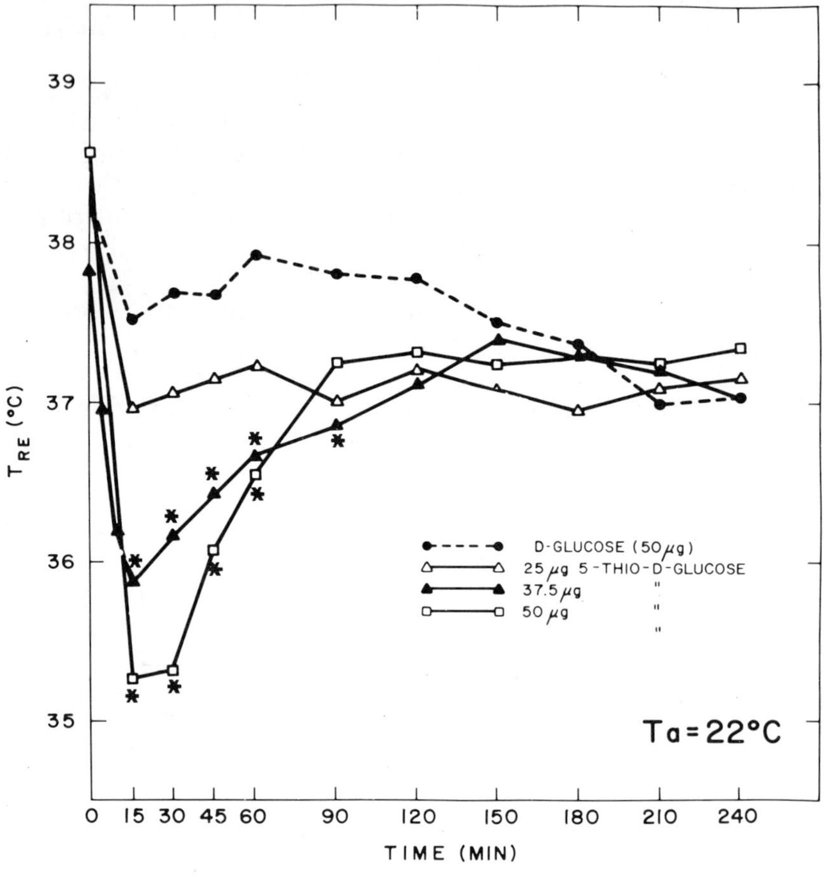

Figure 9-8. Effects of intracerebroventricular administration of 5-TG on the T_{re} of mice at an ambient temperature of 22°C. (From Francesconi and Mager [20].)

dosage (20 mg) effected T_{re} below 26°C and resulted in the deaths of several of the experimental animals. At 22°C, the higher dosages effected significant hypothermia that had not normalized even after 4 hr.

Figure 9-11 demonstrates that the nutritional condition of the animals affected the intensity of the hypothermic response to analogue administration. The results from this experiment show that the food-deprived animals manifested a significantly greater hypothermic response to 5-TG adminisrration. This, again, would be commensurate

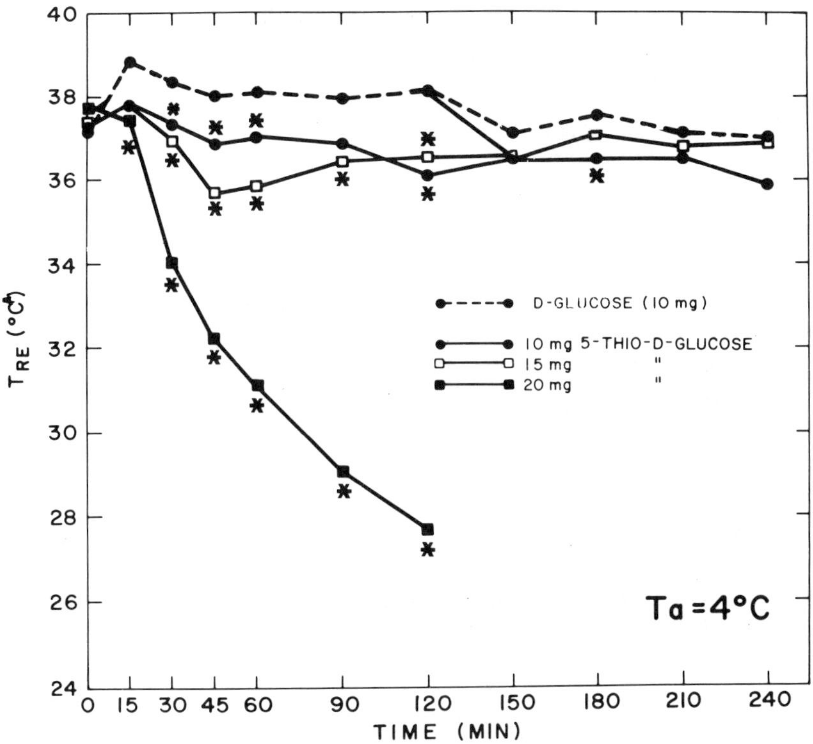

Figure 9-9. Effects of intraperitoneal administration of 5-TG on the T_{re} of mice at an ambient temperature of 4°C. (From Francesconi and Mager [207].)

with the hypothesis that levels of endogenous carbohydrate reserves are an essential determinant of the intensity of the hypothermic response to cold challenge, which is consistent with Estler's (4) earlier data.

Figure 9-12 demonstrates the magnitude of the hyperglycemic responses that occurred 60 min after the injection of 5-TG in cold-exposed mice. Again, control mice were administered physiological saline in equivalent volumes. The adminisration of 5-TG resultd in significantly increased plasma glucose levels in both fed and food-deprived mice. However, it is noteworthy that food-deprived animals manifested significantly lower levels than their fed counterparts. As Figure 9-11 shows, the food-deprived animals suffered the greater degree of hypothermia, also.

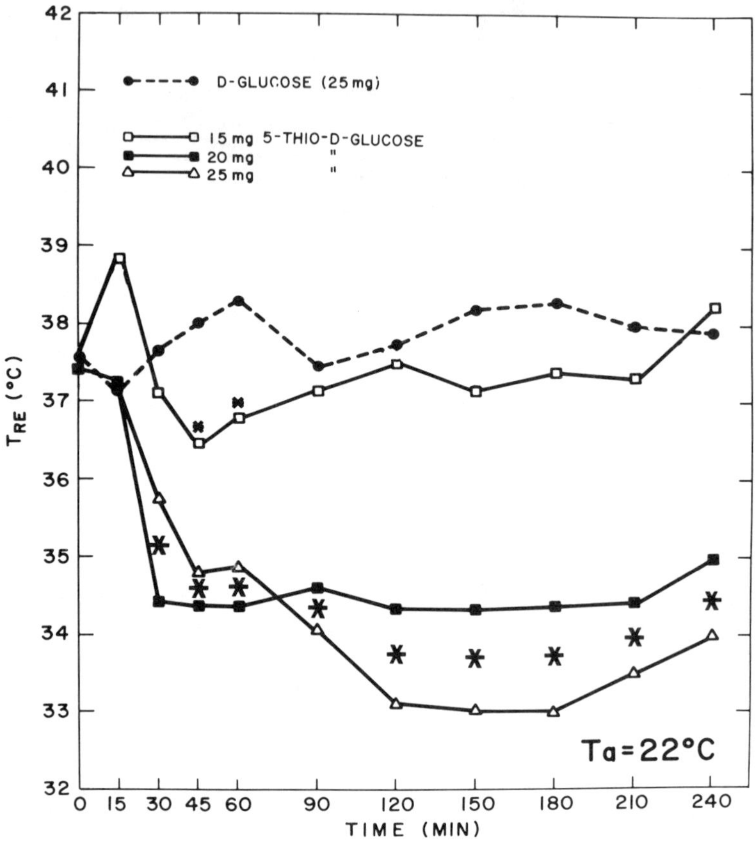

Figure 9-10. Effects of intraperitoneal administration of 5-TG on the T_{re} of mice at an ambient temperature of 22°C. (From Francesconi and Mager [20].)

The authors concluded from these experiments that normal carbohydrate metabolism is requisite for the maintenance of body temperture in the face of acute cold stress. This conclusion seems particularly valid in the rapidity and magnitude of the hypothermia elicited when 5-TG was administered intracerebroventricularly intraperitoneally in the 4°C environment. The mechanism of action of 5-TG appears to be similar to that reported earlier for 2-DG (11, 14, 15). Both compounds elicited circulatory hyperglycemia, cellular glucopenia, and hypothermia at ambient temperatures below thermoneutral; of the two analogues, 5-TG appears to be the more effective agent, with

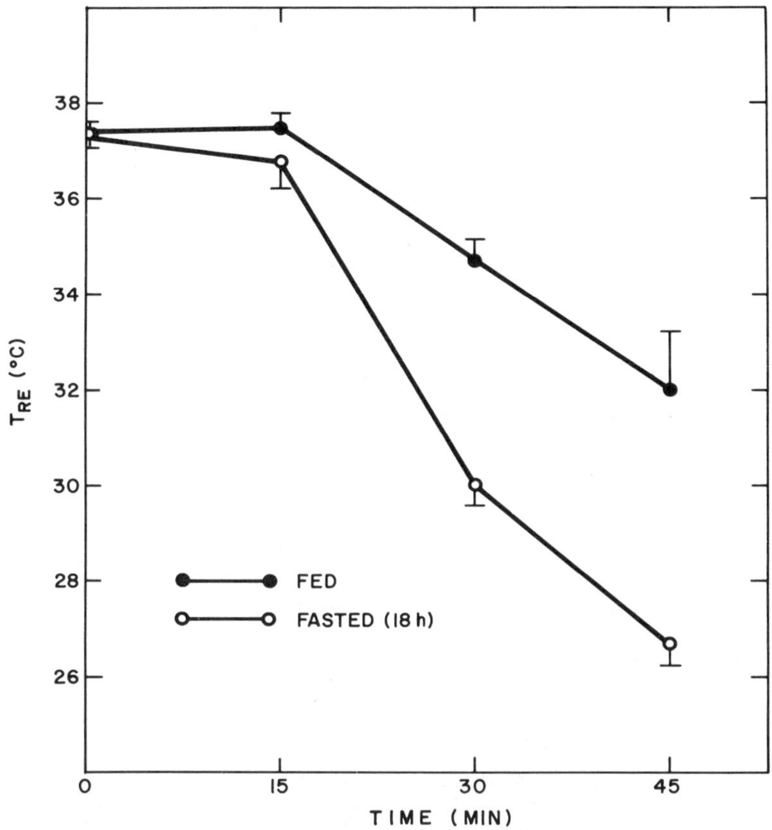

Figure 9-11. Effects of 18 hr food deprivation on the hypothermic response of mice to 5-TG at an ambient temperature of 4°C. (From Francesconi and Mager [20].)

consistently greater thermoregulatory responses and hyperglycemia. Once again, the evidence seems to favor a catecholaminergic response to glucose-analogue administration, since an intense and rapid release of norepinephrine and epinephrine has been reported as a result of 2-DG administration (11, 21, 22).

The authors have attributed the profound hypothermic response to a depletion of tissue glycogen followed by glucose efflux peripherally at the sites of heat production and centrally at the sites of thermoregulatory control. All of the data reviewed are consistent with the hypothesis that the reduced availability of carbohydrate elicits

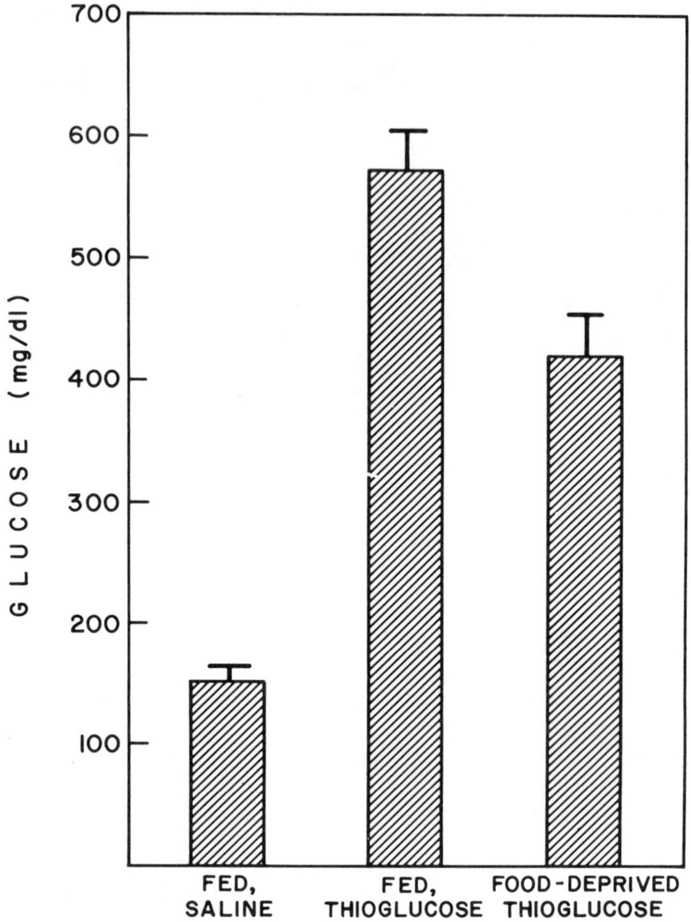

Figure 9-12. Effects of 18-hr food deprivation on the hyperglycemic response of mice to 5-TG administration at 4°C environmental temperature. (From Francesconi and Mager [20].)

a proportional decrement in heat production or thermogenesis necessary to maintain core temperature at normal levels. This is true whether the decrease in available substrate is caused by food deprivation, pharmacological intervention, or decreased sensitivity to metabolic stimulants (as in advancing age).

Sensitivity of Hypothalamic Sites to Glucopenia

To identify the central sites that are sensitive to glucose deprivation and are involved in the peripheral control of heat production, microamounts of 2-DG were stereotaxically injected into 21 sites

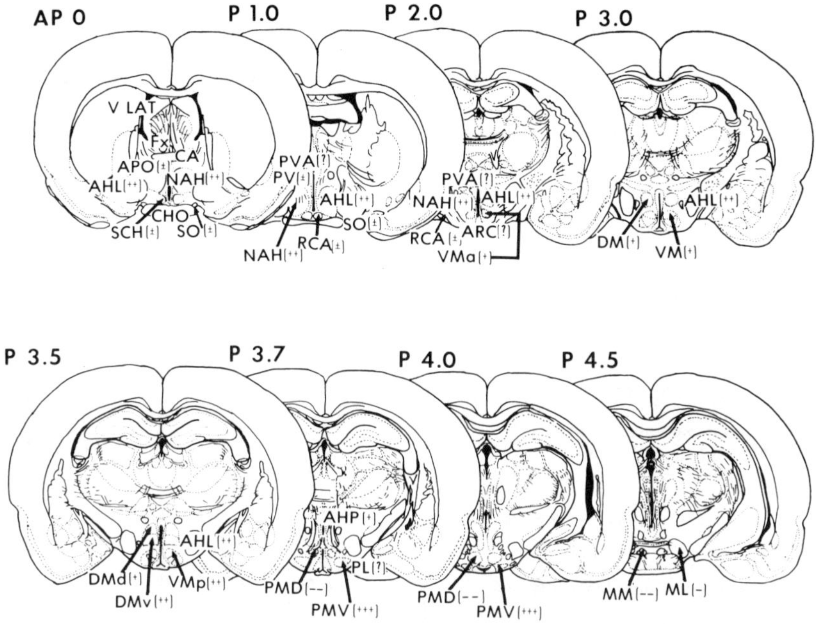

Figure 9-13. Summary of the effect on body temperature of the microinjection of 2-DG into selected hypothalamic areas, as depicted in a series of coronal rat brain sections. (Abbreviations are defined in Table 9-2 except for CA: anterior commissure; CHO: optic chaisma; Fx: fornix; V LAT: lateral ventricle.)

of the hypothalamus of the rat and T_{re} was monitored (23); the ventral premammillary nucleus (PMV) was the most sensitive to glucoprivation. Figure 9-13 summarizes the result of these injections in a series of coronal rat-brain sections that locate the various sites. Maximum response (+++) with 2-DG was observed in the PMV; however, the adjacent nuclei PMD, ML, PL, and MM elicited no alteration in T_{re}. A tabulation of these areas in the anterior and posterior hypothalamus is given in Table 9-2, along with their abbreviations and an explanation of the plus and minus symbols in the legend.

In Figure 9-14 are shown the dose responses to injected 2-DG into the PMV as reflected in changes in T_{re}. This nucleus displayed maximum sensitivity of all of the sites studied; sensitivity was arbitrarily defined by the rapidity of the fall in T_{re} and the comparatively faster return to basal values.

In an experiment to determine whether PMV-lesioned and hypothalamic-deafferentated rats thermoregulated at levels similar to intact animals when exposed to hot (35.5°C) and cold (5°C) environments,

Table 9-2
Summary of the Effect on Body Temperature of the Microinjection of 2-DG into 21 Selected Hypothalamic Areas

Microinjected Area	Abbr.	Response
Lateral hypothalamic area	AHL	+ +
Posterior hypothalamic area	AHP	+
Preoptic area	APO	±
Arcuate nucleus	ARC	?
Dorsomedial nucleus	DM	+
Dorsal subdivision of DM	DMd	+
Ventral subdivision of DM	DMv	+ +
Lateral mammillary nucleus	ML	–
Medial mammillary nucleus	MM	——
Prelateral mammillary nucleus	PL	?
Anterior hypothalamic nucleus	NAH	+ +
Dorsal premammillary nucleus	PMD	——
Ventral premammillary nucleus	PMV	+++
Paraventricular nucleus	PV	±
Anterior periventricular nucleus	PVA	?
Retrochiasmatic area	RCA	±
Suprachiasmatic nucleus	SCH	±
Supraoptic nucleus	SO	±
Ventromedial nucleus	VM	+
Anterior subdivision of VM	VMa	+
Posterior subdivision of VM	VMp	+ +

Note: Symbols used to denote the temperature response are as follows: +++, intense hypothermia; ++, moderate hypothermia; +, hypothermia; ±, slight hypothermia; -, no change (no hypothermia); —, slight hyperthermia; ?, response not clear.

the animals were maintained at these temperatures for 6 hr and their rectal temperatures were monitored (16). After 2 hr in the heat (Figure 9-15), all the rectal temperatures rose; thereafter, the intact animals were able to maintain their T_{re} while the PMV-lesioned and deafferentated rats' rectal temperatures continued to rise.

When the same group of animals was exposed to cold (Figure 9-16),

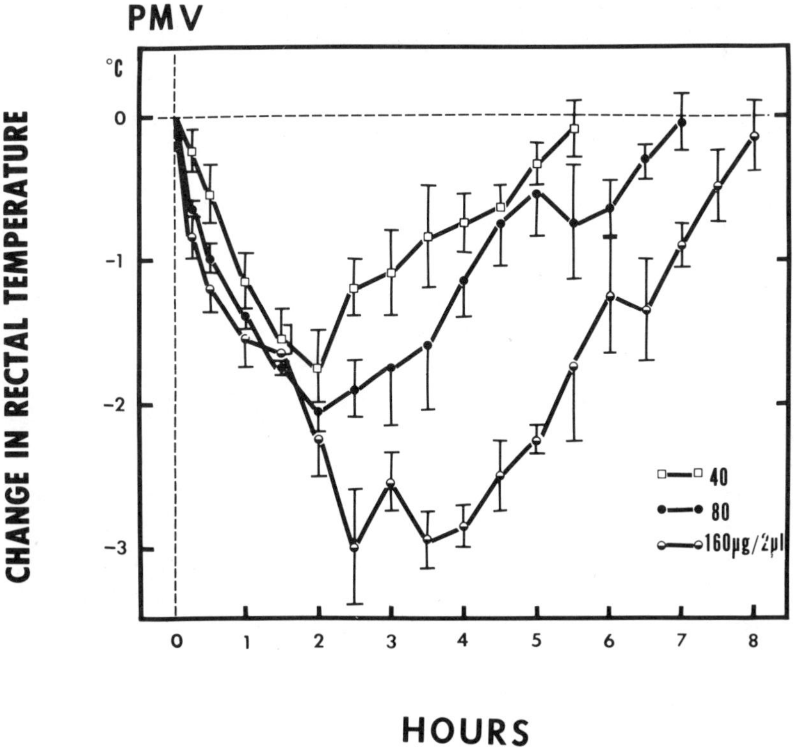

Figure 9-14. Effects on rectal temperature of microinjection of 40 to 160 μg of 2-DG into the ventral premammillary nucleus (PMV) (*n* = 6; each point is mean ± standard error). (From Shiraishi and Mager [16].)

the intact rats maintained their T_{re} for the entire 6-hr period. However, the PMV-lesioned and deafferentated rats were unable to maintain their body temperature, and after 6 hr their rectal temperatures were 1.5°C and 1.8°C, respectively, lower than the intact rats. From these studies, the authors concluded that in the rat an intact PMV nucleus is necessary for normal thermoregulation in a thermoneutral, hot, or cold environment.

References

1. Stolwijk JAJ: Responses to the thermal environment. Fed Proc *36*:1655-1658, 1977.
2. Girardier L: The regulation of the biological furnace of warm-blooded animals. Experientia *33*:1121-1124, 1977.

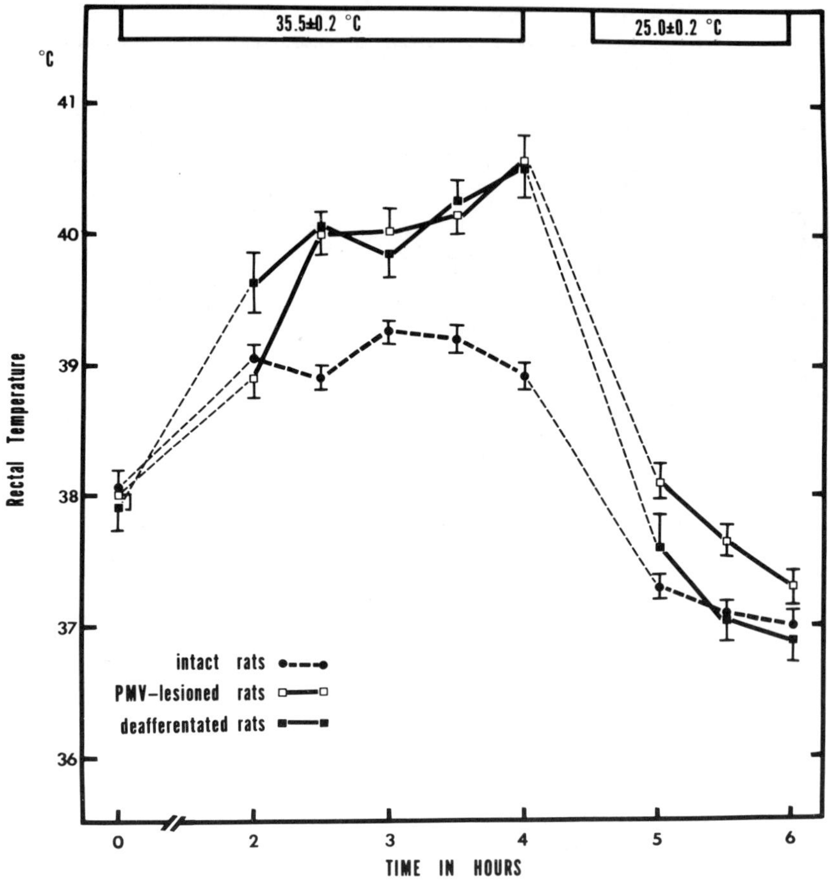

Figure 9-15. Effect of hot environment (35.5°C ± 0.2°C) on rectal temperature of intact (n = 11), ventral premammillary lesioned (n = 14), and hypothalamic deafferentated (n = 13) rats. (Each point is mean ± standard error). Time at each temperature shown by overbars. Gap shows transfer time. (From Shiraishi and Mager [16].)

3. Gale CC: Neuroendocrine aspects of thermoregulation. Ann Rev Physiol *35*:391-430, 1973.
4. Estler GJ: Efficiency of thermoregulation in acutely cold-exposed young and old mice. Life Sci *10*:1291-1298, 1971.
5. Mayer-Gross W, Berliner F: Observations in hypoglycaemia: IV. Body temperature and coma. Jour Ment Sci *88*:419-427, 1942.
6. Freinkel N, Singer DL, Arky RA, et al.: Alcohol hypoglycemia: I. Carbohydrate metabolism of patients with clinical alcohol hypoglycemia and the experimental reproduction of the syndrome with pure ethanol. Jour Clin Invest *42*:1112-1133, 1963.

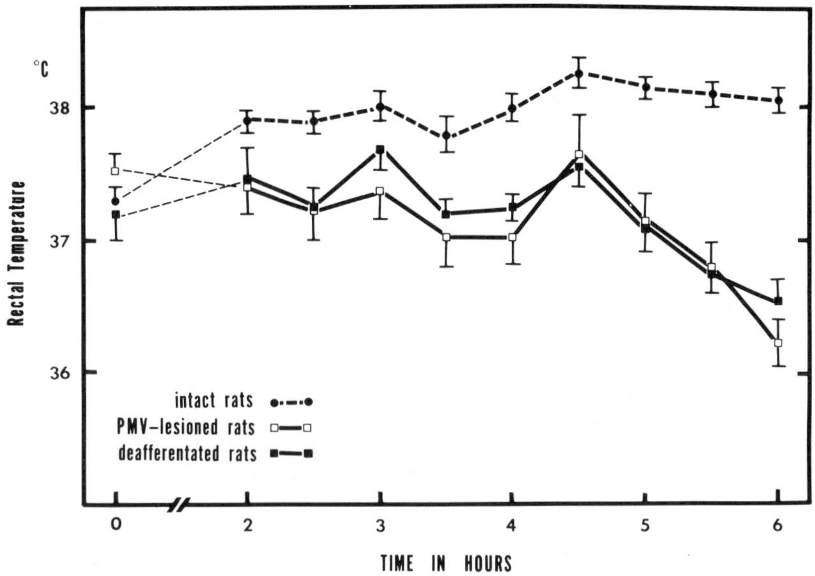

Figure 9-16. Effect of cold environment (5°C ± 0.5°C) on rectal temperature of intanct (n = 11), ventral premammillary lesioned (n = 14), and hypothalamic deafferentated (n = 13) rats. (Each point is mean ± standard error.) (From Shiraishi and Mager [16].)

7. Kedes LH, Field JB: Hypothermia: A clue to hypoglycemia. New Engl Jour Med *271*: 785-787, 1964.
8. Strauch BS, Felig P, Baxter JD, et al.: Hypothermia in hypoglycemia. Jour Amer Med Assoc *210*: 345-346, 1969.
9. Landau BR, Lasz J, Stengly J, et al.: Certain metabolic and pharmacologic effects in cancer patients infusions of 2-deoxy-D-glucose. Jour Natl Cancer Inst *21*:485-494, 1958.
10. Brown J: Effects of 2-deoxyglucose on carbohydrate metabolism: Review of the literature and studies in the rat. Metabolism *11*:1098-1112, 1962.
11. Freinkel N, Metzger BE, Harris N, Robinson S, Mager M: The hypothermia of hypoglycemia: Studies with 2-deoxy-D-glucose in normal humans and mice. New Engl Jour Med *287*:841-845, 1972.
12. Molnar GW, Read RC: Hypoglycemia and body temperature. Jour Amer Med Assoc. *8*: 916-921, 1974.
13. Thompson DA, Lilavivathana U, Campbell RG, Welle SL, Craig AB: Thermoregulatory and related responses to 2-deoxy-D-glucose administration in humans. Amer Jour Physiol (Reg Integ & Comp Physiol) *239*:R291-R295, 1980.
14. Mager M, Robinson S, Freinkel N. Drug modification of hypothermia induced by CNS glucopenia in the mouse. Jour Appl Physiol *41*:559-564, 1976
15. Robinson S, Mager M, Freinkel N: Interrelationship of central nervous system glucopenia and heat production in mice. *In*: Lomax P, Schönbaum E (eds.), The Pharmacology of Temperature Regulation, pp. 112-123. Basel, S. Karger, 1973.

16. Shiraishi T, Mager M: 2-deoxy-D-glucose induced hypothermia: Thermoregulatory pathways in the rat. Amer Jour Physiol (Reg Integ & Comp Physiol) *239*:R270-R276, 1980.
17. Abramson EA, Arky RA, Woeber KA: Effects of propranolol on the hormonal and metabolic response to insulin-induced hypoglycemia. Lancet *2*:1386-1389, 1966.
18. Mager M, Robinson S: Substrate mobilization and utilization in fasting men during cold exposure. Bull NJ Acad Sci, Special Symposium Issue March:26-30, 1969.
19. Chen M, Whistler RL: Action of 5-thi-D-glucose and its 1-phosphate with hexokinase and phosphoglucomutase. Arch Biochem Biophys *169*:392-396, 1975.
20. Francesconi R, Mager M: 5-thi-D-glucose: Thermoregulatory effects in mice at various environmental temperatures. Amer Jour Physiol (Reg Integ & Comp Physiol) *239*: R214-R218, 1980.
21. Wagienka LC, Grasso SG, Forsham DH: Estimation of adrenomedullary reserve by infusion of 2-deoxy-D-glucose. Jour Clin Endocrin Metab *26*:37-45, 1966.
22. Sun CL, Thoa NB, Kopin IJ: Comparison of the effects of 2-deoxyglucose and imobilization on plasma levels of catecholamines and corticosterone in awake rats. Endocrinology *105*:306-311, 1979.
23. Shiraishi T, Mager M: Hypothermia following injection of 2-deoxy-D-glucose into selected hypothalamic sites. Amer Jour Physiol (Reg Integ & Comp Physiol) *239*:R265-R269, 1980.

CHAPTER TEN

The Relationship between Shiver and Respiratory Parameters in Humans

R. S. Pozos, Ph.D.,
and L. E. Wittmers, Jr., Ph.D.

Shivering, an involuntary oscillation of skeletal muscle that is associated with acute and chronic exposure to cold, is a very recognizable aspect of the body's ability to generate additional heat. Although observations concerning shiver are as old as the interaction of humans with the cold, the mechanism of its genesis and control is not well understood.

Shivering is not initially a whole-body response; it develops progressively, and the majority of subjects shiver first in their legs and arms and then in the muscles of their chest and trunk (1). Pozos and Iaizzo's work has quantitated this observation through the use of spectral techniques (2). Shivering has a frequency between 6 and 12 Hz for the hands and legs. One of the important points that arose from studies of shivering is that shiver in neck muscles, which is commonly observed during immersion hypothermia, does not necessarily indicate overall body shiver. Some subjects are shivering in their legs and chest long before the onset of shivering in neck muscles. Shiver is also a very individual response. Some individuals shiver immediately upon entering a cold room or getting into cold water (10°C), while other individuals show a delay in the onset of shivering and/or the amplitude of their shivering is significantly decreased (2). This information is extremely important for cold-water survival, since all wet suits are designed with the assumption that cold water will eventually be warmed by heat production from the body's shivering response.

This chapter is research contribution No. 120. This work is the result of research sponsored by the Minnesota Sea Grant Program, supported by the NOAA Office of Sea Grant, Department of Commerce, under grants NA-79-AA-D-0025, NA-79-AA-D-00134, and NA-80-AA-D-00114 and project R/S-1.

If shivering is absent or of insufficient intensity, then the hypothermic protection of the devices may be reduced. In the authors' experience, approximately 10% of the subject population does not shiver appreciably during cold exposure.

Shiver may be altered either by ethanol ingestion or by the temperature of inspired air. The amplitude of shiver is greatly decreased after ethanol ingestion (3, 4). The mechanism behind alcohol's effect on shiver can be explained in part by the following physiological facts: ethanol promotes a peripheral vasodilatation that inactivates cold receptors, thus decreasing the peripheral input for shiver; ETOH directly decreases the sensitivity of thermal receptors; ETOH directly decreases the sensitivity of muscle spindles, which must be involved in the maintenance of a shiver; and/or ETOH depresses "central" oscillators in the brain or spinal cord. Using surface electrodes to monitor electrical activity in muscles, the authors found some residual activity in intoxicated individuals (blood alcohol level greater than 0.1 g%) who were in a cold chamber. These results indicate that the shiver is reduced but not in all muscles to the same extent. Thus, the effectiveness of shiver in generating body heat may be sharply reduced by ETOH ingestion.

The temperature of inspired air seems to influence the amplitude of shiver (3, 5). Since shiver is related to the respiratory cycle in that its amplitude increases during inspiration (6), the observation that the temperature of the air may play a role in the amplitude of shiver may have some important implications for the design of protective gear. There is a question about whether the response observed is attributable to stimulation of thermal receptors in the upper respiratory tract or whether the warm air stimulates the hypothalamus by way of bone conduction, the latter being less likely due to the quick response time in the alteration of shiver pattern. Present research using pigs and dogs to study the mechanisms behind the decrease of shiver during breathing of warm, humidified air is under way. The results will have important implications for individuals exposed to cold environments, such as divers who are using warm, humidified air in their gas supply. Divers may actually be developing a hypothermic condition in that the warm air may suppress the shiver, thus reducing heat production and removing an important signal of possible danger.

The relationship of shiver to metabolic rate is often questioned. Most investigators assume that an increase in metabolic rate is associated with shiver and/or increased intensity of shiver. There is no documentation for this hypothesis in the literature relative to humans. In fact, there are no reports that correlated shiver intensity to metabolic rates in animals or humans. Using genetically obese mice, Davis and Mayer (7) reported an increase in integrated electromyogram (EMG) activity during cold exposure. However, they did not relate EMG activity with metabolic rate. In order to understand the relationship between shiver and metabolic rate, both should be quantified. Usually, only one parameter is quantified, and the other is given some subjective qualification. Except for some attempts made by Stuart (1) and Jansky, Funke, and Hart (8), there have been few attempts in the literature to quantitate shiver. Some of the research efforts that have attempted to determine a correlation between shiver and metabolism did not adequately quantitate the shiver (8, 9, 10, 11, 12, 13), and so it is difficult to know what they were studying relative to muscle activity. The relationship between shiver and metabolism needs further examination. Many hypothermia experiments measure metabolic rate, and then the investigators make assumptions about how metabolism might be maintained with or without shiver. Shiver is usually measured in the neck (trapezius muscle) with surface electrodes. Metabolic rate has been used as an estimate of overall metabolic substrate utilization. Since a good relationship has been shown to exist between calorimetric data and oxygen consumption, indirect calorimetry—measuring the metabolic activity of O_2 consumption and CO_2 production—is commonly done. Whenever there is an increase in metabolic rate in a cold environment, the assumption is that the organism undergoing the cold stress is shivering. Therefore, the authors decided to study the relationship between shiver and metabolic rate by using the indirect calorimetric method in acute cold-exposure situations.

Materials and Methods

All subjects were selected from the students or staff at the University of Minnesota, Duluth, School of Medicine. Preexperimental evaluation was carried out in order to assess the subjects' health and physical fitness. On the day of the experiment, the subjects reported to the laboratory in a fasted state that included a 24-hr alcohol abstinence. For the testing, subjects were dressed in shorts and cotton socks. A rectal probe was inserted 15 cm past the anus and one or more skin probes were attached. All temperatures were monitored on a Batt 11 system (Bailey Instruments, Inc.).

Electrodes were attached for monitoring the electrocardiogram as well as at least four sets of surface electrodes for electromyogram measurements. An automatic blood-pressure cuff (Vita-Stat model

900-S) was used to obtain systolic and diastolic blood pressures at 2-min intervals.

Respiratory measurements were obtained for minute ventilation ($\dot{V}_E$), tidal volume (V_T), breathing Frequency (f), O_2 consumption ($\dot{V}_{O_2}$), and CO_2 production ($\dot{V}_{CO_2}$). Subjects were fitted with a rubber mouthpiece connected to a one-way valve (modified Douglas type, Warren Collins, Inc.). The inspired air came from the room, and the expired air was carried to a mixing chamber (5 L). The flow velocity of the expired air was monitored with a Fleisch pneumograph (Dynascience Medical Products). The flow signal was electronically integrated to obtain V_T and $\dot{V}_E$. The Oxygen content of the expired air was monitored with an OM-11 oxygen analyzer (Beckman Company), and the expired CO_2 content was monitored with an LB-2 carbon dioxide analyzer (Beckman Company). The sampling tubes for both analyzers were connected in series and placed in the 5-L mixing reservoir.

All the parameters were measured with the subject in a sitting position at normal room temperature (20°C) for a minimum of 10 min (control period). The subject walked into an environmental chamber with a room temperature of between 5°C and 10°C. The monitoring leads were reconnected within 2 min of entering the chamber. The subject remained in the room in a sitting position from 15 to 50 min with all parameters being monitored continuously. In no experiment did the rectal temperatures fall during cold exposure; in fact, there was an average increase of 0.2°C.

For EMG recordings, surface electrodes were placed on the soleus, tibialis anterior, extension digitorum, flexor carpi ulnaris, masseter, pectoralis major, and trapezius. The signals were amplified and then stored on a Hewlett Packard tape recorder for subsequent analysis.

The recorded EMGs were transformed to digital values by playing the recordings through a PDP-12 analog-to-digital converter while an interrupt-driven machine language program sampled the signal at a computer rate in order to obtain the desired bandwidth resolution. The digitized signals were displayed and stored on the disk. These sampled values were then retrieved and displayed on a graphic screen, at which time the operator selected out portions of the shiver data. Once all the segments were chosen, a Fortran-IV program was used to join the segments together, forming a resultant continuous record that was then stored for analysis.

The EMG resultant records were full-wave rectified and demodulated, after which both acceleration and altered EMG records were analyzed for frequency components through the use of autocorrelation and power spectral techniques. The resultant spectral plots of variance in microvolts squared versus frequency were printed for each EMG record. The cutoff frequency was 31.24 Hz, the sampling interval was 0.016 Hz, and the bandwidth resolution was 0.5 Hz. The variance was plotted at every 0.25 Hz.

Results and Discussion

Figures 10-1 and 10-2 represent the recordings of EMG and tidal volume obtained during the experiments. As previously reported, the

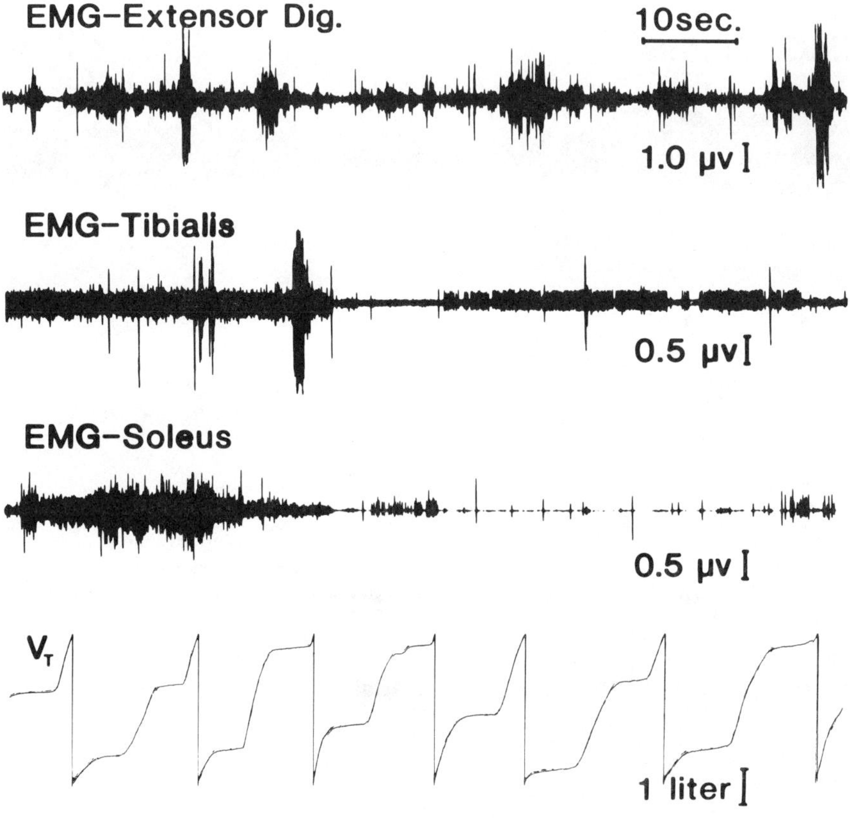

Figure 10-1. An example of the EMG on ventilatory responses upon entering the cold environment. Note the sporadic nature of the electrical activity in the three muscle groups monitored. When compared to control values, there is an increase in motor unit firing in the tibialis and soleus muscles and an increase in ventilatory rate and tidal volume.

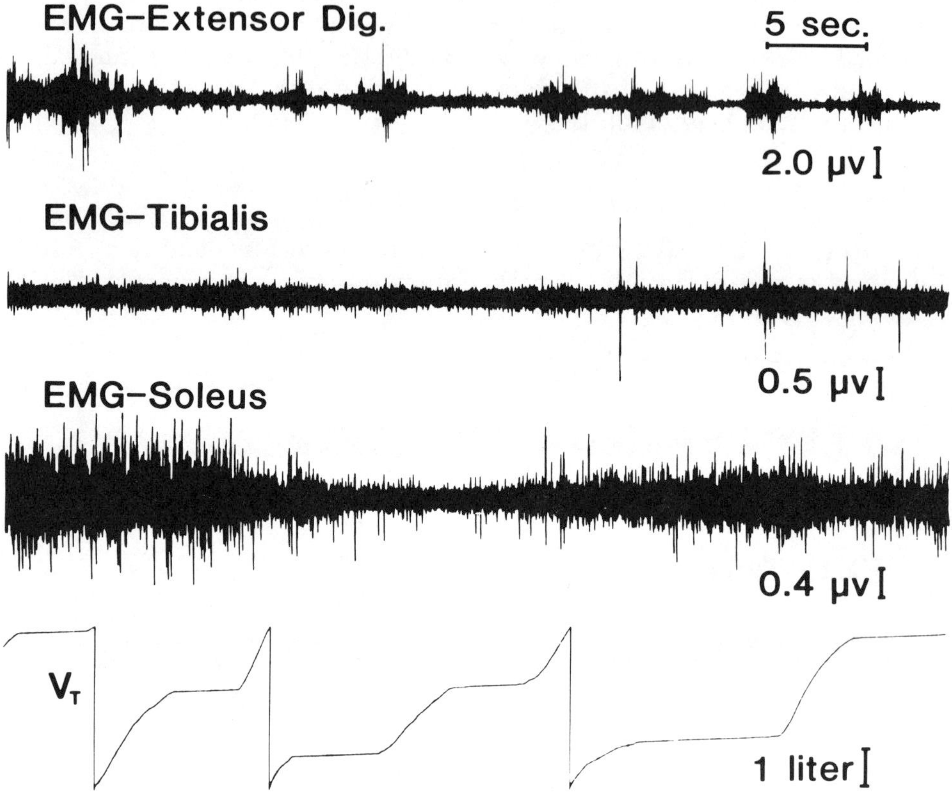

Figure 10-2. An example of the EMG and ventilator responses to prolonged cold exposure associated with shiver. Note the tonic electrical firing in all muscle groups as well as a waxing and waning pattern especially in the extensor digitorum and the soleus. The respiratory rate and tidal volume have decreased from the high values obtained upon entering the cold environment.

initial stages of shiver indicate an initial tensing of the musculature. This initial stage is evident from the increase in motor-unit firing illustrated in the tibialis anterior and soleus. As the cold exposure contiues, there is an increase in motor-unit firing until there are generalized bursts of electrical activity that waxes and wanes. Figure 10-1 also shows a change in the amount of electrical activity to the ventilatory cycle. Figure 10-2 demonstrates frank shiver and its possible coupling to ventilation rate. Figures 10-3 and 10-4 illustrate the respiratory and cardiovascular responses that occur when the subject enters the cold room and remains there for 36 min. There is an immediate increase in $\dot{V}_E$, $\dot{V}_{O_2}$, and $\dot{V}_{CO_2}$, which is followed by a plateau

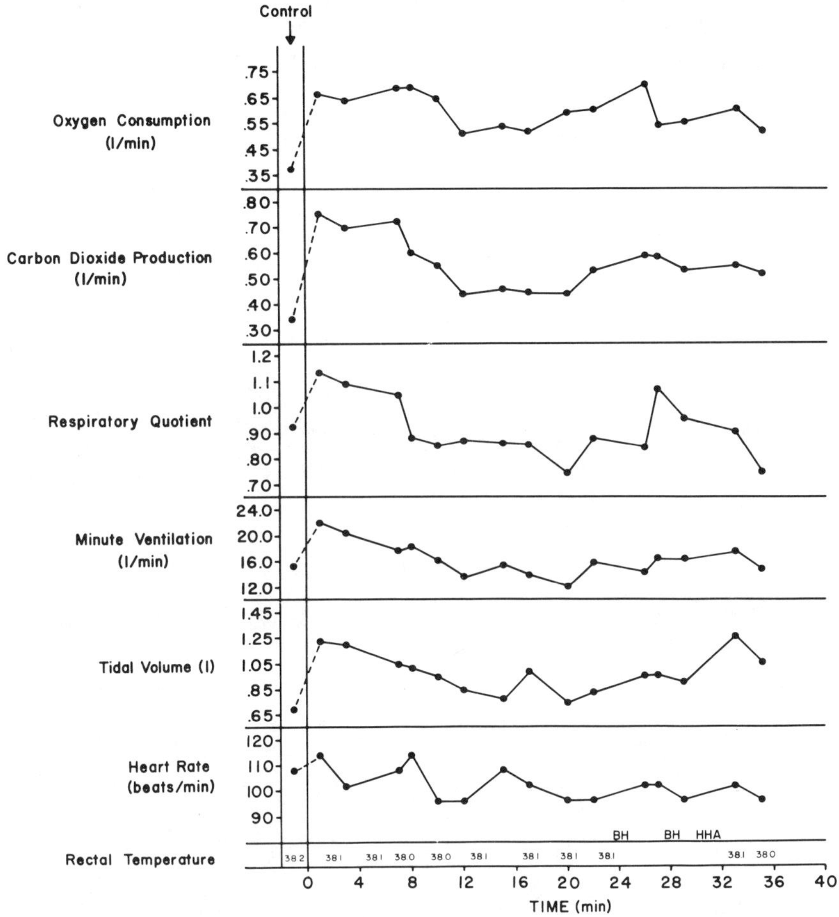

Figure 10-3. An example of an experiment illustrating the metabolic, respiratory, and cardiovascular responses to a 35-min cold exposure. Note that the data in Figure 10-1 and 10-2 were obtained during this type of experiment. The control (room temperature) values are 5-min averages. The rectal temperatures are in °C. BH indicates that a breath-holding maneuver was done at that time; therefore, some of the data points are not included. HHA indicates that the subject was breathing hot, humidified air. When the control value for any parameter is off scale, it is included in digital form in the lower left-hand corner and is not connected to the first experimental point. In this subject there is an initial increase in all parameters, except the respiratory quotient, followed by a second rise with onset after 20 min of cold exposure.

or decreasing phase (8 to 16 min in cold chamber). After 16 to 20 min of exposure, these parameters start to rise again. Initial observations concerning these changes and EMG indicate that the overall EMG amplitude activity varies in a similar fashion.

The authors' initial hypothesis was that there had to be some

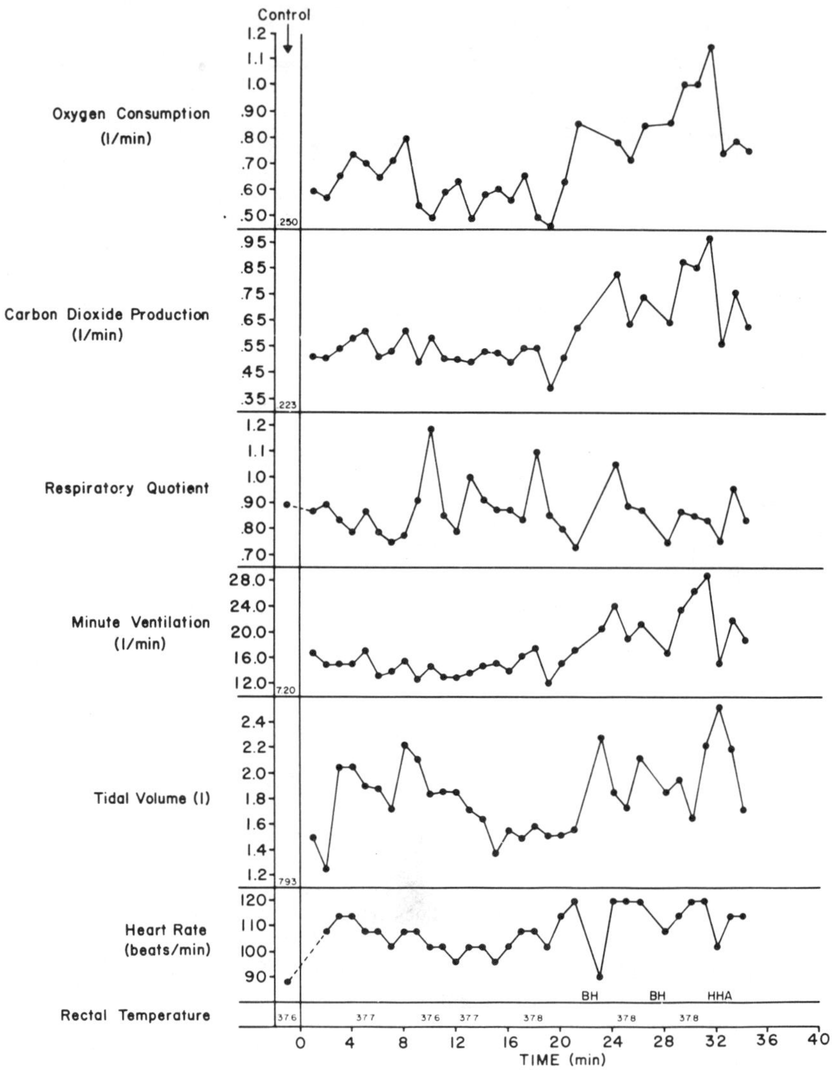

Figure 10-4. The same experimental protocol as in Figure 10-3. This subject is included here to show that different subjects respond with a variety of changes. Again, all parameters show an initial rise but one of smaller magnitude. However, throughout the cold exposure the values return toward control levels and do not show a second rise.

overall relationship between the level of shiver and increased metabolic rate during acute cold exposure. Since shiver obviously increases metabolic rate, one should see a positive relationship between the two. Initial observation indicates that the level of metabolic activity using indirect calorimetry roughly parallels shiver-amplitude levels recorded from a number of different muscles. The amplitude of shiver from the arms seems to be a better indicator of shiver than shiver from neck muscles.

However, long-term, integrated EMG activity may be a better measurement of the body's overall response to acute cold, since the authors only related shiver-amplitude changes at various 16-sec intervals to metabolic rate. In order to measure the overall body's response more accurately, it may be better to suspend the subject in a chair with accelerometers attached to the chair. Thus, one could get an overall value of the body's total shivering response to an acute cold stress and relate those values to metabolic rate.

As previously reported, the spectral analysis of the EMG activity showed a major peak at 6 to 12 Hz during shiver. The major peaks did not shift significantly during cold exposure, but the amplitude did. Whether these observations remain constant when the shiver becomes more accentuated, as the core temperature drops to 35°C, remains to be investigated. These studies on shiver may have a beneficial spin-off. It is well known that shiver stops at about 30°C rectal temperature, but the reason for this change is not understood. It is further known that once shivering stops death does not occur until the body reaches a temperature of 20°C to 25°C. If the mechanism for maintaining shiver could be better elucidated, the information might be extremely useful in warding off hypothermia for longer periods of time. Experiments studying the relationships among shivering, metabolism, and the hormones that regulate both shiver and metabolism are needed in order to understand human responses to cold and possibly to lead to some new hypothermia-preventive measures.

References

1. Stuart D, Ott K, Ishikawa K, Elred E: The rhythm of shivering: II. Passive proprioceptive contributions. Amer Jour Phys Med *45*:75-102, 1966.
2. Pozos RS, Iaizzo P, Petry R: Phsyiological action tremor of the ankle. Jour Appl Physiol *52*:226-230, 1982.
3. Pozos RS: Frequency analysis of shiver in humans and to alteration by the temperature of inspired air. *In*: Kuehn LA (ed.), Thermal Constraints in Diving, pp. 55-80. Undersea Medical Society, 1980.
4. Fox GR, Hayward JS, Hobson JN: Effect of alcohol on thermal balance of man in cold water. Can Jour Physiol Pharmacol *57*:860-865, 1979.

5. Cort JH, McCane RD: The neural control of shivering in the pig. Jour Physiol *120*: 115-121, 1953.
6. Hemingway A: Shivering. Ann Rev Physiol *4*:397-422, 1963.
7. Davis TRA, Mayer J: Nature of the physiological stimulus for shivering. Am Jour Physiol *181*:669-674, 1955.
8. Jansky L, Funke E, Hart JS: Analysis of electromyograms in shivering rabbits. Physiol Bohemoslovaca *19*:397-402, 1970.
9. Blatteis CM, Gilbert TM: Hypoxia and shivering thermogenesis in cold-acclimatized miniature pigs. Jour Appl Physiol *36*:453-456, 1974.
10. Lim, T: Central and peripheral mechanisms of shivering and its effect on respiration. Jour Appl Physiol *15*:567-574, 1966.
11. Baker P, Farrington PJ: Relationship between body fat and shivering in air at 15°C. Jour Appl Physiol *16*:421-425, 1961.
12. Marshall HW, Stoner HB: Catecholaminergic α-receptors and shivering in the rat. Jour Physiol *299*:27-34, 1978.
13. Mott JC: The effect of baroreceptor and chemoreceptor stimulation on shivering. Jour Physiol *166*:563-586, 1963.

PART III. The Treatment of Hypothermia

CHAPTER ELEVEN

Cardiac Function during Accidental Hypothermia

Bruce C. Paton, M.D.

Efficient functioning of the cardiovascular system is essential for the maintenance of body homeostasis and the equilibration of body temperature. But this system, like all others in the body, only works at maximum efficiency within a remarkably small temperature range. As the body cools, cardiovascular function deteriorates and eventually ceases.

The restoration of normal cardiovascular function is of equal importance during rewarming, for without good circulation the body cannot rewarm itself. During both cooling and rewarming, specific malfunctions of the system occur that may seriously or totally affect the recovery of a victim from accidental hypothermia. Although these malfunctions manifest themselves as cardiac arrhythmia or cardiac standstill, they are probably the end result of an inability of human energy systems and enzymes to adapt rapidly to a reduction in temperature, with a failure of essential metabolic activities and a loss of cellular energy.

Cardiovascular Function during Cooling

Most observations from which our knowledge of carciovascular function during cooling are derived were made either during experiments on animals or during cardiac operations under tightly monitored circumstances with general anesthesia and physiological and pharmacological control. In addition, observations have been made on volunteers whose body temperatures have been reduced a degree or two by exposure or immersion (1). These findings confirm those made under more vigorous circumstances in which body temperature is reduced by 10°C or more.

In a conscious person, the initial response to cooling is a rise in blood pressure, an acceleration of the pulse rate, shivering, increased oxygen and energy consumption, peripheral vasoconstriction, and an increase in systemic vascular resistance. Cardiac work is increased.

If cooling is rapid, as after falling into ice-cold water, hyperventilation, a reduction in arterial pCO_2, difficulty in breathing and muscular rigidity further compound the problem. When body temperature has fallen 2°C to 4°C, shivering stops. Blood pressure, heart rate, and cardiac output start to fall in a linear and progressive manner. Oxygen consumption is reduced during cooling by about 7% per °C reduction in temperature. Cardiac output, however, falls more rapidly, and this lack of perfect correlation results in an ischemic acidosis that is corrected slowly during rewarming as cardiac output once again increases. Around 30°C, cardiac arrythmias become increasingly likely, atrial fibrillation being the most usual. Electrocardiographic changes with a pathognomonic J wave may sometimes be seen (2). As temperature falls further, the likelihood of ventricular fibrillation increases, or the heart may become progressively slower and finally arrest (3).

The temperature at which cardiac function ceases is highly variable and, to some extent, species specific. Rats, mice, and cats die between 12°C and 17°C; the lethal temperature for dogs is around 23°C. The lethal temperature for humans is extremely variable. A woman found with a rectal temperature of 18°C survived, and there have been many reports of patients who survived after being found with body temperatures below 25°C. The cessation of cardiac function, however, is probably the terminal event in all victims of accidental hypothermia. Obtundation of central nervous system function and unconsciousness, peripheral anesthesia, and slowing or even cessation of respiration all occur before the heart stops, but all are restorable to normal when cardiovascular function is adequate for rewarming.

The initial peripheral vascular response is constriction. Blood is thereby shunted away from the skin and the biological shell, heat loss is reduced, and the temperature equilibrium of the core is maintained. But as cooling proceeds vasodilatation may occur and the skin becomes bright pink. Later, constriction returns, the skin becomes cyanosed and pale, and the victim may appear to be dead.

The peripheral vasodilatation that develops may be the cause of a terminal feeling of extreme warmth that causes the victim to throw off his or her clothes (4). In several instances recorded in Sweden, victims were found dead and naked or partially clothed in circumstances that immediately raised the question of criminal sexual assault. But it is now recognized that, for whatever reasons, hypothermic people may remove much or all of their clothing, thus accentuating their predicament.

Accidental hypothermia is common among the elderly (4, 5), especially in countries such as Britain where central heating is not universally available. There is evidence that temperature control in the elderly is impaired. Shivering may not always develop as body temperature falls, and so the normal mechanisms for preserving or restoring body temperature are ineffective and hypothermia develops slowly without unusual discomfort or warming signs. Concomitant heart disease constitutes an additional problem. When an elderly person sustains a myocardial infarct in a cold apartment, the reuction in cardiac output following the infarct greatly increases the chances of hypothermia being superimposed upon cardiac failure.

Cardiovascular Function during Rewarming: Temperature Afterdrop

It has long been recognized that, after a hypothermia victim is removed from the cold, the core body temperature may continue to fall even though rewarming has begun. Several explanations have been offered for this phenomenon, the commonest being that, as rewarming starts, "stagnant" cold blood from the periphery is released by peripheral vasodilatation and enters the core circulation. This seems an unlikely explanation because the intense peripheral vasoconstriction ensures that there is little or no peripheral pooling of blood: the peripheral vessels are empty.

A countercurrent system of heating and cooling exists between the arteries and veins. In the limbs, there are two venous systems, superficial and deep, and the deep veins run alongside the arteries. Warm arterial blood from the core runs in close proximity and counter to a flow of colder blood from the periphery. The warmer arterial blood gives up heat to the venous blood, warming it as it flows centrally. When arterial blood reaches the periphery, it relinquishes heat to the tissues as it flows through the smaller arterioles and capillaries. The coldest blood, therefore, is that flowing through the postcapillary venules. The blood in these vessels has given up a maximum amount of heat but has not begun to be rewarmed by the arterial countercurrent system.

Temperature gradients between peripheral and central tissues can be very great. A subcutaneous temperature of 36°C to 4°C can occur at the same time the core temperature is 31°C to 33°C. The venous blood returning from such a cold extremity is very cold, not because it has been stagnant or pooled, but because it has perfused cold tissues. When a person is removed from a very cold environment, there is a skin-to-core temperature gradient unless the duration of exposure has been long enough to equalize these temperatures. As external warming begins, the most superficial layers of skin warm first, but the deeper subcutaneous layers remain cold.

The gradients in a cold body can be represented as follows:

(i) $T_S < T_{SC} < T_C$, where
T_S = skin temperature,
T_{SC} = subcutaneous temperature, and
T_C = core temperature.

During the initial phase of external rewarming, the gradients change:

(ii) $T_S > T_{SC} > T_C$.

In a later phase of rewarming, the gradient may change again:

(iii) $T_S > T_{SC} > T_C$.

As a result, the blood being warmed in the most superficial skin layer may be cooled again by flowing through a deeper, cooler layer before returning to the core. Such a concept relies only on temperature gradients to account for the continuing drop in core temperature as rewarming starts, and it does not postulate unmeasured pools of blood suddenly rejoining the circulation (6). The phenomenon of afterdrop is well recognized, but it does not occur in every case. The longer the period of exposure, and therefore the smaller the skin-core temperature gradients, the less likely is afterdrop.

Soon after hypothermia was first used for cardiac surgery, cardiac failure associated with rewarming was recognized. Blair, Montgomery, and Swan (7) studied dogs cooled by immersion in ice water to below 30°C and then rapidly rewarmed. He found that the animals developed circulatory failure that persisted for at least 3 hr. It was postulated that the failure was due to inadequate blood volume and myocardial depression.

A similar phenomenon has been observed in humans rewarmed rapidly from accidental hypothermia without adequate monitoring of intravascular pressures and without adequate fluid replacement. While the patient is cold, cardiac output is reduced and peripheral resistance elevated. As peripheral warming occurs, vasodilatation reduces peripheral resistance, increases peripheral blood volume, and decreases central blood volume. These changes may occur while the heart is still cool and unable to respond by increasing its output.

Volume replacement is then needed to restore cardiac output. Changes in the oxyhemoglobin dissociation curve affecting the ability of hemoglobin to relinquish oxygen are important in determining whether or not tissues are adequately supplied with oxygen.

As blood becomes colder, the ability of hemoglobin to give up oxygen diminishes (8). Cold blood perfusing warmer cells may not be able to give up enough oxygen for metabolic leads. Part of the acidosis of rewarming may be due to this phenomenon. If a victim is immersed in warm water, superficial cells are warmed directly by conduction and may be warmer than the blood circulating around them. Cellular oxygen demand increases, while oxygen availability remains unchanged or lags behind oxygen demand, and acidosis may ensue.

Hypoventilation further aggravates the problem. The respiratory rate slows and ventilation is decreased by cold. A hypothermia victim might be breathing 8 to 10 times per minute when found. While he or she is rewarmed, the respiratory rate and ventilation may not increase in proportion to the oxygen needs of the body and relative hypoxia may develop.

Cardiac arrythmias, especially atrial fibrillation, often start during cooling. In many instances, an arrhythmia does not pose a significant problem, because the arrhythmia reverts spontaneously to normal sinus rhythm as the patient warms. But atrial fibrillation can reduce cardiac output by 20% to 25%; therefore, during a physiologically important phase of warming, the heart may not be producing a maximal output, thus further accentuating the problems caused by fluid shifts, hypoxia, and oxygen availability.

Clinical Management of Rewarming

The methods available for rewarming are classifiable as active and passive, internal and external, complex and simple (9). An ideal method for rewarming would be noninvasive and rapid; would allow total access to the patient for support, sampling, and resuscitation; and would be equally appropriate for all types of hypothermia. No such method exists, and methods such as extracorporeal circulation that are extremely useful in situations of dire emergency are not suitable for moderately hypothermic patients.

Methods of Rewarming

1. *External insulation:* Surrounding the patient with dry blankets and clothing provides no heat, but it diminishes heat loss. It is an essential first-aid measure (in conjunction with providing shelter from

the wind), and it is applicable in cases of mild hypothermia with conscious patients capable of rewarming themselves.

2. *External heating:* External heating of the victim with warm blankets, "sarongs," and hot-water bottles provides heat slowly, depending on the surface area exposed to warmth. The technique is good in mild to moderate cases and provides good access for resuscitation.

3. *Hot-water tub:* Rewarming in a hot-water tub is very effective and good in all cases. However, it is difficult to manage with unconscious, intubated patients, and it is impossible to continue rewarming if cardiopulmonary resuscitation becomes necessary. The equipment needed for the technique is readily available outside the hospital.

4. *Heated inhaled air:* Rewarming through heated inhaled air is moderately effective (10). But it requires specialized equipment. It is applicable to unconscious patients and permits access for resuscitation (it warms the core). The technique is appropriate for field use.

5. *Hydraulic sarong (warm-water blanket):* This method also is moderately effective (11). It requires special equipment, is applicable to unconscious patients, and permits limited access for resuscitation. It can be applied in the field.

6. *Peritoneal dialysis:* The use of peritoneal dialysis is suitable only in a hospital setting (12). The technique is effective, relatively simple, but invasive. It allows access to the patient.

7. *Diathermy:* Diathermy therapy must be performed in a hospital. Although it is effective, expensive equipment is required, and it may cause burns. The patient is accessible during its use.

8. *Thoracic or gastric lavage:* This technique is rarely used, invasive, and moderately effective. It warms the body's core. Access to the patient is limited.

9. *Extracorporeal circulation:* Femoral-artery-to-femoral-vein perfusion is the most effective method of rewarming (9). It permits rapid, controlled rewarming in unconscious patients and supports circulation even during ventricular fibrillation. It requires specialized equipment, operating room facilities, and a cardiovascular surgical team.

Clinical Management

1. *Mild cases (33°C to 35°C):* If the patient is conscious although perhaps confused, wet, cold clothing should be removed, and the body should be surrounded with warm blankets or a heating blanket. The patient could be immersed in a warm bath (45°C). Rectal temperature and vital signs should be monitored.

2. *Moderate cases (30°C to 33°C):* The victim may be unconscious

or very drowsy. External warmth should be applied by blanket or in a tub. Temperature, electrocardiogram, central venous pressure, blood gases, biochemical changes, and vital signs should be monitored. The medical team should be prepared to replace fluids, to control arrhythmias, to support circulation with pressors, and to administer oxygen.

3. *Severe cases (below 30°C):* The patient is usually unconscious and must be handled gently in order to avoid inducing arrhythmias. External warming, hot-water warming, hot inhaled oxygen, and extracorporeal circulation should be instituted. Arterial pressure (with an indwelling catheter), central venous pressure or pulmonary artery pressure (via Swan-Ganz catheter), cardiac output, urinary output, arterial gases, biochemical changes, and rectal temperature should also be monitored. The medical staff should be prepared to intubate, to restore fluid volume, to support circulation, to correct cardiac arrhythmias, and to institute cardiopulmonary resuscitation.

Cardiac Problems during Rewarming

1. *Atrial arrhythmias:* Atrial fibrillation, atrial flutter, and intermittent conduction defects are common. In most instances, they can be corrected by warming the patient to 30°C to 32°C. If the patient is elderly or has underlying cardiac disease, the arrhythmia may have preceded the hypothermia and so may be permanent, in which case it must be treated with appropriate medication.

If fast atrial fibrillation (more than 140 beats per minute) develops during rewarming, it may be necessary to administer digoxin (0.5 to 1.5 mg) intravenously in order to control the heart rate and to improve cardiac output. Prolonged treatment should not be necessary.

2. *Ventricular arrhythmias:* Premature ventricular contractions (PVCs) should be treated as though the patient were not hypothermic. Biochemical and blood gas abnormalities should be identified and corrected. As an immediate treatment, lidocaine intravenously given as a bolus of 50 to 75 mg may prevent aberrant beats. Warming is essential for final stabilization, and attempts at rewarming should be maintained as fully as possible in spite of difficulties in giving medication at the same time.

Ventricular fibrillation may develop spontaneously as the patient cools, or it may be induced during warming by rough handling, intubation, or insertion of central venous catheters. The possibility of inducing ventricular fibrillation should not deter the physician from intubating a patient in order to facilitate ventilation and oxygenation, unless equally good ventilation can be obtained with a mask and manual ventilation. Because continued ventilation may be necessary for several hours, manual ventilation may be impractical.

When a patient is admitted with ventricular fibrillation, the most rapid rewarming technique available should be instituted. Extracorporeal circulation is ideal because by this means circulation can be restored and supported much better than by external cardiac massage and, while the body is rapidly rewarmed, acid-base and biochemical abnormalities are corrected.

Cardiac arrest or ventricular fibrillation is extremely difficult to correct in a hypothermic patient if the patient cannot be warmed. If the patient's temperature is less than 28°C, it is extremely unlikely that electrical defibrillation will be successful, although it should certainly be tried. Cardiopulmonary resuscitation with external massage and controlled ventilation can, at best, produce a cardiac output equal to about one-third of normal resting output. Therefore, such a low cardiac output is not likely to be adequate for rewarming.

The most efficient noninvasive method for rewarming is immersion in warm water, but it is virtually impossible to conduct cardiopulmonary resuscitation on a patient in a hot-water tub. The patient is likely to be intubated, and warm, moist oxygen can be used for ventilation. Intravenous fluids can be warmed before infusion. Peritoneal dialysis could be used. The patient should be placed on a warming blanket during resuscitation.

It is important that acidosis be corrected, with the appropriate allowances for blood temperature, that all biochemical abnormalities be corrected, and that blood volume be restored as necessary.

The brain is protected by cold, but this safety factor should not be relied upon too heavily. A brain at 30°C tolerates 6 to 8 min of total ischemia; at 20°C, 30 min may be tolerable. The duration of tolerable ischemia, however, is extremely variable. Children can withstand longer periods of cerebral ischemia than can adults, and young adults can tolerate more than the elderly. It is not safe to think that because a patient is cold and develops ventricular fibrillation that attempts at rescuscitation can be delayed for relatively long periods because the brain is cold and "protected." The emergency should be treated with the usual urgency.

The mortality rate in hypothermic patients depends on the patient's health and many other circumstances (13, 14, 15). In healthy, young adults not intoxicated or drugged but only exposed to a cold environment, the mortality rate may be as low as 8% to 10%. In those who become hypothermic as a result of drug overdoses, the outcome depends more on the severity of intoxication than on the severity of hypothermia. Likewise, in the elderly, survival depends greatly on the presence or absence of underlying diseases—cardiac, endocrinological, or neurological. The mortality in these latter groups may be 50% to 80%.

Summary

Efficient functioning of the cardiovascular system is essential for the maintenance of a stable body temperature, for survival during developing hypothermia, and for resuscitation and rewarming. Cardiac function decreases with cold at a rate somewhat greater than the diminution in oxygen demand resulting in a slowly developing metabolic acidosis. The method chosen for resuscitation and rewarming should be appropriate to the degree of emergency. Mildly hypothermic patients require only simple, noninvasive methods for rewarming, but unconscious, severely hypothermic victims may need support by extracorporeal circulation. Cardiac problems should be treated much as in a normothermic patient, although many arrhythmias correct themselves as the patient warms. Energetic rewarming is essential but difficult in cold patients with ventricular fibrillation if normal cardiac action is to be restored. The mortality rate depends on the victim's age and the presence of intoxication by alcohol or drugs and underlying diseases. It may vary from 10% to 80%.

References

1. Marcus P: Laboratory comparison of techniques for rewarming hypothermic casualties. Av Space Environ Med *49*:692-697, 1978.
2. Emslie-Smith O: Accidental hypothermia: A common condition with a pathognomonic electrocardiogram. Lancet *2*:492-496, 1958.
3. Lloyd EL1, Mitchell B: Factors affecting the onset of ventricular fibrillation in hypothermia. Lancet *2*:1294-1296, 1974.
4. Wedin B, Vangaard L, Hirvonen J: Paradoxical undressing in fatal hypothermia. Jour Forensic Sci *24*:543-553, 1979.
5. Editorial. Accidental hypothermia in the elderly. Jour Amer Med Assoc *239*:1888, 1978.
6. Golden FS, Hervey GR: The mechanism of after-drop following immersion hypothermia in pigs. Jour Physiol *272*:26-27, 1977.
7. Blair E, Montgomery AV, Swan H: Posthypothermic circulatory failure: I. Physiologic observations on the circulation. Circulation *13*:909-915, 1956.
8. Callaghan PB, Lister J, Paton BC, Swan H: Effects of varying carbon dioxide tensions on the oxyhemoglobin dissociation curves under hypothermic conditions. Annals Surg *154*:903-910, 1961.
9. Reuler JB: Hypothermia: Pathophysiology, clinical settings and management. Ann Intern Med *89*:519-527, 1978.
10. Lloyd EL1: Accidental hypothermia treated by central rewarming through the airway. Brit Jour Anaesth *45*:41-47, 1973.

11. Dayton LB, Arnold JW: Hydraulic sarong: Emergency treatment for hypothermic casualties. Off Belay *21*:2-4, 1975.
12. Soung LS, Swank L, Ing TS, et al.: Treatment of accidental hypothermia with peritoneal dialysis. Can Med Assoc Jour *117*:1415-1416, 1977.
13. Ledingham I Mc A, Mone JG: Treatment of accidental hypothermia: A prospective clinical study. Brit Med Jour *280*:1102-1105, 1980.
14. Weyman AE, Greenbaum DM, Grace WJ: Accidental hypothermia in an alcoholic population. Amer Jour Med *56*:13-21, 1974.
15. Hudson LD, Conn RD: Accidental hypothermia: Associated diagnoses and prognosis in a common problem. Jour Amer Med Assoc *227*:37-40, 1978.

CHAPTER TWELVE

Emergency Treatment of Hypothermia

G. Patrick Lilja, M.D.

The emergency treatment of the hypothermic patient has received increased attention in recent years. This is probably due to the increasing number of cases in which patients have reportedly survived after periods of profound hypothermia with very few neurological sequelae. The improved likelihood of survival is primarily related to the more aggressive treatment of hypothermia, which begins when the patient is found by rescue personnel and continues through the hospital stay.

Degree of Hypothermia

A mildly hypothermic patient is one who has a core temperature of 34°C to 35°C (95°F to 97°F). Such patients are fully awake unless some other injury is present. They generally are shivering and very uncomfortable.

In a case of moderate hypothermia, the core body temperature is 30°C to 34°C (86°F to 94°F). Such patients are generally obtunded secondary to their hypothermia, but shivering is still present.

In severe hypothermia, the core body temperature is lower than 30°C (86°F). Such patients generally are obtunded or unconscious. Shivering at this temperature has ceased or has markedly diminished. Respirations and pulse may be depressed, or one may not be able to auscultate them. The extremities are generally rigid, as in rigor mortis. The distinction between life and death at these low temperatures at times may be difficult.

Prehospital Treatment

The management of the hypothermic patient should begin before the patient's arrival at a medical facility. Patients with mild hypothermia should first be removed from the cold environment if at all possible. Warm fluids can be administered by mouth, and warm clothing should be wrapped around the patient. It is imperative that any wet clothing be removed as soon as possible. Since a significant amount of heat is lost through the scalp, a cap or other covering should be placed over the patient's head as soon as possible. It should be stressed that alcohol in any form should not be administered because it will cause peripheral vasodilatation and may actually increase heat loss.

The treatment of the patient with moderate hypothermia must be aggressive in the prehospital phase. Like the mildly hypothermic patient, the moderately hypothermic patient should be removed from the cold environment. Warm clothing and/or blankets are certainly useful and the patient's head should be covered as soon as possible. In addition, the patient should be started on oxygen by mask. If a heating unit is available and humidity can be added to the oxygen unit in the field, using warm, humidified oxygen certainly may be of some advantage in helping to maintain the patient's body temperature (1). If respirations are shallow, the use of the bag valve mask to assist ventilation may be of importance. In caring for this type patient, one must be very careful to avoid excess stimulation since this can result in the development of ventricular fibrillation. If electrocardiograph monitoring is available during the prehospital phase, it can be attempted, but often the patient's shivering causes too much interference for a reliable tracing to be obtained. The moderately hypothermic patient should then be transported to an emergency facility capable of taking care of hypothermic patients.

The prehospital care of the severely hypothermic patient presents a challenge to any community rescue service. The first challenge that ambulance and rescue personnel face is identifying the hypothermic patient, who may appear to be dead. The most important point in the prehospital care of severe hypothermia is that resuscitation must be attempted for *any* patient who *may be* hypothermic. The absence of pulse and/or spontaneous respiration does not necessarily mean that a victim is beyond help. Therefore, the dictum of "don't assume a patient is dead until he is warm and dead" (2) must be strictly observed by ambulance and rescue personnel. What, then, is the treatment for a patient who is found without pulse or respirations and who clinically appears dead but may by hypothermic?

There is some controversy in the literature over the initial treatment of such individuals. Some authorities recommend that CPR should not be started since this may precipitate ventricular fibrillation if a rhythm is present (3). Others, however, feel that CPR should be started when there is no pulse or respiratory activity. There are numerous case reports (4, 5, 6, 7) in which CPR was administered to hypothermic victims with successful resuscitation. The author's current opinion is that CPR should be started when there are no pulse and respirations. In all other instances, the author feels that CPR should be started and can be continued to the hospital. In addition, if the prehospital personnel are authorized to use intravenous therapy, an intravenous with lactated Ringer's or normal saline should be started and 1 amp of sodium bicarbonate can be administered during transportation. Defibrillation and cardiac drugs are not routinely indicated in the prehospital management of the profound hypothermic patient since they will be ineffective.

If a profoundly hypothermic patient has a pulse, he or she must be handled extremely gently in order to avoid inducing ventricular fibrillation. The patient's head should be covered, and blankets should be applied to his or her body in order to prevent further temperature drop as much as possible. In addition, oxygen by mask should be begun. If the rescue crew is authorized to start an intravenous procedure, an intravenous solution with lactated Ringer's or normal saline should be started and 1 amp of sodium bicarbonate administered during transport.

Ambulance and rescue personnel should always remember that patients who have hypothermia may present with other illnesses or injuries as well. Sometimes hypothermia victims may have underlying diseases that have contributed to the development of hypothermia. Traumatic injuries can disable a patient, who may later succumb to hypothermia. Patients found outdoors in cooler temperatures must always be suspected of having some degree of hypothermia. It should be stressed, of course, that the treatment of other injuries and/or conditions must be carried out concomitantly with the treatment of the hypothermia. In addition, any history that can be obtained, either from the scene where the patient is picked up or from witnesses, is extremely helpful in the later in-hospital management of the patient.

Emergency-Department Treatment

Patients presenting with mild hypothermia to the emergency department primarily require warm blankets and warm fluids by mouth. It is very important that a thorough history and physical exam be conducted to search for predisposing factors that may have resulted in hypothermia. Patients should be carefully checked for frostbite and treated when necessary.

Patients with moderate or severe hypothermia present a greater challenge to emergency-department personnel. Just as in the prehospital phase, oftentimes the greatest difficulty for emergency-department personnel is recognizing that hypothermia exists. This condition must be anticipated and diligently sought in any patient with a history of having been found obtunded or unconscious. An absolute must for any modern emergency department is an electronic rectal temperature probe. All patients admitted for emergency treatment certainly must have their temperatures taken routinely. If the patient's temperature does not register on a standard thermometer or if the patient is unconscious or obtunded, the rectal temperature probe should be used. It must be emphasized again that patients presenting with other injuries or illnesses are often hypothermic and, conversely, hypothermic patients often have other injuries or underlying illnesses.

In general, several types of rewarming have been advocated by different authorities. These methods primarily take the form of external rewarming (passive or active) or active internal rewarming. There is much debate in the literature over the pros and cons of each type.

External Rewarming

Methods for external rewarming include passive environmental rewarming, rewarming with blankets, rewarming with radiant lamps, rewarming with a heating mattress, and warm-water immersion. The easiest form of external rewarming is passive rewarming, simply placing the patient in a warm room. Although this was once the method of choice, the high mortality rate associated with the use of this method in cases of profound hypothermia limits its utility.

A form of active external rewarming uses warm blankets or a combination of warm blankets and radiant lamps to rewarm the body. The heat sources should be applied primarily to the trunk of the body and not to the extremities in order to prevent so-called rewarming shock and afterdrop, which may result from the cooler blood in the extremities flowing into the central core. Peripheral rewarming may also result in a drop in blood pressure secondary to vasodilatation with insufficient volume on board. A third device that could be utilized for active external rewarming is a hyperthermic mattress. All of these methods have been used with success in warming patients with moderate hypothermia (8, 9, 10, 11, 12).

Another form of active external rewarming, which utilizes rapid rewarming, is to immerse the patient in a warm bath, either a standard bathtub heated to 48°C to 50°C or a Hubbard tank. This method has been used successfully, and it is recommended by some as the method of choice for rewarming hypothermia victims (1, 13, 14).

The prime advantage of most external rewarming methods is that they are relatively easy to start and, unless one has to purchase a Hubbard tank, relatively inexpensive. The major disadvantage is that it may lead to rewarming shock. An additional disadvantage in using a warm bath is that it may be more difficult to monitor the patient. Also, performing CPR in a tub is not easily accomplished. Despite these disadvantages, all forms of active external rewarming have been successful in a number of patients.

Internal Rewarming

The main types of internal rewarming described in the literature include inhalation of warm air, intravenous administration of prewarmed fluids, gastric lavage with warm fluids, and peritoneal lavage with warm fluids. (Cardiopulmonary bypass is discussed in the following section.) The use of warm air has been advocated as a very convenient way of rewarming patients who are hypothermic. It has been shown to be faster than simply placing the patient in a warm room (1, 15). However, the degree of temperature rise in the profoundly hypothermic patient is very slow when only warmed humidified oxygen is used as a rewarming therapy. Probably the method's main usefulness is in preventing a further drop in temperature. In some areas of the United States, prehospital equipment has been adapted to provide warm, humidified oxygen in the field.

Prewarmed intravenous fluids have some benefit. Still, the rewarming provided by their use alone is still relatively slow.

Gastric lavage and peritoneal lavage have been described by numerous authors as ways to rewarm profoundly hypothermic patients, including some who have been successfully resuscitated from cardiac arrest (16, 17, 18). There is a significant increase in core body temperature when both gastric and peritoneal lavage are used. Peritoneal lavage probably raises body temperature somewhat faster, but it has the disadvantage of being an invasive procedure. However, this factor may also be an advantage in that peritoneal lavage provides the opportunity to ascertain whether or not there is any intraabdominal bleeding. This is important in that the absence of any reliable history is a problem in treating any obtunded or unconscious hypothermic patient. The possibility that a hypothermic patient may have sustained an earlier injury resulting in intraabdominal hemorrhage must be strongly considered, and peritoneal lavage is probably indicated in all hypothermic patients for diagnostic reasons. Therefore, it would seem to be a reasonable approach to utilize peritoneal lavage as an extension of diagnostic lavage.

Cardiopulmonary Bypass

Partial cardiopulmonary bypass has been advocated by some authorities as the best way of treating profound hypothermia (19). Others have been more conservative but have described the usefulness of partial bypass in the resuscitation of profoundly hypothermic patients or hypothermic patients who are in cardiac arrest (20, 21, 22). In addition, Wickstrom and associates (2) described one patient with solidly frozen extremities who suffered only limited frostbite damage after bypass was used, and they speculate that bypass may also be the method of choice for rewarming frozen extremities.

The advantage in utilizing core-rewarming techniques may be that they warm the core first and so prevent rewarming shock. The problem with using peritoneal lavage and especially bypass is that many hospitals in the country do not have the staff or the equipment required to initiate these invasive procedures.

It is clear that each method of rewarming has been shown to work in certain types and groups of patients. In addition, both active external rewarming and active internal rewarming have been effectively used in patients suffering cardiac arrest secondary to hypothermia. The question, therefore, is: what type of rewarming techniques should be made available within the emergency department?

Emergency-Department Treatment Protocols

The hypothermia treatment protocol that is described here would be easy to use in most emergency rooms. First, one must remember to suspect hypothermia in all patients and to use an electronic rectal temperature probe when no other temperature is easily ascertained or when the patient is unconscious.

For cases of mild hypothermia, continuing the prehospital treatment by providing a warm environment and warm fluids is all that is needed in the emergency department. This can be accomplished by placing warm blankets over the patient or by placing him or her on a warm heating pad. The patient must be carefully checked for signs of frostbite, and predisposing factors leading to hypothermia must be diligently sought out.

For cases of moderate and severe hypothermia, the followng treatment protocol should be executed.

1. The patient should be ventilated with 100% oxygen. If there is forewarning of the patient's arrival, a system for delivering heated, humidified oxygen should be set up; otherwise, the system should be set up as soon as possible after the patient arrives. If the patient is unconscious, his or her airway should be protected by intubating the patient very gently in order to avoid triggering ventricular fibrillation. At this time, sputum cultures should be obtained, if possible.
2. The patient's circulation should be supported as necessary. Frequent blood-pressure and vital-sign readings must be obtained. It is important to remember that some degree of hypotension can be tolerated in hypothermic states.
   a. An intravenous line should be started with prewarmed lactated Ringer's at 42°C as soon as possible.
   b. A central-venous-pressure line is very helpful in determining the shifting fluid states that often result as patients are rewarmed.
   c. Blood samples should be obtained for CBC, electrolytes, BUN, glucose, clotting studies as indicated, CPK and cardiac isoenzymes, and SGOT. In addition, blood typing should be done.
3. It is essential that blood gases be obtained and corrected for temperature. It is good to remember that some degree of acidosis may be helpful in increasing the degree of oxygen dissociation.
4. A Foley catheter should be placed in order to monitor kidney function.
5. A chest X ray should be obtained as soon as possible.
6. Antibiotics should not be administered until signs of sepsis and causative organisms are identified. In addition, when hyperglycemia is present, it should not be treated aggressively at first, unless it is causing hyperosmolar problems. Hyperglycemia often relents somewhat just with rewarming.
7. Frequent monitoring of vital signs, including the central venous pressure, is necessary throughout the rewarming process.

In addition, the treatment for rewarming currently recommended by the author is as follows. For a core temperature of 30°C to 34°C (86°F to 93°F), active external rewarming, such as radiant heat or a heating mattress, is applied to the trunk, and frostbite is treated if necessary. Though deep-bath therapy may be useful, this method does not offer any significant advantage because it is difficult to monitor patients easily while they are in a water environment and immersion has no clearcut advantage over other forms of external heat. For patients with a core temperature of less than 30°C (86°F), active rewarming is the method of choice. This is especially true until the danger of ventricular fibrillation has passed (core temperature warmer than 28°C). According to the author's preferences, these patients would be started with a heated blanket and radiant heat to the trunk of the body as soon as possible. Gastric lavage with lactated Ringer's or normal saline heated to 42°C should be instituted as soon as possible. When there are no surgical scars in the abdomen, peritoneal lavage with two lavage catheters placed in the lower abdomen is begun. Warm lactated Ringer's at 42°C, alternated with 1 L of 5% dextrose every fourth or fifth bottle, is used. Peritoneal lavage is not only a therapeutic method, it is a diagnostic method for determining whether any intraabdominal hemorrhage exists.

If the patient is in cardiopulmonary arrest, cardiopulmonary bypass is the rewarming method of choice when the hospital's facilities are adequate. Bypass offers the advantage of rapid rewarming, thus allowing earlier conversion to a perfusing rhythm. It also guarantees that oxygen will be available to meet the body's needs during the rewarming. In addition, it may offer some advantage when the patient's extremities are fozen solid. When the facility does not have the capability for cardiopulmonary bypass, core rewarming utilizing gastric and peritoneal lavage should be continued, together with other forms of active rewarming. It must be reiterated that cardiopulmonary resuscitation should be continued until a perfusing rhythm is obtained or until the patient has reached an adequate temperature for conversion to a spontaneous rhythm.

When these guidelines are followed, a number of patients who were thought to be dead can be successfully resuscitated from profound hypothermic states. No patient should be pronounced dead until an adequate attempt at resuscitation and rewarming has been undertaken.

References

1. Collis ML, Stinman AM, Chaney RD: Accidental hypothermia: An experimental study of practical rewarming methods. Av Space Environ Med *48*:625-632, 1977.
2. Reuler JB: Hypothermia: Pathophysiology, clinical settings and management. Ann Intern Med *89*:517-519, 1978.
3. Accidental hypothermia. Pediatrics *63*, 1979.
4. Lilja GP, Hill M, Ruiz E, Clinton J: Clinical assessment of patients undergoing CPR in the emergency department. Jour Amer Coll Emer Phys *8*:81-83, 1979.
5. Pickering BG, Briston GK, Craig DB: Core rewarming by periotoneal irrigation in accidental hypothermia with cardiac arrest. Anesth Analg *56*:574-577, 1977.
6. Sekar TS, MacDonnell KF, Namsirikul P, Herman RS: Survival after prolonged submersion in cold water without neurologic sequelae. Arch Intern Med *140*:775-779, 1980.

7. Southwick FS, Dalglish PH: Recovery after prolonged asystolic cardiac arrest in profound hypothermia. Jour Amer Med Assoc *243*:1250-1253, 1980.
8. Atukorale DP: Accidental hypothermia coma at Adams Peak. Ceylon Med Jour *16*: 100-103, 1971.
9. Chinard FP: Hypothermia treatment needs controlled studies (letter). Ann Intern Med *90*:990, 1979.
10. Fernandez JP, O'Rourke RA, Ewy GA: Rapid external rewarming in accidental hypothermia. Jour Amer Med Assoc *212*:153-155, 1970.
11. Hamilton G, Rosen P: Hypothermia (letter). Ann Intern Med *90*:721-722, 1979.
12. Ledingham IM, More JG: Treatment of accidental hypothermia: A prospective clinical study. Brit Med Jour *280*:1102-1105, 1980.
13. Davies L: Treatment of hypothermia (letter). Lancet *2*:656, 1978.
14. Frank DH, Robson MC: Accidental hypothermia treated without mortality. Surg Gyn Obst *151*:379-381, 1980.
15. Morrison JB, Conn ML, Hayward JS: Thermal increment provided by inhalation rewarming from hypothermia. Jour Appl Physiol *76*:1061-1065, 1979.
16. Coniam SW: Accidental hypothermia. Anesthesia *34*:250-256, 1979.
17. Jessen K, Hagelsten JO: Peritoneal dialysis in the treatment of profound accidental hypothermia. Av Space Environ Med *49*:426-429, 1978.
18. Reuler JB, Parker RA: Peritoneal dialysis in the management of hypothermia. Jour Amer Med Assoc *240*:2289-2290, 1978.
19. Welton DE, Mattox KL, Miller RR, Petmecky FF: Treatment of hypothermia. Jour Amer Med Assoc *240*:2291-2292, 1978.
20. Kugelberg J, Schuller H, Berg B, Kallum B: Treatment of accidental hypothermia. Scand Jour Thor Cardiovasc Surg *1*:142-146, 1967.
21. Truscott DG, Firor WB, Clein LJ: Accidental profound hpothermia: successful resuscitation by core rewarming and assisted circulation. Arch Surg *106*:216-218, 1973.
22. Wickstrom P, Ruiz E, Lilja GP, Hinterkopf JP, Haglin JJ: Accidental hypothermia: core rewarming with partial bypass. Amer Jour Surg *131*:622-625, 1976.

CHAPTER THIRTEEN

Submersion Hypothermia and Near-Drowning

A. W. Conn, M.D., G. A. Barker, M.B., J. F. Edmonds, M.B., and D. J. Bohn, M.B.

"Submersion hypothermia" and "near-drowning" are terms of relatively recent origin, and some clarification may be helpful. "Hypothermia has been defined as a state of body temperature which is below normal in a homeothermic individual" (1). This definition cannot be faulted, but less agreement exists for other definitions and classifications in the field of hypothermia.

A classification of hypothermia based on depth and duration is essential in clinical practice. Although a reduction in body temperature must be 2°C or more to be of much significance (2, 3), greater reductions are frequently observed. The following description is related to the depth of hypothermia, with each level graded according to a specific temperature range (4): mild hypothermia (36°C to 34°C), moderate hypothermia (34°C to 28°C), deep hypothermia (28°C to 17°C), and profound hypothermia (17°C to 10°C). A classification based on duration (5) includes: acute hypothermia (measured in minutes), prolonged hypothermia (measured in hours), and chronic hypothermia (measured in days).

A separate classification of hypothermia is based on etiological factors. "Induced hypothermia" is defined as deliberate hypothermia in humans or animals that is produced by either surface cooling or blood-stream cooling (6). "Accidental hypothermia" is defined as hypothermia that has not been induced deliberately (6). Body cooling can result accidentally from exposure to low ambient temperatures in air, in water, or under water. By common usage, "accidental hypothermia" is the term usually applied to body cooling resulting from exposure to cold air. "Immersion hypothermia" is defined as a reduction in body temperature resulting from immersion in cold water. In most reports, "partial immersion" is implied when only the trunk and extremities are involved when the victim was swimming or using a flotation device. Hypothermia varies greatly in depth and can be acute or prolonged in duration, but asphyxia is not an immediate complication in most circumstances. A new term, "submersion hypothermia," has been introduced for cases of hypothermia suffered under water (7). It is defined as the well-recognized process of acute asphyxia during drowning from total immersion, but it includes the simultaneous development of acute hypothermia, which can occur with great rapidity, especially in children and in very cold water. This refinement in terminology seems appropriate since it emphasizes the concept of a brief but critical race, run concurrently, between the progressively destructive effects of increasing asphyxia and the beneficial protective effects of increasing hypothermia.

Since water temperature is almost always lower than body temperature, most drowning victims show evidence of submersion hypothermia to some extent. In Table 13-1, a temperature trend is evident between increasing hypothermia and increasing neurological injury (from asphyxia), both resulting, presumably, from increasing submersion time.

Table 13-1
Neurological Injury and Hypothermia Level (as Measured in the Emergency Room) in Cases of Near Drowning

Temperature Range	Hypothermia Level	Neurological Category				
		A	B	C 1	C 2	C 3/C 4
36°C or less	Normal	18	4	0	2	2
36°C-34°C	Mild	7	5	1	3	7
34°C-28°C	Moderate	0	2	0	6	10
28°C-17°C	Deep	0	0	0	0	7
Unknown/unrecordable		19	6	3	1	12
Total (125 cases)		54	17	4	12	38

Note: See Table 13-3 for explanation of neurological categories.

In summary, submersion hypothermia includes the two pathological processes interacting simultaneously for a brief period during the act of drowning that could have important clinical implications. A simple comparison of immersion hypothermia with submersion hypothermia is given in Table 13-2.

Accidental drowning causes approximately 140,000 deaths per year throughout the world (8), including 7,000 per year in the United

Table 13-2
A Comparison of Various Factors in Immersion Hypothermia and Submersion Hypothermia

Factor	Immersion Hypothermia	Submersion Hypothermia
Immersion	Partial	Total
Onset of cooling	Immediate	Immediate
Onset of asphyxia	Delayed	Immediate
Cooling versus asphyxia	Sequential	Simultaneous
Hypothermia rate (versus air)	Rapid	Very rapid
Duration of hypothermia	Prolonged	Acute
Level of asystole in hypothermia	Moderate to deep	Mild to moderate
Cerebral death (from initial exposure)	Delayed (hours)	Delayed (minutes)
Resuscitation efforts (vary with temperature)	2 to 6 hr	1 to 2 hr

States (9) and 1,300 per year in Canada. "Drowning" is defined as death by suffocation under water (10), but many humans now survive a severe drowning incident because of emergency resuscitation. This development has led to the invention of the term "near-drowning," which is used to describe a submersion incident in which the victim is successfully resuscitated and survives 24 hr (11). This definition excludes those who "drowned" but refers to the clinical course following rescue, which ignores the degree of subsequent recovery. It is the authors' firm belief that a victim's failure to recover completely can be a tragedy worse than death (12). This chapter discusses the relationship between submersion hypothermia and recovery from near-drowning, especially with reference to children, and describes the results from aggressive resuscitation in reducing the incidence of neurological injury.

Submersion Hypothermia

Submersion hypothermia, as limited by definition, is a specific entity in the field of immersion hypothermia. Immersion hypothermia was a common cause of death at sea during the Second World War and has been exhaustively studied (13). A brief review of immersion hypothermia with reference to drowning follows.

It is well known that, when an inadequately clothed person suffers prolonged exposure to cold, accidental hypothermia may develop. Immersion hypothermia is an accelerated version of the same process (the thermal conductivity of water is 20 times that of air) (13). The physiological regulation of body temperature is controlled by balancing heat production with heat loss across the skin surface. Since heat production can only be increased by exercise or shivering to a limited extent, reducing heat loss is the prime method of control. No amount of shivering or exercise can compensate for the great heat loss that invariably occurs when one is immersed in icy water and is unprotected by suitable clothing.

Many factors can contribute to the rate at which acute immersion hypothermia develops. Heat loss is increased with an increase in exposed surface area or cutaneous blood flow, especially when associated with a limited layer of insulating fat. Dominating all other factors is the temperature of the surrounding water. Keatinge (13) reported that for all persons immersed in water at a temperature of 0°C death usually occurs within 1 hr whereas at 15°C most die within 6 hr. However, when the temperature is 20°C or higher, almost all persons can survive indefinitely. Therefore, warm water temperatures are crucial for survival. At water temperatures below 10°C to 12°C, the vascular smooth muscle is paralyzed and heat loss accelerates (14). With increased body activity such as swimming or panicky movements, the rate of cooling increases as a result of skeletal muscle vasodilatation and additional heat loss from the extremities. It is obvious that acute hypothermia is a potential hazard in all accidental immersion incidents.

Death from immersion hypothermia can occur in at least three different ways. Rarely, the sudden shock of entering ice-cold water causes death from immediate ventricular fibrillation (the immersion syndrome) (15) before preliminary cooling has occurred. This syndrome may be involved in some reported cases of good swimmers who after falling into icy water never regain the surface. Others may simply drown immediately from the reflex involuntary gasping of ice-water submersion. In this situation, immersion hypothermia and cerebral ischemic anoxia (drowning?) are separate and unrelated entities for clinical purposes.

Most commonly, the sequence of events is a relentless reduction of core temperature, with delirium at 35°C and unconsciousness at approximately 32°C followed by cessation of swimming and subsequent drowning. Death is preceded by moderate levels of immersion hypothermia so that prolonged submersion (10 to 30 min) can be compatible with complete recovery even when cardiopulmonary arrest is present at rescue. An analogy can be made in adult surgical practice requiring bilateral carotid occlusion or cardiac standstill. Induced moderate hypothermia prior to surgery provides an extended "safe" period for circulatory arrest without neurological injury.

When a person is properly supported by a life jacket, his or her head remains above the water; therefore, asphyxia should not occur immediately unless caused by waves or an obstructed airway. Progressive hypothermia results in a loss of consciousness at approximately 32°C and spontaneous ventricular fibrillation at a core temperature less than 28°C or cardiac asystole at 22°C (deep hypothermia). Deep hypothermia precedes the development of bradycardia and subsequent cardiac arrest without asphyxia. A similar surgical analogy can be made from elective pediatric cardiovascular operations, in which extracorporeal circulation induces profound hypothermia (i.e., 12°C) followed by total circulatory arrest for up to 60 min and subsequent complete recovery. It is not surprising therefore that a person can make a complete neurological recovery after much longer periods of immersion and submersion hypothermia with cardiac arrest than previously thought possible. These three mechanisms producing circulatory arrest indicate that cooling and drowning may occur separately, simultaneously, or sequentially, but each process is distinct and may require different treatment.

Although immersion hypothermia can cause death in several ways, paradoxically, it protects the brain from asphyxia for a time. But the exact limits are always unknown. If rescue occurs within 10 to 40 min, complete recovery is possible. Therefore, treatment (CPR) must be instituted immedately in all cases, and resuscitation must be continued regardless of the time required. Only when the victim remains unresponsive after 1 to 2 hr of continuous CPR and when he or she has a body temperature exceeding 30°C should cerebral death be diagnosed and treatment discontinued.

Circulatory arrest represents the "great divide" separating those patients with a potentially better chance of recovery from those with an exponentially diminishing chance in spite of hypothermia. If cardiorespiratory arrest has *not* occurred, then the chances of complete recovery are much improved. Rewarming the patient to correct the total metabolic effects of immersion hypothermia is urgently required. However, if the patient has suffered cardiac arrest or prolonged submersion, the effects on the brain of excessive fluid infusion with rapid rewarming may be disastrous. In this latter situation, treatment should follow the guidelines recommended for the treatment of comatose cases in category C, as outlined below. Core temperatures as low as 30°C are amenable to both treatment regimes and are consistent with full recovery. The best method of rewarming patients with immersion hypothermia remains controversial, and it must be determined by whatever means available.

In contrast to immersion hypothermia, submersion hypothermia is always associated with immediate asphyxia occurring simultaneously with acute hypothermia. The risk of death or brain damage is consequently much greater, and the maximum submersion time consistent with full recovery is correspondingly shorter. Nevertheless, the rate of cooling in the whole body is very rapid, especially in cold (less than 15°C) or very cold (less than 5°C) water (16). In addition to the relevant factors mentioned in the preceding discussion of immersion hypothermia, submersion increases the rate of heat loss by additional surface cooling from the head with its extensive blood flow (17) and by core cooling when associated with involuntary swallowing (18) or pulmonary aspiration.

In small children, the rate of cooling may be proportionately faster because of their relatively large surface area and reduced fatty insulation. In addition, the "diving reflex" is very active up to at least the age of 2 or 3 yr (17) and can maintain circulation for a prolonged period. The "diving reflex" is a circulatory reflex (19, 20) triggered neurologically by apnea and immersion of the face in cold water that shunts blood and available oxygen from the lungs to the heart and brain and is accompanied by severe bradycardia. This reflex can produce a minimal but vital perfusion for considerable time that permits acute hypothermia to develop and delays permanent organ and tissue damage.

Involuntary aspiration of cold fresh water in the late stages of drowning can be compared to an intravenous injection with direct delivery to the heart and brain (21). In recent studies at the Anesthesia Laboratories at the University of Texas, San Antonio, the author noted a falling brain temperature rate of up to 1°C per minute during agonal respirations of drowning animals submerged in fresh water (20°C to 22°C). Asystole may have occurred just prior to the recovery of the victim and so, regardless of the clinical condition, treatment must be started at the time of rescue and continued during transportation to the hospital. Unfortunately, the risk of residual brain damage in children is much higher than in adults because a healthy child's heart can be restarted after a much longer asystolic period than that of most adults (22).

Near-Drowning

Near-drowning victims survive for at least 24 hr after a drowning episode, but a relationship between submersion hypothermia and near-drowning with intact recovery is difficult to verify. Five different groups of independent variables have been described that may affect cerebral recovery (23). These factors include physiological features: age, sex, "diving reflex," activity, oxygen content at submersion, resistance to asphyxia, et cetera; immersion hypothermia: time of onset, level, duration, independent organ cooling, et cetera; submersion time (often unknown and impossible to estimate when repeated surfacing and sinking occurred); initial cardiopulmonary resuscitation (CPR): efficiency and unbroken continuation, uncertain, especially with untrained personnel; and critical care (prompt in-hospital application of an aggressive cerebral resuscitation program shown to be significantly effective [24] but not always possible). It is apparent that for any given drowning case most of these factors are uncontrolled and uncontrollable, but they play a major role in the patient's subsequent course. Therefore, at the time of rescue, it is important to assume that full recovery is possible even when the situation is apparently hopeless and to treat the patient aggressively until the clinical course becomes obvious. This philosophy is the result of practical experience derived from the authors' study of 125 children who had suffered a submersion accident and were seen at the Hospital for Sick Children in Toronto from 1970 to August 1981.

Management in the Intensive Care Unit

After the rescue, successful cardiopulmonary resuscitation, and hospital admission of the near-drowning victim, the clinician often faces an acute dilemma over the patient's future management (24). The selection of appropriate treatment can be very difficult when, for example, the duration of submersion is uncertain (unknown, erroneous, or contradictory) and the asphyxial effects of a submersion time of 20 sec versus 20 min are contrasted. Since complete cerebral recovery is of paramount importance and requires neurological priorities in treatment, the most appropriate therapeutic guide is based on the patient's level of consciousness. A simple neurological classification was devised by Dr. J. Modell and his colleagues (24, 25); it consists of three main categories—A (awake), B (blunted), C (comatose)—with some modifications (Table 13-3). The patient's category is determined by his or her state of consciousness within approximately 60 min after rescue or upon reaching a hospital emergency room. Cerebral resuscitation measures are unnecessary in categories A and B and must be restricted to those patients in category C (comatose).

The rationale (24) for aggressive therapy to improve cerebral salvage is as follows. Any acute brain injury, including asphyxia from near-drowning, causes abolition of neuronal function, edema, vasomotor

Table 13-3
A "Triage" Neurological Classification of Near-Drowning Victims
(Assessed within 1 Hour after Rescue)

Category	Description
A (awake)	Alert, fully conscious
B (blunted)	Obtunded, stuporous but rousable; purposeful response to pain; normal respirations
C (comatose)	Comatose, not rousable; abnormal response to pain; abnormal respirations
C subcategories (comatose)	
C 1	Flexion response to pain, Cheyne-Stokes respiration (decorticate)
C 2	Extensor response to pain, central (?) hyperventilation (decerebrate)
C 3	No response to pain, apneustic or "cluster" breathing (flaccid)
C 4	Flaccid, apneic, no detectable circulation (deceased)

paralysis, hyperemia, and tissue acidosis (26). It is now believed that neurons that have survived the primary brain insult and could recover often die secondarily from the effects of raised intracranial pressure as a result of acute brain swelling. Therapeutic measures are primarily directed at the control of intracranial pressure, but a direct neuronal effect by hypothermia and barbiturate coma is possible. The onset of contracranial hypertension is variable in time, but the more severe the injury, the earlier the onset. The lethal effects on the brain of a continuously high intracranial pressure are too well known to require further comment (27). In instances of severe asphyxia, this process is predictable, often preventable, and usually controllable. Since a damaged brain is extremely susceptible to hypoxia, and pulmonary edema with hypoxemia is usually present, this complication must also be rigorously controlled. It should be assumed that the brain injury is reversible, and aggressive therapeutic measures should be initiated.

HYPER Therapy

The authors' therapeutic regimen has been given the acronym HYPER (28) on the basis of the common clinical state of the deeply comatose near-drowned patient following successful CPR (i.e., these patients are hyper*h*ydrated and hyper*v*entilated with hyper*p*rexia, hyper*e*xcitability, and hyper*r*igidity). These five factors dictate corresponding measures for critical cerebral care and may be considered therapeutic "overkill," but they seem justified by the authors' results.

Aggressive therapeutic measures (HYPER) for neurological purposes are summarized as follows: mild dehydration, controlled hyperventilation, induced moderate hypothermia, and induced barbiturate coma and skeletal muscular paralysis for up to 4 d continuously. Details of this protocol have been reported elsewhere (12, 23, 24). Possible complications of induced chronic hypothermia (moderate) such as neutropenia and immune suppression are currently under investigation.

The introduction of single or sequential methods of treatment is not currently recommended, since all measures to achieve these goals should be implemented and must take priority over the treatment of other body systems. The twin goals of cerebral salvage are preserving those neurons that are viable but nonfunctioning and preventing a significant rise in intracranial pressure.

The results of cerebral salvage efforts following neurological classification and comparing routine and aggressive therapy were reported in a recent retrospective review of 96 patients (24). It is important to note that in that series cases were classified neurologically after their arrival in the intensive care unit (not in the emergency room) and results reported. All patients in categories A (51 cases) and B (6 cases) recovered completely after routine medical management.

In category C (39 comatose patients), there was an overall mortality of 33.3% and normal recovery in 43.6%. When the results of treatment were reviewed, two subcategories (C 1 and C 2) were combined for comparative purposes. The results in 14 cases receiving routine therapy revealed a mortality of 21.4%, a morbidity of 42.8%, and an intact survival rate of 35.7%. By comparison, 11 patients who received aggressive (HYPER) therapy had no mortality, a morbidity of 9.0%, and a significant 90.9% incidence of intact survival.

In the most severely asphyxiated group, subcategory C 3, there were 14 patients but only 4 survivors, with 1 patient in each treatment group surviving intact (14.2%) This group of C 3 cases had temperatures in the emergency room ranging from 36.4°C to 25°C, but there was no relationship of temperature to outcome (Table 13-4). During the decade 1970 through 1979 there were only 14 cases in subcategory C 3, but during the subsequent 18 months 24 additional cases were admitted. This change in the patient population resulted from more aggressive initial resuscitation and led to an expansion of the neurological classifications to include an additional subcategory C 4 (deceased?).

The practice of initially recording the temperature and neurological-category of the patient in the intensive care unit is unsatisfactory for some practical reasons. It is essential for uniformity and comparative

Table 13-4
Outcome of Patients in Category C3/C4 Related to Temperature
(as Measured in Emergency Room)

Level of Hypothermia (Temperature)	Number of Cases	Outcome of Cases		
		Dead	Damaged	Normal
Unknown	12	6	4	2
Normothermia (36°C)	2	1	0	1
Mild hypothermia (36°C-34°C)	7	3	2	2
Moderate Hypothermia (34°C-28°C)	10	5	2	3
Deep hypothermia (28°C-17°C)	7	5	0	2
Totals	38	20 (52.6%)	8 (21.1%)	10 (26.3%)

purposes that upon the arrival of the victim at the emergency room of the primary hospital the body temperature and neurological category are recorded instantly. Appropriate therapy should commence immediately and should produce significant changes in the patient's condition before the patient is examined in an intensive care unit. For example, major alterations in body temperature have been observed as a result of circulatory changes, therapeutic measures, and transport conditions. More important, improvement in the patient's neurological category is a frequent finding. In the authors' series of 125 cases, there were 38 cases diagnosed as C 3 category (in the emergency room) of whom 15 cases (39.5%) had improved by one or two subcategories by the time they arrived at the intensive care unit. These observations dictate that the first determination of the patients' neurological category must be made upon the arrival at the hospital's emergency room.

In this current updated report reviewing 125 cases, there were 38 cases in category C 3/C 4. From this group the most serious brain injury from prolonged submersion and a high incidence of deep hypothermia with possible recovery might be anticipated. The authors' findings (Table 13-4) show no direct relationship. However, as might be expected, these retrospective results are equivocal and inconclusive due to small numbers of patients, body temperatures reported at random, and measurement difficulties at low temperatures. Finally, at least 3 cases in this group died of pulmonary or other complications while developing sigificant neurological improvement. This matter is unlikely to be resolved by clinical studies, and controlled animal investigations are needed. Nevertheless, the value of aggressive resuscitation of patients in this severely asphyxiated group of near-drowning victims is evident.

Conclusions

It may be impossible to confirm clinically a relationship between submersion hypothermia and subsequent intact recovery. It is tantalizing to assume a causal relationship when studying some isolated reports of prolonged submersion with complete recovery (Table 13-5) in which all cases are associated with hypothermia. In 1968 Cahill stated, "Obviously, if the submersion has been over 15 minutes, little hope is warranted unless the temperature of the water was near freezing " (39). Numerous other cases have been reported in which submersion time could not be estimated but in which the victims were asystolic and in deep or profound hypothermia and still recovered fully. Nevertheless, such anecdotal evidence, surgical analogies, and hypothetical causes have not been confirmed by the authors' clinical series. Hypothermia is only one factor among many that affect the patient's course. Until further information is available, aggressive treatment of all comatose patients must be recommended, regardless of body temperature, as providing the best chance of recovery. When hypothermia is present at rescue, it may contribute to a successful outcome!

Table 13-5
Near-Drowning Cases Prolonged Submersion with Full Recovery

Authors	Sex	Age	Submersion Time	Body Temperature	Result
Derbyshire/ Clark (29)	M	26 mo	45 min	28°C	Normal (7 d)
Siebke and others (30)	M	5 yr	40 min	24°C	Normal (1.3 mo)
Nemiroff (31)	M	18 yr	38 min	(Waters <5°C)	Normal
Posthumus (32)	F	40 yr	40 min	(?)	Normal
Hunt (33)	M	5 yr	30 min	27°C	Normal (3 mo)
Anderson (1978) (32)	M	6 yr	25 min	30.4°C	Normal (24 d)
Kvittingen/Naess (34)	M	5 yr	22 min	24°C	Normal (6 mo)
Cooke (32)	F	24 yr	25 min	24.5°C	Normal (2 wk)
Imbach (32)	M	2 yr	20 min	<32.5°C (4 hr)	Normal (1 yr)
Green (35)	F	3½ yr	20 min	34°C	Normal
Conn (36)	M	22 mo	20 min	27.5°C	Normal (1 mo)
King Webster (38)	M	21 yr	17 min	32°C (4 hr)	Normal (1 mo)
Sluiter (37)	F	6 yr	16 min	(Water <5°)	Normal
Conn (36)	M	6 yr	15 min	35.7°C (2 hr)	Normal (1 mo)
Young (32)	M	7 yr	15 min	27°C	Normal (6 mo)

References

1. Virtve RW: Hypothermic Anesthesia. Springfield, Ill., Charles C. Thomas, 1955.
2. Questions and Answers: Proceedings of Cold Water Symposium, p. 43. Royal Life Saving Society of Canada, May 8, 1976.
3. Miller JW, Daniel DF, and Thomas DM: Urban accidental hypothermia: 135 cases. Ann Emerg Med *9*:456-461, 1980.
4. Hypothermia. Therapeutic Notes *10*:15, 1965.
5. Popovic V, Popovic P: Hypothermia in Biology and in Medicine. New York, Grune and Stratton, 1974.
6. MacLean D, Emslie-Smith D: Accidental Hypothermia. Oxford, Blackwell Scientific Publishing, 1977.
7. Conn, AW: Near-drowning and hypothermia (editorial). Can Med Assoc Jour *120*:397-400, 1979.
8. Clarke EB, Niggermann EH: Near-drowning. Heart Lungs, *4*:946-955, 1975.
9. Giammona ST: Drowning: Pathophysiology and management. Curr Prob Paediatr 7:1-33, 1971.
10. Shorter Oxford English Dictionary, 3rd ed. London, Oxford University Press, 1964.
11. Schuman SH, Rowe JR, Glazier HM, and Redding JS: The iceberg phenomenon of near-drowning. Soc Crit Care Med *4*:127, 1976.
12. Conn AW, Edmonds JF, and Barker GA: Cerebral resuscitation in near-drowning. Pediatr Clin N Amer *26*:691-703, 1979.
13. Keatinge WR: Survival in Cold Water. Oxford, Blackwell Scientific Publishing, 1969.
14. Keatinge WR: The concept of hypothermia. Proceedings of Cold Water Symposium, p. 16. Royal Life Saving Society of Canada, May 8, 1976.
15. Segarra F, Redding RA: Modern concepts about drowning. Can Med Assoc Jour *110*: 1057-1059, 1974.
16. Golden F St C, and Rivers JF: Thoughts on immediate care: The immersion incident. Anesthesia *30*: 364-373, 1975.
17. Hayward JS: Personal communication, 1981.
18. Banting FG, Hall GE, Janes JM, Leibel B, Lougheed DW: Phsyiological studies in experimental drowning. Can Med Assoc Jour *39*:226-228, 1938.
19. Hunt PK: Effect and treatment of the diving reflex; Can Med Assoc Jour *111*:1330-1331, 1974.
20. Editorial. Drowning and the diving reflex. Can Med Assoc Jour *108*:1209, 1973.
21. Kylstra JA: Lavage of the lung. Acta Physiol Pharmacol Neerl 7:163-221, 1958.
22. Modell JK: Personal communication, 1980.
23. Conn AW, Edmonds JF, Barker GA: Near-drowning in cold fresh water: Current treatment regimen. Can Anaes Soc Jour *25*:259-265, 1978.
24. Conn AW, Montes JE, Barker GA, Edmonds JF: Cerebral salvage in near-drowning: Following neurological classification by triage. Can Anaes Soc Jour *27*:201-210, 1980.
25. Modell JH, Graves SA, and Kuck EJ: Near-drowning: Correlation of level of consciousness and survival. Can Anaes Soc Jour *27*:211-215, 1980.
26. Alexander SC, and Lassen NA: Cerebral circulatory response to acute brain disease. Anesthesiology *32*:60-68, 1970.
27. Marsh ML, Marshall LF, and Shapiro HM: Neurosurgical intensive care. Anesthesia *47*: 149-163, 1977.
28. Conn AW: The role of hypothermia in near-drowning. Proceedings of the Cold Water Symposium, pp. 33-35. Royal Life Saving Society of Canada, May 8, 1976.

29. Derbyshire DR, and Clark RG: Cerebral recovery after prolonged global brain ischemia. Lancet *2*:637, 1980.
30. Siebke H, Rod T, Breivik H, Lind B: Survival after 40 mins submersion without cerebral sequelae. Lancet *1*:1275-1277, 1975.
31. Nemiroff: Personal communication, 1980.
32. Young RSK, Zalneraitis EL, Dooling EC: Neurological outcome in cold water drowning. Jour Amer Med Assoc *244*:1233-1235, 1980.
33. Hunt PK: Effect and treatment of the diving reflex. *111*:1330-1331, 1974.
34. Kvittingen TD, Naess A: Recovery from drowning in fresh water. Brit Med Jour *1*: 1315-1317, 1963.
35. Green J: The Daily Colonist, Victoria B.C., March 10, 1979.
36. Conn AW: Cases included in Hospital for Sick Children Series, May 1980.
37. Sluiter HJ: Survival after submersion. Lancet *2*:513, 1975.
38. King RB, Webster IW: A case of recovery from drowning and prolonged anoxia. Med Jour Aust June 13, 1964:919-920.
39. Cahill JM: Drowning: The problem of non-fatal submersion and the unconscious patient. Surg Clin N Amer *48*:423-430, 1968.

CHAPTER FOURTEEN

Clinical Management of Elderly Hypothermic Patients

Ian McA. Ledingham, M.D.

"Accidental hypothermia" is the term used to describe the pathophysiological state in which an unintentional reduction in central temperature to below 35°C has occurred (1). It is distinguished from hypothermia induced for the safer conduct of major cardiovascular surgery or for other therapeutic purposes. Accidental hypothermia may arise as a result of (a) exposure to adverse climatic conditions (2); (b) immersion in cold water (3, 4), and (c) drug ingestion, intercurrent illness, and impaired thermoregulation (5). The author's personal experience relates to a prospective study of patients presenting with accidental hypothermia in an urban environment. Particular reference is made in this chapter to the cardiorespiratory disturbances revealed during the course of the study and to the effect of an aggressive approach to treatment on the patient's outcome.

Mortality among elderly patients suffering from accidental hypothermia is high, from 40% to more than 80% (6). Although some advances have been made within the past decade, there is still no generally agreed-upon treatment policy (7). A number of key issues remain unresolved, including the optimum rate of rewarming, the requirement for intravenous fluids, the role of oxygen administration and positive-pressure ventilation, and the indications for drug therapy. The treatment program to be described owes its evolution to earlier laboratory studies of induced hypothermia modified in the light of experience with patients suffering from accidental hypothermia. The effect of treatment has been to eliminate mortality during the rewarming period. Overall mortality is also lower than that reported in a previously published series, and it is related to underlying precipitating factors or disease in the victims rather than to hypothermia.

During the period of the prospective study, a number of hypothermic patients were treated by others in the same institution along conventional (i.e., less aggressive) lines. This group of patients did not constitute a properly planned control group, but the opportunity was taken to determine their fate on a retrospective basis.

Materials and Methods

During the period from 1963 to 1978, 44 patients suffering from accidental hypothermia were referred from the medical units and the accident and emergency department of the Western Infirmary, Glasgow, Scotland. After 1968, the patients received their initial treatment in the intensive therapy unit.

Initial Assessment and Measurement

On admission, preliminary assessment was made of the patient's general condition. Arterial blood samples were withdrawn for measurements of sodium, potassium, chloride, calcium, urea, creatinine, amylase, glucose, and enzymes and osmolality, in addition to hemoglobin, hematocrit, white cell and platelet counts, and (on occasion) coagulation screen. Blood-gas analysis was performed through the use of standard electrodes at 37°C, and the usual convention of correcting for the difference in temperature between the electrodes and the patient was followed (8). A chest X ray and full-lead EKG were performed. Radial artery and central venous catheters were inserted for measurement of heart rate and systemic arterial and central venous blood pressures; thermocouples were placed in the rectum and on the great toe for measurement of central and peripheral temperatures; heart rate, arterial pressure, temperatures, and lead II of the EKG were continuously displayed on a bedside monitor. Respiratory rate and inspired oxygen concentration were recorded in spontaneously breathing patients and more detailed information in those being ventilated. Bladder catheterization permitted accurate measurement of urine output. No exhaustive investigation was carried out at this stage to uncover the cause of the hypothermia.

Occasionally, more sophisticated measurements were performed (including cardiac output, mixed venous pO_2 and pulmonary artery pressures) and were used in conjunction with the more routine measurements to calculate such derived data as systemic vascular resistance, pulmonary vascular resistance, oxygen consumption, intrapulmonary shunt, and alveolar/arterial pO_2 difference. A Swan-Ganz catheter (9, 10) passed via a peripheral vein into the pulmonary artery was used to make the primary measurements.

Standard Treatment

Rewarming was achieved in all but two of the patients by means of a radiant heat cradle applied over the torso (Figure 14-1); the skin of the torso was protected by a thin sheet. Active rewarming was discontinued at about 35°C in order to allow for the usual spontaneous further rise in temperature of 2°C to 3°C. The two patients not rewarmed by this method were treated with thoracotomy and mediastinal irrigation with warmed fluids. Intravenous fluids were administered in order to reduce hemoconcentration; to restore circulating blood volume; and to maintain arterial pressure, central venous pressure, and urine output at satisfactory levels. Any fluids thus administered were warmed before infusion. Oxygen was administered in order to maintain arterial pO_2 (corrected for temperature) within the normal range; indications for intermittent positive-pressure ventilation (IPPV) included (a) a combination of hypoxemia and arterial pCO_2 in excess of about 35 mm Hg (corrected for temperature), (b) evidence of deteriorating pulmonary gas exchange, (c) coma, and (d) cardiovascular instability. Throughout rewarming, careful observation was made of the cardiovascular and respiratory parameters outlined above, and appropriate action was instituted when required; biochemical and hematological disturbances were also detected early and remedied. No special consideration was given to the fact that the patient was hypothermic other than that hypotension was more frequently tolerated without recourse to pharmacological agents and arterial pCO_2 was maintained at levels below the normal range in patients being ventilated.

The patients were "followed up" for a period of a month after the episode of hypothermia. Postmortem examinations were performed on 9 of the 12 patients who died.

For the purpose of the retrospective study, the hospital coding system was utilized. A total of 89 patients appeared to fulfill the required diagnostic criterion. Adequate case records of 77 were recovered; from these a preliminary analysis was made.

Central Rewarming

A new method of rewarming hypothermic subjects has undergone laboratory investigation and has been used successfully in one patient

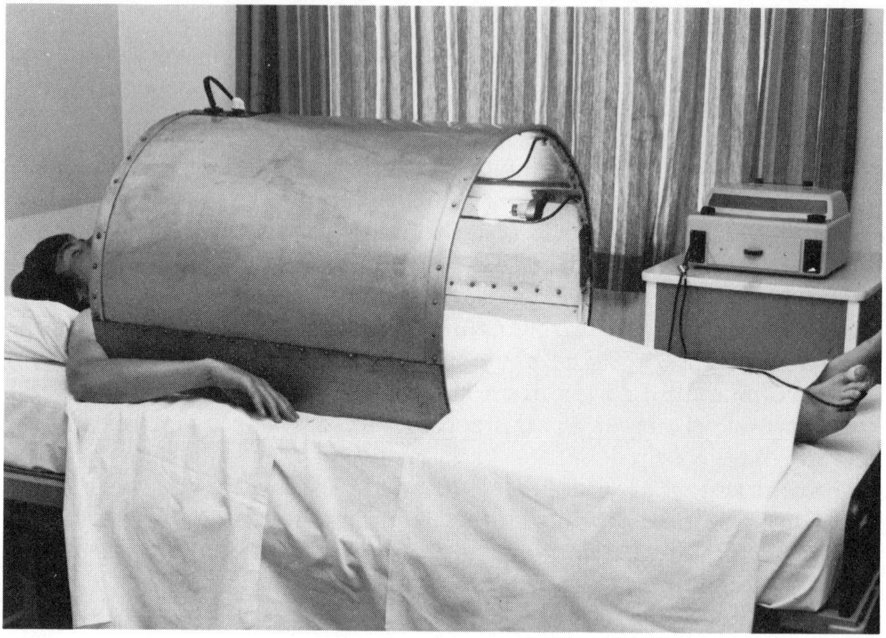

Figure 14-1. Heat cradle applied over torso, with limbs left unheated.

(11). The system consists of a modified Sengstaken tube through which Ringer's lactate solution is recirculated in the esophageal and gastric balloons at 41°C. In this way, the central organis are rewarmed before the peripheral tissues.

Eight greyhounds were anesthetized and ventilated with oxygen-enriched air in order to achieve normal blood-gas values. Central (rectal) and blood peripheral (skin) temperatures were monitored; the electrocardiagram (EKG) and arterial pressures were continuously displayed, and cardiac output was measured intermittently by a dye-dilution technique. The dogs were cooled in ice water until their final rectal temperature was below 25°C. Six dogs were rewarmed through the use of the modified tube (Figure 14-2), and a 100-W radiant heat bulb was used to provide surface heat over the chest. The remaining two dogs were rewarmed with surface heat alone.

Results

The mean age of the 44 patients was 60 ± 3 yr (mean ± standard error of the mean), and the majority were in their fifth to seventh

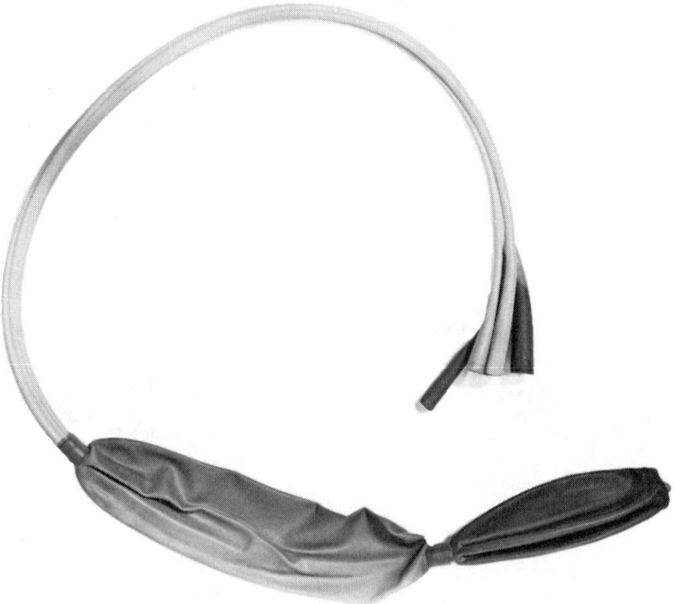

A

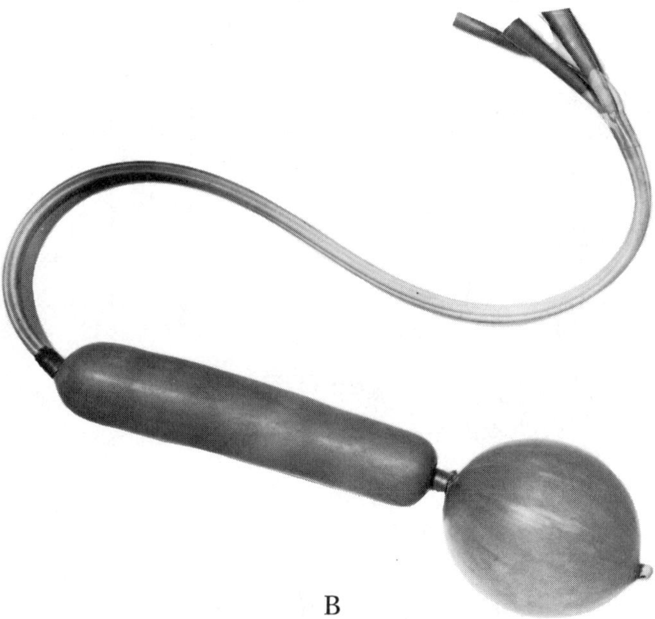

B

Figure 14-2. Central rewarming tube: (A) deflated for passage via esophagus and (B) with esophageal and gastric balloons filled with fluid.

decades of life. Of the 44 patients, 24 were female and 20 male. The most common months for admission were December and March. The lowest individual recorded core temperature ranged from 20.0°C to 34.3°C (Figure 14-3); all but 7 (84%) were below 32.2°C. The precipitating factors in the elderly patients' hypothermia are listed in Table 14-1; drugs appeared to be predominant in 57% of the patients. In the remainder, an assortment of acute and chronic medical ailments was found, with cardiovascular accidents and endocrine diseases being most common.

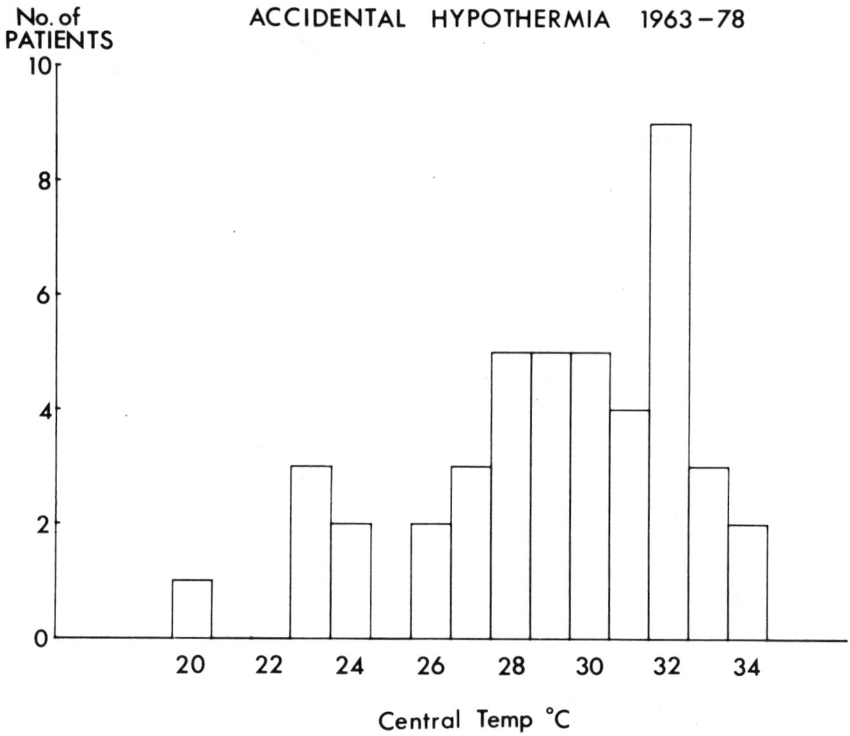

Figure 14-3. Lowest recorded core temperatures.

Cardiovascular and Respiratory Aspects

The patients' heart rates tended to be slower at lower temperatures, but the relationship was not as striking as might have been expected. There was no consistent relationship between arterial blood

Table 14-1
Precipitating Factors in Accidental Hypothermia

Factor	Number of Patients
Long-acting barbiturate poisoning	2 + NI, PH
Other barbiturate poisoning	8 + A, TRI
Other drug poisoning	8 (T/A, PH, M, F, TRY, D, T)
Alcohol poisoning	4 + P
Coal-Gas Poisoning	3
Total	25
Cardiovascular accident	4
Endocrine disease	4
Malnutrition/dehydration	3 + A
Malignancy	2
Myocardial infarction	1
Pneumonia	1
Old age	1
Injury	1
Skin disease	1
Mentally defective	1
Total	25

Abbreviations: A = alcohol; D = diazepam; F = fluphenazine; M = meprobamate; P = pentobarbitone; NI = nitrazepam; PH = phenothiazine; T = tryptazole; TRI = trichloral; TRY = tryptophan; + = additional drugs involved.

pressure and temperature, although in 10 of the early patients initial blood pressure on admission was found to be unrecordable. (Such incidents occurred before intraarterial pressure measurement became routine.) Of the 34 patients whose admission EKG record has been retained, almost 56% had dysrhythmias (Table 14-2); 2 of the 3 patients with ventricular fibrillation survived.

Of the 44 patients, 39% had obvious respiratory inadequacy on clinical examination; 9 were apneic and 8 were nearly apneic. On

Table 14-2
Prevalence of Dysrhythmias on Admission for Accidental Hypothermia

Dysrhythmia	Number of Cases
Total number of EKG recordings	34
Dysrhythmias	19
Sinus bradycardia (less than 60 beats per min)	9
Atrial fibrillation	7
Ventricular fibrillation	3

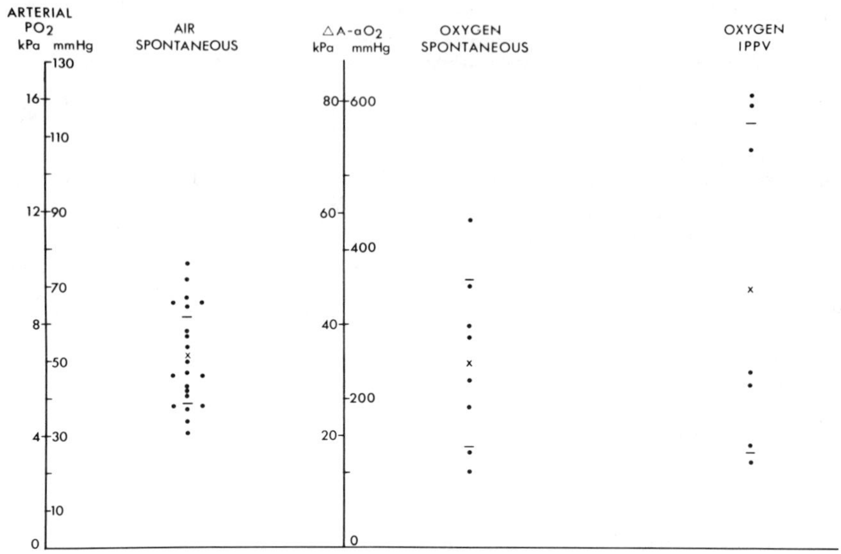

Figure 14-4. Arterial pO_2 in patients breathing (air) spontaneously, and alveolar-arterial pO_2 difference (Δ A - aO_2) in patients breathing (oxygen) spontaneously and receiving ventilation (IPPV) at lowest temperature; crosses indicate means and bars, standard deviation.

initial chest X ray, 12 of 30 patients (40%) had patchy opacification (usually bilateral), and 5 more (for a total of 57%) developed radiological changes during the ensuing days. Blood-gas analysis confirmed the frequency and severity of disturbances in pulmonary gas exchange. The majority of the patients in whom analyses were performed during spontaneous air breathing had arterial oxygen tension values of less than 55 mm HG (Figure 14-4), and in those breathing oxygen spontaneously or via a ventilator the mean aveolar/arterial oxygen tension differences were 250 and 350 mm Hg, respectively. Mean arterial carbon dioxide tension for the whole group was 32 mm Hg, which accounted for a normal arterial pH of 7.38 units in the presence of a mean base deficit of −9 mmol per liter.

The endocrine and metabolic disturbances observed among this group of patients with accidental hypothermia were similar to those that have been described by other investigators (12). The hemoglobin values of 20% of the patients were less than 10 mg per deciliter. Patients who were oliguric on admission amounted to 16%, but only one subsequently developed acute renal failure. There was a remarkably low incidence of peripheral vascular disturbance, and local cold injury was uncommon.

Treatment

No patient was adversely affected by any of the maneuvers instituted for the purposes of monitoring or treatment. Neither reflex cardiac slowing nor induced arrhythmia was observed.

Rewarming was achieved at a mean rate (± standard error of mean) of 1.13°C ± 0.09°C per hour, and the mean duration of rewarming was 8.03 ± 0.85 hr. The course of an uneventful rewarming procedure is illustrated in Figure 14-5; The patient breathed spontaneously throughout. Most patients received some intravenous fluids during the rewarming period, and the mean volume infused was 2.1 ± 0.2 L (Table 14-3). Dextrose (5%) and saline were the fluids most frequently used, but on occasion plasma and blood were given; potassium was administered as indicated by sequential biochemical analyses; calcium was not usually given. Oxygen (in high concentration) was administered to all but four of the patients, and mechanical ventilation was instituted in 48% of the cases. At the end of rewarming, the standard criteria for weaning a patient from the ventilator were observed, and adequate spontaneous ventilation was usually achieved without difficulty.

The most troublesome problem during rewarming was hypotension, which caused alarm in 14 of the 44 patients (32%). Of these 14 patients, 7 received drugs aimed at increasing the blood pressure and thereby improving perfusion to the vital organs. Of the 14, 4 were given vasoconstrictors; of these, 1 appeared to respond well, another had a variable response, and 2 showed no response. Three of the patients received drugs with a major inotropic action on the heart; all responded well, and the improvement in the urine output was marked in the 2 patients given dopamine. One patient was given the alpha-adrenergic blocking agent thymoaximine because of persistent

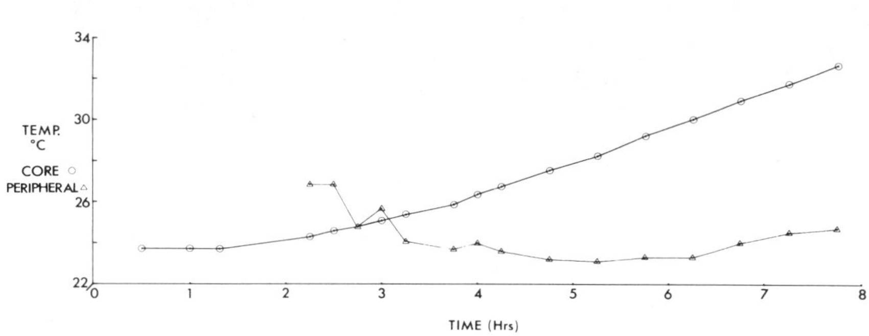

Figure 14-5. Core and peripheral temperature changes in response to heat cradle in a 48-y-old male suffering from barbiturate and alcohol overdose (lowest core temperature 23.6°C)

Table 14-3
Summary of Treatment for Accidental Hypothermia

Factor		Number of Cases		
Total number of patients		44		
Active rewarming		44		
Oxygen (mean maximum concentration		40		(65%)
IPPV/warm air humidifier		21		
IV fluids (liters)		41		(2.1 ± 0.2)
Antibiotics		24		
Steroids		7		
Vasoactive agents	metaraminol	4	8	
	dopamine	2		
	isoprenaline	1		
	thymoxamine	1		

vasoconstriction toward the end of rewarming; and a moderate response was noted.

Steroids had been administered on 7 patients on occasions prior to their referral, but only small doses had been given and their effect was impossible to judge. Antibiotics were not administered on a prophylactic basis, but 24 patients (55%) received a variety of antibiotics when infection of clinical significance (usually of respiratory origin) was confirmed from bacteriological examinations.

The data relating to the mortality rates of patients in the two studies are presented in Table 14-4. In the prospective study, the overall motality rate was 27%. Only 2 patients died during rewarming, and both deaths occurred during the early years of the study period, one from premature discontinuation of mechanical ventilation and the other from premature discontinuation of mechanical ventilation and the other from inadequate fluid replacement. The other 10 patients died after regaining normal body temperature (3 to 19 d), usually from cardiovascular accidents or causes unrelated to the hypothermia.

Analysis of the data from the retrospective study revealed that the mean age of the patients was slightly higher than that of the

Table 14-4
Mortality in Cases of Accidental Hypothermia

Mortality	Prospective Study	Retrospective Study
Total number of patients	44	77
Mortality		
During rewarming	2 (5%)	36 (47%)
Overall	12 (27%)	46 (60%)

prospective study, but there was no significant difference in the mean central temperature. Of the 77 patients, 19 (25%) were hypothermic as a result of drug abuse, the remainder having some serious underlying illness or no obvious cause for the hypothermia. The overall mortality was 60%, the majority of patients (78%) dying during the first three days following admission.

Central Rewarming

The pattern of rewarming consistently observed in the actively rewarmed group of animals is illustrated for one animal (Figure 14-6). The main features are these. During the first hour of rewarming, the blood temperature rose from 21.6°C ± 0.2°C (mean ± standard error) to 2.5°C ± 0.3°C. During the same period, central temperature rose by 2.2°C ± 0.4°C, while peripheral temperature rose by 1.2°C ± 0.3°C. Thereafter, central temperature continued to rise more rapidly than peripheral temperature (3.1°C ± 0.3°C per hour and 2.1°C ± 0.2°C per hour, respectively).

Transient cardiac arrhythmias were observed during hypothermia in several dogs, although none was attributable to the passage of the tube. During rewarming, these arrhythmias disappeared.

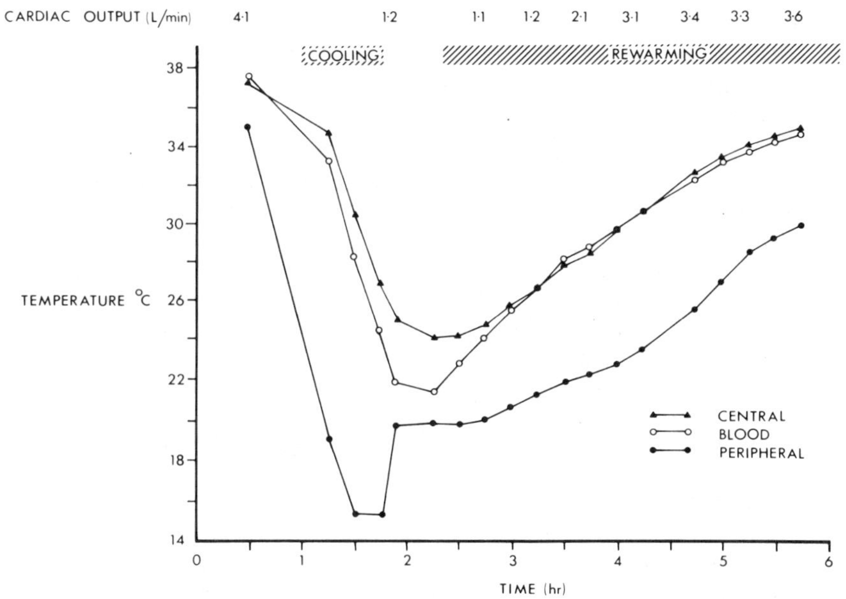

Figure 14-6. Changes in rectal, blood, and skin temperatures during the cooling and rewarming phases in one of the centrally rewarmed animals.

In the animals not centrally rewarmed, temperature failed to rise throughout the 4 hr of study, and cardiac output remained at hypothermic levels (circa 1 L per minute).

Clinical Case Report: A 63-year-old woman was admitted deeply unconscious, areflexic, and with no localizing neurological signs. There was a history of recent heavy drinking and evidence of a head injury. The patient was hypotensive (blood pressure 90/60 mm Hg) with sinus rhythm (100 beats per minute). Rectal temperature was 29.5°C. The blood alcohol level was 280 mg%.

Shortly after admission, spontaneous ventilation ceased. Although progressive brain damage was probable, brain death could not be confirmed in the presence of hypothermia and alcohol intoxication. Resuscitation therefore was instituted, and conservative passive surface rewarming was started.

Twelve hours after admission, the central temperature had risen to only 31°C. Active central rewarming by the method described above was instituted. The rewarming tube was passed into the stomach, and the balloons were filled with Ringer's lactate solution. No EKG or other cardiovascular disturbance was observed throughout this maneuver.

Rewarming to normothermia was completed in 6 hr at a rate of 1.0°C to 1.3°C per hour. Since another blood-alcohol measurement was negative at that time, all the criteria for the validity of brain-death testing were fulfilled; no brain-stem activity was demonstrable. Spontaneous hypothermia ensued as soon as central rewarming was discontinued, and asystole occurred 10 hr later, when the core temperature had fallen to 33°C.

Postmortem examination confirmed severe, irreversible brain damage. There was no evidence of mucosal damage to the esophagus or stomach.

Discussion

Cardiovascular and Respiratory Aspects

The cardiovascular and respiratory abnormalities in patients suffering from accidental hypothermia derive from a number of factors, including the past medical history, the precipitating cause, the circumstances of the hypothermic episode, and the effects of reduced body temperature. The relative contribution of each clearly influences the condition of the patient on admission to hospital and his or her subsequent response to resuscitation.

The cardiovascular effects of hypothermia in this study were similar to those previously reported. Systemic arterial blood pressure tends to fall, principally because of a decrease in cardiac output; systemic vascular resistance increases as a consequence of vasoconstriction and increased blood viscosity. The fall in cardiac output is attributed mainly to a decrease in heart rate (13); changes in stroke volume occur later, when venous return is reduced. Cardiac work and myocardial oxygen consumption decrease progressively with temperature, but the relative magnitude of these changes varies such that the effects on cardiac efficiency are difficult to predict. Myocardial blood flow is reduced in response to a reduction in body temperature, although in the normal heart oxygen availability to the cooled myocardium is generally believed to be adequate for metabolic requirements. It is unlikely that the same assertion can be made in the presence of coronary artery disease or when the duration of hypothermia is prolonged but detailed information is lacking. The EKG changes of hypothermia have been detailed before (14, 15), and the present study confirmed the usual uniform and progressive depression of myocardial conductivity with an increased frequency of dysrhythmias below 32°C.

McNicol and Smith (16) were among the first to draw attention to the frequency of hypoxemia among patients suffering from accidental hypothermia, and they believed that "anoxia was related to the high mortality" associated with this condition. They considered the possibility of "cold injury" to the lungs as a cause of the increased alveolar/arterial oxygen tension gradients found in all of their patients. In a later study made by Hedley-White and his colleagues (17) on patients subjected to induced hypothermia, however, no evidence for such a mechanism could be demonstrated. It is probable that hypothermia's only effect on the lungs per se is bronchodilatation. Neither carbon dioxide excretion nor oxygen uptake is impaired, and pulmonary mechanics are not destroyed. The main explanation for hypoxemia of accidental hypothermia is a reduction in ventilation and a depression of coughing predisposing to collapse of alveolar units and larger segments of the lungs. Acidosis and infection may accelerate deterioration in lung function.

It may reasonably be concluded from this study that, although the oxygen supply may be adequate at low temperatures for *normal* tissue requirements, the presence of preexisting disease (or other factors) may adversely affect the oxygen balance in patients with accidental hypothermia. Coronary artery disease, pulmonary disturbances, and anemia may reduce oxygen transport critically and lead to a fatal outcome—if not while the patient is hypothermic, then during subsequent rewarming when the oxygen demand increases. Greater awareness of the importance of these observations during recent years has led to a reappraisal of the methods of resuscitation used on hypothermic patients.

Treatment

The value of different forms of treatment of accidental hypothermia can be assessed in relation to the time and the circumstances of the deaths of the nonsurvivors. After using conservative ward management, MacLean and Emslie-Smith (12) reported that in their series of 100 consecutive patients 41 died while still hypothermic. Others have reported similar experiences. Since restoration of normal body temperature through the use of this technique may take 24 hr or considerably longer when there are cardiorespiratory complications, it can be assumed that the majority of the patients in the present retrospective study also died during rewarming; hypothermia per se, therefore, cannot be excluded as a significant cause of death in these patients. Indeed, it is notoriously difficult to make unequivocal diagnoses (particularly of cardiovascular, respiratory, and neurological conditions) in the presence of hypothermia.

By contrast, in the prospective study, of the patients who died, all but two failed to return to normal body temperature and most of the deaths occurred some time after rewarming from causes that were readily explained on other grounds. It was not, of course, possible to exclude hypothermia as a contributing factor in the early acute cardiovascular deaths, since vascular occlusions are believed to be a common postmortem finding in hypothermia (18). It can be concluded, however, that the treatment program that evolved at the Western Infirmary in Glasgow has effectively eliminated deaths that are directly attributable to hypothermia and by decreasing the duration of recovery has probably reduced the number of deaths indirectly attributable to this cause as well.

One of the more controversial aspects of the treatment of accidental hypothermia concerns the rate and technique of rewarming. Rapid external rewarming has been used largely although by no means exclusively for younger patients suffering from hypothermia of relatively brief duration, and rapid internal rewarming has usually been reserved for patients with profound hypothermia whose resuscitation by simpler methods proved to be difficult or impossible. Rapid external rewarming, particularly in the elderly, fell into some disrepute after early reports of sudden deaths associated with the use of this technique

(5). The deaths were attributed to rapid release of intense vasoconstrictor tone resulting in hypotension and circulatory failure. Since then, with few exceptions, those concerned with the management of urban hypothermic patients have opted for the method known as passive external rewarming, which consists of nursing the patient in an ambient temperature of 25°C to 32°C (12).

Comparison of the results of rapid and slow rewarming is a largely unrewarding exercise, since no clinical study has been designed to examine the two techniques while other factors in treatment were kept constant. The fact that no clear-cut difference in efficacy between the two techniques has yet emerged therefore is not surprising. What is clearer is that before about 1970, and apparently for good reason, the general approach to treatment was conservative, with passive rewarming and minimal disturbance of the patient in order to lessen the risk of arrhythmia. During the past few years, a more aggressive attitude has begun to emerge as our understanding of the underlying pathophysiological mechanisms of hypothermia has increased. The conservative approach tends to be adopted in general medical wards; the aggressive approach, with continuous and often invasive monitoring and treatment techniques, is more frequently practiced in intensive therapy units.

Several facts have emerged from the newer aggressive approach to treatment. Perhaps the most obvious from the present prospective study is that invasive monitoring and treatment maneuvers are not in themselves harmful. It appears that, in cases in which ventricular fibrillation was precipitated by these maneuvers in past studies, factors other than hypothermia per se were responsible (e.g., hypoxia, hypotension, or acidosis). The awkward or sudden movement of a hypothermic patient may cause cardiac arrest or cerebral hypoxia (19), but the same may be true when any critically ill patient is moved in this fashion. Clearly, the frequency of such movements is lessened during a shorter period of rewarming.

The frequency of dehydration and hypoxemia among hypothermic patients has become increasingly appreciated during recent years, and it is not surprising that obvious benefit has derived from the careful, controlled administration of intravenous fluids together with oxygen by mask or, if necessary, via a mechanical ventilator. The present study has shown that high concentrations of oxygen are often required to restore normal oxygenation. Mechanical ventilation was considered to be justified as an aid to oxygenation in half the patients, most frequently in those with drug-induced hypothermia. In the critically ill patient, the use of mechanical ventilation reduces immediate anxiety about poor lung function and allows more concentration on the potentially life-threatening cardiovascular disturbances.

The interaction between drugs and hypothermia is complex and variable (20). For this reason, it has seemed appropriate to restrict the use of all drugs during the rewarming phase. Adoption of such a policy in the present study has not been regretted, although on occasions the use of vasoactive agents has seemed warranted. In the latter context, two points are worthy of note. The first is that low blood pressure in the hypothermic patient may be more apparent than real; this observation has been confirmed with the more frequent use of intravascular pressure monitoring. The second is that hypotension usually responds to fluid infusion and may only require pharmacological support when there is associated evidence of organ or tissue hypoperfusion.

It is clear from the prospective study that patients suffering from accidental hypothermia can ben consistently and safely rewarmed to normal body temperature irrespective of the cause of hypothermia. Normothermia can be achieved as rapidly as is compatible with adequate tissue perfusion and oxygenation. Surface rewarming of the torso is perhaps the simplest technique available at present, but more efficient and noninvasive methods need to be developed. The increasingly widespread application of these principles should reduce the mortality directly attributable to hypothermia.

Central Rewarming

Although a similar technique was suggested by Khalil and MacKeith in 1954 (21), its successful use in treating hypothermia has not been described previously. The author's studies suggest that the technique is safe and effective, with no adverse cardiovascular effects. A rapid increase in central temperature to above 28°C reduces the risk of sudden ventricular fibrillation and leads to early improvement in myocardial performance. The peripheral temperature rise lags behind, thus avoiding hypotension due to vasodilatation commonly seen with surface-rewarming techniques.

This new technique will probably have most use for patients with central temperatures below 32°C. Active surface rewarming (22) is a suitable method for patients with temperatures between 32°C and 35°C, and heat exchange using cardiopulmonary bypass offers the best chance of survival for patients with ventriuclar fibrillation.

References

1. BMA Special Committee: Accidental hypothermia in the elderly. Brit Med Jour *2*: 1255-1258, 1964.
2. Pugh LGCE: Accidental hypothermia in walkers, climbers, and campers: Report to the Medical Commission on Accident Prevention. Brit Med Jour *1*:123-129, 1966.
3. Keatinge WR: Survival in Cold Weather. Oxford, Blackwell, 1969.
4. Golden F St C: Recognition and treatment of immersion hypothermia. Proc Roy Soc Med *66*:1058-1061, 1973.
5. Duguid H, Simpson RG, and Stowers JM: Accidental hypothermia. Lancet *2*:1213-1219, 1961.
6. Mills GL: Accidental hypothermia in the elderly. Brit Jour Hosp Med *2*:691-699, 1973.
7. Gregory RT, and Doolittle WH: Accidental hypothermia: Part II. Clinical implications of experimental studies. Alaska Med *15*:48-52, 1973.
8. Severinghaus JW: Blood gas calculator. Jour Appl Physiol *21*:1108-1116, 1966.
9. Swan HJC, Ganz W, Forrester J, Marius H, Diamond G, and Chonette D: Cardiac catheterization with a flow-directed balloon tipped catheter. N Engl Jour Med *283*: 447-451, 1970.
10. Swan-Ganz catheters. Lancet *2*:357-358, 1978.
11. Ledingham I. McA, Routh GS, Douglas IHS, and MacDonald AM: Central rewarming system for treatment of hypothermia. Lancet *1*:1168-1169, 1980.
12. MacLean D, and Emslie-Smith D: Accidental Hypothermia. Oxford, Blackwell, 1977.
13. Bigelow WG, Lindsay WK, and Greenwood WF: Hypothermia: Its possible role in cardiac surgery; an investigation of factors governing survival in dogs at low body temperatures. Ann Surg *132*:849-866, 1950.
14. Hook WE, and Stormont RT: Effect of lowered body temperature on heart rate, blood pressure and electrocardiogram. Amer Jour Physiol *133*:334-335, 1941.
15. Emslie-Smith D, Sladden GE, and Stirling GR: The significance of changes in electrocardiogram in hypothermia. Brit Heart Jour *21*:343-351, 1959.
16. McNicol MW, and Smith R: Accidental hypothermia. Brit Med Jour *1*:19-21, 1964.
17. Hedley-White J, Pontoppidan H, Laver MB, Hallowell P, and Bendixon HH: Arterial oxygenation during hypothermia. Anesthesiology *26*:595-602, 1965.
18. Mant AK: The post-mortem diagnosis of hypothermia. Brit Jour Hosp Med *2*:1095-1098, 1969.
19. Freeman J, and Pugh LGCE: Hypothermia in mountain accidents. Inter Anes Clin 7: 997-1007, 1969.
20. Blair E: Generalized hypothermia. Fed Proc *28*:1456-1462, 1969.
21. Khalil HH, and MacKeith RC: A simple method of raising and lowering body temperature. Brit Med Jour *2*:734-736, 1954.
22. Ledingham I McA, and Mone JG: Treatment of accidental hypothermia: A prospective clinical study. Brit Med Jour *208*:1102-1105, 1980.

CHAPTER FIFTEEN

Accidental Hypothermia

William J. Mills, Jr., M.D.

Accidental hypothermia is a year-round hazard in the state of Alaska. The Arctic Ocean on the north and the Bering Sea and the Gulf of Alaska on the west and south constitute potential sources of heat-stealing water for downward aircraft passengers and shipwreck victims. Heat transfer is immediate in cold water unless the victims are protected by immersion suits, clothing that has catapulted the longevity of victims of accidents at sea from a few hours or less to 5 or more days.

The temperature on Alaska's mountain slopes above the 6,000-ft level is in the arctic range during the whole year. The dangers of hypothermia there are increased by the possibility of high-altitude hypoxia and by severe winds. The hazards of snowfields, mountain crevasses, and avalanches await the unwary and the foolhardy.

During the winter months, cold temperatures await the dog musher whose team runs off and leaves him or her stranded in the wilderness and the snow-machine traveler whose vehicle breaks down miles from the road. In the towns and villages, insidious slow loss of heat brings a hypothermic state to the victim of accident, drug abuse, alcoholic stupor, or assault. Such victims are found in the vacant lots, alleys, and byways. The number of hypothermia victims are not yet counted officially on a yearly basis in Alaska, but official records and newspaper reports in the state indicate that, for whatever cause, more victims of exposure are discovered dead beneath the snow than are discovered soon after injury and brought to hospitals for resuscitation and treatment.

Management by Total Physiological Control

Recently, a department of high altitude to be established at the University of Alaska, Anchorage, was funded by the legislature. Its concern is with all the medical problems of the Far North, particularly the problems of freezing injury, hypothermia, immersion injury, drowning, and high-altitude illness. Plans are being made to review the numerous case histories of generalized hypothermia and freezing and nonfreezing injuries throughout the state in the federal and civilian hospital system. A segment of that study, 66 case histories, has been reviewd for this report. The time covered is from 1956 through 1981. The patients' age range is from 24 hr to 90 yr. The geographical area covered is from Point Barrow to Ketchikan, from Fairbanks to Kodiak, and from Kotzebue through Nome and Bethel to Anchorage.

Accidental hypothermia generally is associated with a core temperature of 34.4°C (94°F) or lower. Since most clinical thermometers register no lower than 34.4°C, this level of body temperature has been charted in patient records as the temperature of many Alaskan victims of cold (12), even when they have presented as cold, cyanotic, and lifeless. Even more interesting is the fact that the obvious signs of developing hypothermia (i.e., numbness, fatigue, dyscoordination and stumbling, and dysarthria) are found to be present at or near the temperature of 34.4°C. In this sense then, the choice of 34.4°C is logical (12).

The Glossary Committee of the International Union of Physiological Sciences (14) has defined "hypothermia" as the condition of a temperature-regulating animal in which the core temperature is more than one standard deviation below the main core temperature of the species in resting conditions in a thermoneutral environment. The chairman of this committee stated that his interpretation of the definition indicates that the level of hypothermia for a human would be in the neighborhood of 35°C (96°F).

The loss of heat may be rapid as in cold-water immersion, or insidious as in alcoholic stupor, or even more gradual as in wandering through the wilderness. The victim lost in the wilderness is usually fatigued, without food, and generally dehydrated.

Not all hospitals in Alaska use low-reading thermometers. In addition, because geographical isolation and unpredictable weather are not unusual, some victims of deep hypothermia cannot be safely transported to larger hospitals for care, even if that were desirable. In some areas, it is necessary that the rescue, the rescue care, the diagnosis and immediate emergency care and resuscitation, and the postcare warming all be handled at or near the site where the victim was discovered, regardless of the sophistication of the rescue unit and hospital.

Not uncommonly a call from an outlying area reports that a patient has just arrived in the receiving unit, said to be cold, cyanotic, pulseless, and without heart sounds. The victim demonstrates no respiratory movements and is apprarently lifeless. Often, the extremities are reported to be "frozen"; sometimes all four extremities are truly frozen, occasionally even beyond the wrist and ankle level. The patient's rectal temperature is usually reported to be 34.4°C, the lowest reading on most rectal thermometers. This description fits a hypothermic victim's temperature level of 18.3°C to 24°C (65°F to 75°F), even allowing for the likelihood of changes secondary to drug abuse, alcohol intoxication, head injury, or other trauma, rather than a level of 34.4°C.

Confronted with such a history or presented with a patient at a rescue site or in an emergency room who has an actual core temperature of 21°C to 23.8°C (70°F to 75°F), what should medical personnel do? Many find this event catastrophic. The patient is apparently lifleless, the methods of rewarming are numerous, the pitfalls are many, and there are disagreements and controversy among authorities regarding management. Generally, the first responder or initial physician is a lone practitioner in an isolated area. Occasionally, the rescue dilemma can be solved by helicopter evacuation or aircraft transport to a regional hospital where emergency and intensive care units are available.

Almost immediately one element of controversy is apparent either in the field or in the emergency unit, namely, should or should not cardiopulmonary resuscitation be instituted. Some authorities on hypothermia have recently challenged the use of CPR in hypothermia at low levels of temperature.

There is no fault to be found with mouth-to-mouth resuscitation or the use of airways or warm, moist inspired air to prevent further heat loss (3, 11). But if trauma, rough handling, bouncing about in the rescue sled, and rattling stretchers do often precipitate ventricular fibrillation (10) (as most agree that they do), how can thoracic thrusts and rib-rattling compression with or without fracture in a patient with a cold, unresponsive heart be defended?

Also, the use of CPR, which has without question saved thousands of arrest victims, was designed for sudden arrest in a normothermic patient. The cold heart, perhaps in asystole, is unable to respond to cardiac compression or defibrillation until warmed. Some authorities feel that cardiac compression should be reserved for the heart still arrested or in a state of ventricular fibrillation at temperatures of 29.4°C (85°F) or higher and that attempts at cardioversion by electric defibrillation should be begun at 32.2°C (90°F).

This problem is under study at the University of Alaska's Institute of Arctic Biology and elsewhere in the United States. Numerous aspects of the resuscitation of a cold heart are under scrutiny, including the proper use of cardiopulmonary resuscitation in hypothermia cases.

Further information on the subject of hypothermia and the many methods of care and treatment for it can be found in several excellent papers in the literature (2, 4, 5, 6, 7, 8, 9, 13).

Other factors are important in the recovery of hypothermia victims. It is now known that the first consideration in treating hypothermia should be the assessment of the total patient, as in any emergency. The degree of hypothermia present is of prime concern. General body cooling and loss of heat with exhaustion of caloric reserve and severe depression of core temperature can lead to death. Homothermic control is unstable and is often lost at temperatures below 34.5°C (94°F). Continued cooling and unrelieved heat loss can result in coma and eventually in cardiorespiratory failure.

Many hospitals and rescue units do not have thermometers or temperature probes that read below 34.5°C (94°F). This lack of equipment often delays or prohibits proper diagnosis.

Most patients in a state of hypothermia are dehydrated and are often hypovalemic and demonstrate mild to severe acidosis. This was true of most of the 66 patients studied for whom such records of electrolytes and blood gases were available (12).

Many of the patients with atrial or ventricular arrhythmias (fibrillation) demonstrated prewarming acidosis and lowered pH levels. At least from the eight deaths reported it appeared that as the result of postwarming hyperkalemia some cases developed arrhythmias and heart block.

Observation of the arrival and subsequent management of the hypothermia victim in any emergency area reveals that—without a preplanned approach, without a standard but flexible protocol for care, and without a good leader—the result is chaos. The victim appears cold and lifeless, without respirations and with a heart that will not respond and pupils that are fixed and often dilated. The rescuer or physician may feel a need to "do something," to get the treatment moving. With a slow response to warming, drugs such as epinephrine have been injected into the cold heart; calcium chloride may be given intravenously; lidocaine bolus may be administered when arrhythmias are present; cardiopulmonary resuscitation may be utilized frequently and throughout; the ventilator may be applied; defibrillation procedures may be attempted with more injections of drugs through intravenous lines or into the heart itself and with various quantities of electrolytes of sodium, potassium, and chloride given as well. All these measures in a cold patient may yield little result since the drugs are not properly absorbed or effective. But, as rewarming continues and circulation improves, the accumulation of these drugs, given in desperation during the "cold period," suddenly takes effect, sometimes with disastrous results.

Such chaos can be controlled when a team is trained to work together with the smoothness and discipline of a race-car crew at a pit-stop at Indianapolis. All members of the team should be interested in hypothermia and familiar with the problem. In Anchorage, orthopedic surgeons, internists, and anesthesiologists have formed the hypothermia-treatment groups. Trained intensive care nurses, emergency physicians, and emergency room medical personnel provide the initial care.

From the review of the 66 records from Alaska, some interesting facts emerge. Of the cases with actual recorded temperatures (including 16 cases of temperature equal to 94°F), 14 had a core temperature from 66°F to 80°F; 7 of the 8 deaths that occurred were in this group. The other 52 patients had temperatures from 81°F to 97°F upon their admission; in this group only 1 death occurred. If the same 66 patient records were studied for comparisons with actual recorded temperatures as above and corrected estimated (94°F) temperatures (i.e., converting the reported 94°C temperature to match its clinical level), then 20 patients had core temperatures varying from 66°F to 80°F with 8 deaths in that group and 46 patients had core temperatures varying from 81°F to 97°F without a death.

Mortality increased in a direct linear fashion as the core temperature fell. The line of safety seems to level off at 81°F (27.2°C). The average temperature of those who died was 76.8°F (24.8°C). Moderate to severe freezing injury of the extremities effected 33 of the patients; of this group (Table 15-3) 6 (or 18%) died. Of the 66 patients, 12 had extremity-immersion injury; there were no deaths in this group. Of the 66 patients, 23 were drug or alcohol intoxicated; of this group 4 died. Therefore, 50% of the deaths were alcohol or drug related (Table 15-1).

Of the eight deaths, three occurred during uncontrolled management, two being the first patients treated in 1964 by me in Anchorage.

Table 15-1
Events Causing the Hypothermic State

Causal Event	Number
Alcoholic stupor	15
Psychotic episode	3
Drug abuse	4
Child abandonment in snow	2
Victim of assault while intoxicated	4
Victim of assault while not intoxicated	1
Attempted suicide	2
Vehicle accident	3
Aircraft accident on land	2
Aircraft accident in seawater	5
Found in home or cabin	2
Saltwater immersion including shipwreck	11
Freshwater immersion	4
Lost in blizzard or storm	3
Lost in wilderness	2
Mountain accident or avalanche	3
Total	66
Disrobing syndrome or paradoxical undressing	5

The death of one was sudden. Blood gases and electrolytes were not obtained in that case, but one EKG taken prior to death was flat line. The severity and depth of freezing injury present, with the deep

Table 15-2
Results by Method of Rewarming

Method of Rewarming	Number Treated	Result
Uncontrolled, spontaneous rewarming, K-thermia pad, warm blankets, dry heat	7	6 survived 1 died
Controlled spontaneous rewarming	21	21 survived 0 died
Uncontrolled rapid rewarming, warm-water water bath or whirlpool (external wet heat)	5	3 survived 2 died
Controlled rapid rewarming, warm-water bath or whirlpool (external wet heat 90°F to 106°F)	21	21 survived 0 died
Controlled peritoneal dialysis	9	4 survived 5 died
Total control in surgery, gradual rewarming with warm fluids (IV), and use of anesthetic breathing apparatus	3	3 survived 0 died
Total patients	66	58 survived (87.9%) 8 died (12.1%)

Table 15-3
Results of Mixed Insult, Hypothermia, and Extremity Freezing Injury

Method of Warming	Anatomical Function Result		Amputation		Died
	Good	Poor	Minor	Major	
Uncontrolled spontaneous rewarming, K-thermia pad, warm blankets, dry heat	—	—	—	3	—
Controlled spontaneous rewarming	2	—	2	—	—
Uncontrolled rapid rewarming, warm-water bath or whirlpool (external wet heat)	—	1	2	—	2
Controlled rapid rewarming, warm-water bath or whirlpool (external wet heat) (90°F to 106°F)	10	1	1	—	—
Controlled peritoneal dialysis	1	—	2	—	4
Total control in surgery, gradual rewarming with warm fluids (IV), and use of anesthetic breathing apparatus	—	—	2	—	—
Total (33 patients)	13	2	9	3	6

Note: Anatomical function result: good = no anatomical loss, useful range of motion of digits; poor = no amputation, intrinsic muscle loss, limited range of motion. Amputation: minor = amputation distal to M-P junction; major = amputation proximal to M-P junction.

hypothermia managed by uncontrolled rapid rewarming resulted in excess of potassium (hyperkalemia), and heart block, as the cause of death. In two other patients, tourniquets had been applied to the extremities in order to keep "cold blood" from striking the core until the core itself had been properly rewarmed. The release of the tourniquets resulted in sudden death, presumably as a result of potassium overload. Two other patients demonstrated sudden death after the thawing of massive freezing injury to all four extremities without total physiological control (Table 15-3). Thus, in five patients it is likely that the sudden release of potassium from seriously ischemia- and anoxic-damaged celluluar compartments in the extremities caused death. In two other patients, tourniquets had been applied to the extremities in order to keep "cold blood" from stiking the core until the sium, is of vital importance.

The combination of problems from trauma, alcohol abuse, drug overdose, and severe frostbite and hyperkalemia contributed to the eight deaths. It is interesting to note that in the process of rescue and transport of the group that died, initial CPR, sometimes vigorous,

Table 15-4
Results of Mixed Insult, Hypothermia, and Extremity Immersion Syndrome (Wet Foot)

Method of Warming	Anatomical Function Result: Good	Anatomical Function Result: Poor	Amputation: Minor	Amputation: Major	Died
Uncontrolled spontaneous rewarming, K-thermia pad, warm blankets, dry heat	1	–	–	–	–
Controlled spontaneous rewarming	7	1	1	–	–
Uncontrolled rapid rewarming, warm-water bath or whirlpool (external wet heat)	1	–	–	–	–
Controlled rapid rewarming, warm-water bath or whirlpool (external wet heat) (90°F to 106°F)	1	–	–	–	–
Controlled peritoneal dialysis	–	–	–	–	–
Total control in surgery, gradual rewarming with warm fluids (IV), and use of anesthetic breathing apparatus	–	–	–	–	–
Total (12 patients)	10	1	1	–	–

Note: Anatomical function result: good = no anatomical loss, useful range of motion of digits; poor = no amputation, intrinsic muscle loss, limited range of motion. Amputation: minor = amputation distal to M-P junction; major = amputation proximal to M-P junction.

was associated with five cases of ventricular fibrillation present upon arrival at the hospital. In these cases, unsuccessful defibrillation was carried out at temperatures of 78, of 85, of 91, and 92°F, all during periotoneal dialysis rewarming (Table 15-3).

While the victim slides quietly into the hypothermic state and stays for a while is in his or her "metabolic icebox" with few aerobic requirements for body function, he or she may or may not develop serious arrhythmias. But clinical evidence shows that, when the victim is handled with care, all his or her body's physiological requirements will be met in rewarming by his or her own "self-adjustment of cardiorespiratory function" and a normothermic state will develop without serious problems. Of course, this occurs only when he or she is under total physiological control, when acidosis, dehydration, and hyperkalemia have been corrected, and when other basic requirements have been met as they developed.

Under total physiological control in the process of rewarming, one may anticipate (if all problems are handled well) in uncomplicated cases of hypothermia that no more serious problems should develop during management than one might expect of the hypothermic patient undergoing cardiac surgery under general anesthetic in full phsyiological control.

Most patients who are dehydrated demonstrate mild to severe acidosis and evidence of hyperkalemia either after or during rewarming. The degree of awareness and consciousness has been correlated with the level of hypothermia in both adults and children, and it is obvious that cerebration, physiological responses, and even shivering ability are present at much lower temperature levels than previously considered likely.

The optimum solution to the problem of hypothermia in the emergency room depends on the amount of time allotted to solving complex metabolic, cardiac, and chemical changes as they appear. Obviously, slow spontaneous rewarming methods require more treatment time (3 to 8 hr) than rapid warming methods (30 min to 2 hr). With controlled rewarming, good results have been demonstrated for all methods (Table 15-2). However, the patient with associated freezing injury appears to receive better anatomical and functional results when rapid rewarming and thawing methods are used in warm water, 35°C to 37.7°C (95°F to 100°F) (Tables 15-3 and 15-4).

The problems presenting in hypothermia are lowered core temperature; decreasing function of metabolic system; dehydration; loss of caloric reserve; enzyme-system dysfunction; hypoxia of tissues and transfer to anerobic metabolism; metabolic acidosis; renal dysfunction; increasing loss of neuroregulation; fluid shifts and electrolyte imbalance; and in the field death from total systems cessation. If found alive by rescue personnel, the victim may essentially be in "a metabolic ice-box," a midlethal state, so that further exposure results in death from cooling of vital organs. Rewarming, if uncontrolled, may result in death because of (a) uncorrected acidosis and the sudden effect of released metabolites, (b) increased serum potassium levels resulting in cardiac excitation, or (c) hypovolemic shock.

It should be noted that a cold heart is in a fragile state and that it is possible that aggressive manipulation using CPR or efforts to cardiovert a heart not metabolically prepared to accept such stimulation may result in irreversible cardiac failure.

Knowing the problem, then, what are we attempting to do? The solution should include the following treatment protocol.

1. Safely, under control, the "cooled" or "cooling" body should be rewarmed so that the core temperature is elevated.

2. The patient should be placed under physiological control through:
   a. Adequate airway control.
   b. Restoration of fluid-electrolyte imbalance.
   c. Correction of dehydration.
   d. Correction of acidosis or alkalosis.
   e. Development of adequate intravenous access (multiple) and use of a central venous pressure line.
   g. Proper monitoring of the heart, vital organs, and fluid intake and output.
   h. Recognition and/or treatment of all conditions prohibiting immediate recovery.

In order to perform these steps, it is necessary that one take immediate control of the patient's rescue environment or rewarming environment and of the rescue and treatment personnel. Depending on the rewarming method, the patient may rapidly come to a responsive state and therein lies his or her greatest danger. While in the field in his or her "metabolic ice box," the patient was for a while at least, unless cooling continued, cold but alive. The likelihood of metabolic and cardiopulmonary failure occurs during the rewarming period either in the hospital or rescue environment.

Therefore, a planned approach to hypothermia treatment is essential, and it is important that physiological control be obtained as soon as possible. In this regard, careful patient handling, establishment of the airway, thorough evaluation of the patient, and early monitoring of temperature, electrocardiogram, and urinary output are essential. The control, as noted above, includes the initiation as soon as possible of intravenous lines the ordering of blood gases and electrolytes, and the repeated monitoring of these values.

The correction of hypovolemia with the administration of glucose and water solutions or physiological saline once baseline blood gases and electrolytes have been obtained is mandatory. With the baseline studies in hand, sodium bicarbonate can be given in order to correct acidosis and mannitol or Lasix® in order to aid in development of renal perfusion. Intravenous fluids should be warmed to physiological levels (98°F to 100°F). It must not be assumed that the patient is always in acidosis because acid-base values may indicate other disease or injury or loss of H^+ ion. If nasogastric suction is instituted, the patient may occasionally be in a state of alkalosis, as a result of loss of H^+ via the gastric tube.

Once the patient is under total system control, rewarming by the method best suited to the emergency room of the hospital facility should be instituted. The methods available include the following:

1. Spontaneous warming, controlled.
2. External rapid rewarming (90°F to 106°F) in warm-water bath or whirlpool bath.
3. Peritoneal dialysis.
4. Both external rapid rewarming and peritoneal dialysis.
5. Extracorporeal (heat circulation) blood, which includes:
   a. Cardiopulmonary bypass.
   b. Hemodialysis.
   c. Other technology.
6. Anesthetic breathing apparatus support with total control.
7. Warm, moist inspired air with total control.
8. Thoractomy: lavage, controlled.
9. Other methods under total control and with total familiarity.

The purpose of the treatment is to:

1. Restore a normal blood volume and overcome dehydration.
2. Restore the acid-base balance.
3. Restore a proper electrolyte balance and avoid a postwarming hyperkalemic state resulting in cardiac excitation.
4. Encourage a normal renal flow.
5. Avoid serious cardiac arrhythmias and arrest of the heart. In this regard, it is recommended that consideration be given to the fact that the cold heart, at very low temperatures, is not responsive to defibrillation procedures and electroshock. The cold heart, in fact, may not be in true cardiac arrest of the pattern familiar in a normothermic state but may represent a very delayed metabolic response to severe cooling. It does not seem logical to stimulate by closed chest massage or electrostimulation a heart that is unable to respond to that stimulation at such low temperatures. This matter is currently the subject of debate and investigation.

At this stage, it appears that the smaller, outlying hospitals need not be concerned that all rewarming methods are not available to them. Those patients who had spontaneous controlled rewarming from the hypothermic state, with or without rapid rewarming of the frozen extremities, with use of a mechanical respirator (or anesthetic gas machine, if available) most likely are utilizing the safest method of recovery. Under physiologically controlled rewarming, there is enough time for continuous correction of any imbalance while the patient approaches a normothermic state.

References

1. Burton, AC, Endholm: OG *Man in a Cold Environment* pp. 8-16, 200-222. London, Edward Arnold Publishers, Ltd., Monograph of the Physiological Society, 1955.

2. Grossheim RL: Hypothermia and frostbite treated with peritoneal dialysis. Alaska Med *15*:53-55, 1973.
3. Hayward J, Steinman A: Accidental hypothermia: An experimental study of inhalation rewarming. Av Space Environ Med *46*:1236-1240, 1975.
4. MacLean D, Emslie-Smith D: Accidental Hypothermia. London, Blackwell Scientific Publishing, 1977.
5. O'Keefe KM: Accidental hypothermia: A review of 62 cases. JACEP *6*:491-496, 1977.
6. Bangs CC, Hamlet MP, Mills WJ: Help for the victim of hypothermia. Patient Care *11*: 132-134, 1977.
7. Reuler JB: Hypothermia Pathophysiology, clinical settings, and management. Ann Intern Med *89*:519-527, 1978.
8. Reuler JB, Parker RA: Peritoneal dialysis in the management of hypothermia. Jour Amer Med Assoc *240*:2289-2290, 1978.
9. Welton D, et al.: Treatment of profound hypothermia. Jour Amer Med Assoc *240*: 2291-2292, 1978.
10. Coniam SW: Accidental hypothermia. Anesthesia *34*:250, 256, 1979.
11. Morrison JB, Conn ML, Hayward JS: Thermal increment provided by inhalation rewarming from hypothermia. Jour Appl Physiol *46*:1061-1065, 1979.
12. Mills WJ: Accidental hypothermia: Management approach. Alaska Med *22*:9-11, 1980.
13. Paton B: Managing the patient in cardiac arrest. Contemp Surg *2*:15-21, 1973.
14. Bligh J, and Johnson KG: Glossary of terms for thermal physiology. Jour Appl Physiol *35*:948, 1973.

CHAPTER SIXTEEN

Rewarming

Frank St. C. Golden, M.B., B.Ch., Ph.D.

The philosophical rationale behind the rapid reversal of abnormal physiological variations, which may be life threatening, is as reasonable as it is logical. One does not hesitate to take immediate steps to reverse hypoxia, hypoglycemia, or acute disorders of fluid and electrolyte balance. This is also true with thermal disorders. It is now well established that the optimum treatment for many such disorders is an attempt at immediate reversal; for example, one cools with ice packs or wetted sheets and forced convection patients suffering from malignant hyperpyrexia, heat stroke, and similar disorders just as one rapidly rewarms frostbitten limbs by immersion in whirlpool baths. However, controversy exists over whether or not one should actively rewarm patients suffering from hypothermia and about the optimum rate of any such rewarming. This chapter reviews the controvery's background and discusses the philosophy of rewarming.

History

A review of the literature reveals many well-documented accounts of a variety of methods advocated for rewarming hypothermic victims. St. Gregory of Nyssa (1), describing the martyrdom of the 40 Christian Roman soldiers at Sebaste in A.D. 320, provided a classic description of a rewarming death in one soldier who was being rapidly rewarmed in a tub of hot water. In 1757 Naucler (2) described the successful rewarming by hot formentations applied to the trunk of an individual who was believed to be dead and who, in fact, was already in his coffin when the author chanced upon the scene! Sir James Lind (3) (the father of maritime medicine and one of the first, if not the first, individual to perform a controlled study in therapeutics with the treatment of scurvy with fresh limes) in his treatise on the "Health of Seamen in the Royal Navy," published in 1762, gave a rather bizarre regime of treatment for people suffering from the effects of cold following immersion (Figure 16-1).

But let us turn our Eyes to thoſe in a State more juſtly demanding the Attention of Humanity; ſuch as have been unfortunately drowned. So ſoon as a Perſon ſuppoſed to be drowned is taken out of the Water, he ought not, as uſual, to be held up long by the Heels; the Continuance in ſuch a Poſture is the moſt likely Means to prevent him from coming to Life. The Head muſt be inclined in a Poſition favourable to empty the Stomach; mean while the utmoſt Diſpatch is uſed to remove all the cold, wet Cloaths, by ſtripping the Perſon quite naked, and immediately expoſing the Body to the Heat of the warm Sun, or a Fire, to prevent Stiffneſs and Cold; or, to regenerate Heat, he may be put in a Bed well warmed, where the Belly, Breaſt, and eſpecially the Pit of the Stomach, muſt be well and conſtantly rubbed with warm Clothes, keeping the Head and Face gently inclined forwards, as in a Perſon under the Operation of an Emetic. At the ſame time, the Limbs muſt be well chafed with hard coarſe Clothes, made very warm, and the whole Body often ſhook or rolled about. All poſſible Attempts muſt be made from the Beginning to bleed; and theſe in different Veins. The temporal Artery may alſo be cut. Warm Bricks, Irons, or Bottles of Hot Water muſt be applied to the Feet; volatile Salts, and ſtimulating Spirits to the Noſtrils; and Air, moderately heated by being near the Fire, blown by means of a Bellows into the Anus and Lungs. Or, a Perſon that chews Garlick may endeavour to blow into the Lungs with his Breath, keeping the Noſtrils of the Patient ſhut for a few Seconds of Time, to prevent its Eſcape: mean while, another Perſon, by a gentle alternate Preſſure and Dilatation of the Ribs, with a correſponding alternate Compreſſion of the Contents of the Belly upwards, imitates as near as poſſible the Act of Reſpiration in a living Body. A Clyſter of Tobacco Smoke may alſo be given, and Tobacco moiſtened, or its Juice, may be put into the Mouth, from the Stimulus of which in the Throat and Stomach, a Recovery and Vomiting has ſometimes enſued. Though theſe Means ſhould not ſpeedily produce the deſired Effect, yet the Perſon is not to be relinquiſhed. They muſt be repeated and continued for ſome Hours, keeping the Body all the while warm, or in a hot Place, perſevering in the Concuſſions and Rollings; and laſtly, he may be immerſed and kept for ſome Time in a Bath of luke-warm Water, after which, the former Means are to be again eſſayed.

Figure 16-1. Extract of pages 40 through 43 from Sir James Lind's treatise (3) on the "Health of Seamen in the Royal Navy," published in 1762.

The first experiments designed to study the effects of immersion in cold water on body temperature, with the subsequent rapid and slow rewarming, appear to be those of James Currie (1798) (4), a Liverpool physician whose interest in the subject was stimulated by witnessing the deaths of some American sailors after the grounding of their ship on a sandbank at the mouth of the Mersey River on December 13, 1790. Currie immersed human volunteers in water at 7°C (45°F) while he monitored their oral temperatures. He observed an initial rise in temperature followed by a continuing fall, which persisted for a period after removal from the cold water—the "after-drop." (See pp. 201-202.) He graphically described the advantages of rapidly rewarming the chilled subject in a tub of hot water rather than allowing passive spontaneous rewarming to take place while the victim was wrapped in blankets.

The dangers of rewarming by radiant heat were illustrated nicely in Sir John Franklin's account (5) of the treatment of his surgeon, Sir John Richardson, by placing him near a "roaring fire" when Richardson had collapsed after an attempt to swim the Coppermine River during Franklin's expedition to the Northwest Territories in 1821. Richardson lost consciousness during the treatment and on recovery found that the side nearest the fire was "deprived of sensation" for some period afterward.

Barron Larrey's vivid description (6) of the decimation of Napoleon's armies by the cold during their retreat from Moscow and the futile attempts at rewarming them are worthy of mention on several counts, not least of which because it probably served as the catalyst for the extensive research on the physiological effect of cooling performed by French physiologists in the mid-19th century.

Gaynard (1828) (7) reported that frozen toads returned to their normal condition and full activity on being thawed. He emphasized that both freezing and thawing must be gradual, an idea contrary to the technique used by more-contemporary researchers (8, 9) who have conducted experiments in freezing and thawing rats and golden hamsters. This technique is not usable with larger animals; regrettably, it was tried on humans during the 19th century with fatal consequences. (The English naturalist Hunter believed that, like some small animals, the lives of humans could be prolonged by their being frozen from time to time. He thought that, if the body was frozen and revived several times in the course of a few years, the limits of life could be considerably extended. Unfortunately, the experiment brought death instead of prolonged life.)

In 1862 Walther (10) found that cooling rabbits to below 20°C abolished their ability to rewarm spontaneously but that they could be revied when they were artificially rewarmed. In humans, the lowest recorded temperature in accidental hypothermia is that of a young woman found unconscious in the snow in Chicago in 1951 (11); she had a rectal temperature recorded 90 min after admission of 18°C (64°F)! She was slowly rewarmed by exposure to room air at about 20°C (68°F) in which she rewarmed at a rate of about 1°C per hour. In accidental hypothermia, death from asystoli or ventricular fibrilation usually occurs at deep-body temperature in the region of 24°C to 26°C (75°F to 79°F).

Lapchinski (1880) (12) is generally credited with the honor of being the originator of the rapid rewarming technique (13), but he was just one of many throughout the ages who have used this procedure. This very brief review of the history of hypothermia treatment demonstrates the fluctuating preferences for rapid and slow methods of rewarming.

The immediate, dramatic improvement in patients unconscious as a result of acute accidental hypothermia when they were placed in a tub of hot water led to the popularity of this method of treatment in an age when such speedy recoveries were frequently regarded as near miracles or at least cases worthy of recording. Reviewers of the literature (14), biased by such reports, popularized this method of treatment, which remained in favor until the outbreak of the Second World War when Talbot, Consolazio, and Pecora (15) reported a fatality in a patient undergoing rapid surface rewarming after a period of induced therapeutic hypothermia.

Subsequently, slow spontaneous rewarming remained in vogue until wartime experience gained from treating aircrews rescued from the North Sea indicated that rapid surface rewarming was the treatment of choice (16). This was substantiated by both practical (17, 18) and experimental (19, 20) evidence from Germany at the end of the war. The experiments carried out by the Nazi researchers in Dachau (20), in which some attempt was made to conduct controlled experiments evaluating different methods of rewarming after chilling (sometimes lethal) immersion in cold water, showed the advantage of rapid rewarming by immersion in a tub of hot water.

The popularity of rapid surface rewarming was further perpetuated by the anesthetic/surgical experience of the 1950s (21, 22, 23, 24) and in particular by the extraordinary case reported by Niazi and Lewis (25) in 1958. Niazi and Lewis "surface cooled" a female patient to 9°C, at which point she developed a cardiorespiratory standstill. After 1 hr, they rapidly rewarmed her, initially with hot packs, until her temperature rose to 20°C before immersing her whole body in water at 45°C. Consciousness returned 10 hr after normal body temperature was restored, and the patient suffered no ill effects from her cooling experience.

The recognition of accidental hypothermia as a common clinical problem in the geriatric population of Great Britain, and reports of the dangers inherent in rapid surface rewarming of such patients (26) again swung opinion away from this form of treatment. Gradually, in the British literature of the 1960s the exponents of both rapid and slow rewarming began to voice their opinions, with several options being offered. Table 16-1 lists various methods of rewarming advocated in the literature and some relevant references.

Table 16-1
Various Methods of Rewarming Proposed for Hypothermic Patients, with References to Some of the Relevant Publications

External	Internal
(a) Slow passive (insulation or exposure to room air) (11, 15, 26, 27, 28)	(k) Inhalation rewarming (42, 43, 44)
(b) Rapid surface (hot tub 41°C) (17, 20, 24, 25, 29, 30, 31, 32)	(l) Extracorporeal cardiopulmonary bypass (47, 48, 49)
(c) Immersing isolated limbs (33)	(m) Peritoneal dialysis (50, 51, 52)
(d) Radiant heat (heat cradles) (34, 35, 56)	(n) Warmed intravenous fluids (35, 52, 53, 54)
(e) Diathermy (36, 37)	(o) Mediastinal lavage (55, 56)
(f) Microwave (8, 38)	(p) Intragastric (lavage or balloon) (14, 57)
(g) Hot fomentations to torso (25, 39)	
(h) Neck coil (40)	
(i) Liquid heated suits (41, 42)	
(j) Water mattress (bed) (45)	

It appears that the method of rewarming chosen is largely based on the degree of expertise, facilities available, and experience of a particular group. Thus, patients being treated by general physicians are more likely to be slowly and passively rewarmed, with the minimum of intervention; patients being treated in an intensive care unit are usually rapidly rewarmed, with any physiological or biochemical abnormalities controlled as they appear. Those whose experience is limited to the immediate care of immersion victims in the field usually favor simple surface rewarming in a hot tub.

Another explanation for the controversy regarding the optimum method of rewarming is the failure of some authors to classify adequately the nature of the hypothermic case being referred to. It should be appreciated that the etiological factors leading to hypothermia may result in totally different pathophysiological disburbances, so that a regime of treatment successful in one particular case may not be relevant to another in which body temperature is comparable.

Classifications of Hypothermia

When the body heat loss continually exceeds body heat production, inevitably deep-body temperature falls. When deep-body temperature has fallen below an arbitrarily defined level of 35°C (95°F), the state of hypothermia is said to exist. Such a lowering of deep-body temperature may occur in individuals with normal thermoregulatory function but in whom the normal function is completely overwhelmed by the extreme nature of the stress, either because the environmental conditions are severe or because the insulating properties of their clothing are impaired by wetting or other damage. Such hypothermia can be classified as primary accidental hypothermia.

Secondary accidental hypothermia, as the name implies, refers to hypothermia resulting from cold exposure in individuals who have

Table 16-2
Accidental Hypothermia

Primary (Normal Thermoregulation but Overwhelming *Cold Exposure*	Secondary (Mild to Moderate Cold Exposure but *Abormal Thermoregulation*)
A. Cold-water immersion	A. Regulatory failure
e.g., shipwrecks, boating accidents,	1. Central
shallow-water accidents, caving,	(a) Hypothalmic disorders
B. Cold, wet climates	(e.g., neoplasms, trauma, degenerative disease, etc.)
(e.g., backpacking accidents, hill-walking accidents, moorland hiking accidents, etc.)	(b) Central circulatory disorders (e.g., thrombosis, hemorrhage, low cardiac output)
C. Cold, dry climates	(c) Drug intoxication
(e.g., mountaineering accidents and avalanches)	2. Peripheral
D. Deep diving	(a) Drug use and drug intoxication
(e.g., respiratory heat loss below 150 m)	(b) Spinal cord lesions
	B. Impaired heat reduction
	(a) Neuromuscular disorders
	(b) Metabolic disorders (e.g., myxo-edema, hypopituitarism)
	(c) Malnutrition
	(d) Drug intoxication
	(e) Inactivity (e.g., result of trauma)
	C. Increased heat loss
	(a) Skin disorders (e.g., erythroderma)
	(b) Drug use and drug intoxication
	(c) Hypercapnea
	(d) Malnutrition

some disorder of the thermoregulatory mechanism, which may impair heat production, increase heat loss, or interfere with central or peripheral control of thermoregulation. Some examples of both types of accidental hypothermia are listed in Table 16-2.

Accidental hypothermia can be further classified as being either acute or chronic, depending on the rate of body-heat loss. Acute accidental hypothermia entails the development of the hypothermic state in a period of less than 6 hr. When hypothermia has been present for more than 6 hrs, the condition is said to be chronic. This time scale is purely arbitrary and is based on the assumption that major fluid and electrolyte changes have not occurred or at least that specific corrective treatment for such changes is not required. Homeostasis returns to normal upon the restoration of normal body temperature. Primary accidental hypothermia is usually of the acute variety, whereas secondary hypothermia is usually of the chronic variety.

Treatment of Hypothermia

The aim of the treatment of primary hypothermia, which is essentially a physiological disorder, is to ensure that the patient's body temperature returns to normal while the development of any adverse complications is avoided. In cases of secondary hypothermia, one is concerned with the management of the underlying pathological disorder of which the hypothermia may be only one of several undesirable complications. Obviously, there is a subtle difference in emphasis of treatment, but in both situations a decision must be made about whether or not active rewarming should be undertaken.

Reasons for Rewarming

The reasons usually advanced for active rewarming of hypothermic patients are these: (1) the incidence of complications is directly related to the duration of hypothermia, (b) the hypothermic patient is unable to generate sufficient metabolic heat to rewarm spontaneously, and (c) active rewarming reduces the magnitude of the afterdrop and its associated complications.

Complications Related to Duration of Hypothermia: It has been claimed by some authors (27, 46, 58) that the incidence of complications and late mortality in hypothermia is related to the time spent at hypothermic temperatures. Although this is certainly true of peripheral tissue damage resulting from cold injury, within the confines of the controlled environment of a hospital with adequate patient monitoring available, one should be able to detect the prodromal signs of any adverse complications and act accordingly at that stage. Certainly in patients in whom hypothermia was induced and maintained over several days for therapeutic purposes (15, 59, 60), the incidence of complications does not appear to be related to the time spent in a hypothermic state but rather to the subsequent rate of rewarming.

Because of the proclivity of the "cold" myocardium to fibrillation and the difficulty of defibrillating when cardiac temperatures are below 28°C (82°F), the most feared complication in profound hypothermia is ventricular fibrillation. Consequently, reducing the time spent by the patient in this temperature zone (deep-body temperature less than 30°C or 86°F) is a valid justification for instituting rewarming procedures, provided that the methods adopted do not in themselves increase the risk of ventricular fibrillation or that facilities are readily available to manage the cardiac arrest if it should develop.

Inability to Rewarm Spontaneously: It is commonly believed that as body temperature falls below 35°C metabolism declines proportionately. This theory, which is in accordance with the predicted Q_{10} effect, is supported by the evidence from the anesthetic and surgical literature (37) for cases of induced hypothermia. However, it is not true for cases of primary accidental hypothermia (61) until very profound cooling has occurred.

Provided that metabolic heat production is greater than heat lost from the core into the heat sink of the surrounding cooler peripheral tissues and that surface heat loss is minimized by adequate insulation, the body does rewarm spontaneously. When heat production is not adequate, as evidenced by a continuing fall or a stabilization of deep-body temperature, measures must be instituted to rewarm the patient actively.

The Afterdrop: One of the most frequently quoted reasons for rapidly rewarming a hypothermic casualty or for employing some particular method of rewarming (41, 42, 44) is the reduction of the magnitude of the afterdrop and its associated complications (13, 32). This fear, which originated from the experimental work of the Nazis at Dachau (20), applied particularly to immersion hypothermia. It was believed by the Nazi researchers that the initial continued fall in rectal temperature, the afterdrop, observed when the victim was removed from the cold environment was caused by cold venous blood returning centrally from the cooler peripheral tissues. It was postulated that this cold blood further lowered the cardiac temperatures below the fibrillatory threshold and that this was the most probable explanation of the phenomenon of "postrescue death" reported so frequently by rescuers of immersion survivors (13).

Placing the cooled victims in a tub of hot 45°C [113°F]) water immediately after they were removed from the cold water not only speedily reversed the afterdrop but also improved the survival chances when compared with other methods of treatment (20). However, recent animal experiments (62) subsequently confirmed by mechanical and mathematical computer models (63) show that it is not necessary to invoke a hemodynamic mechanism in order to explain the afterdrop. Indeed, on rewarming anesthetized pigs cooled to 31°C, there was no evidence of an afterdrop in the central venous circulation, although one was recorded in the rectum. As Figure 16-2 illustrates, the temperature of the central venous blood is rising at a time when the rectal temperature is still falling. Thus, if cold blood in the hemorrhoidal or pelvic veins is the explanation for rectal afterdrop, some mechanism must exist to alter the temperature of that blood dramatically between the pelvis and the right heart; even if such a mechanism does exist, clearly cold blood returning to the heart cannot be the explanation for rewarming deaths.

Further evidence to suggest that the afterdrop is more typical of a physical than a physiological phenomenon can be found in Cooper and Ross (23), who showed that changing the method of rewarming may alter the speed of the reversal of the afterdrop but not its magnitude. Finally, when one rewarms a subject who is maintaining heat balance by shivering hard while immersed in water at 12°C (i.e., zero rate of cooling), one does not observe an afterdrop on rewarming (63).

Taking all the available evidence into consideration, this author is confident that the afterdrop is not a significant consideration in rewarming but is simply a crude indication of the rate of cooling that has taken place during cold exposure.

Rewarming by Immersion in Hot Water

The coincidental association between the nadir of the afterdrop and the anecdotal stories of postimmersion collapse and death misled the Dachau researchers into assuming a causal relationship. The beneficial effects of rapidly reversing the afterdrop by immersing the victims in hot water and the "associated" (coincidental) improved survival rates compounded the erroneous deductions. Nevertheless, it is an inescapable fact that immersing these victims in a tub of hot water bestowed some beneficial effect and improved their survival rates.

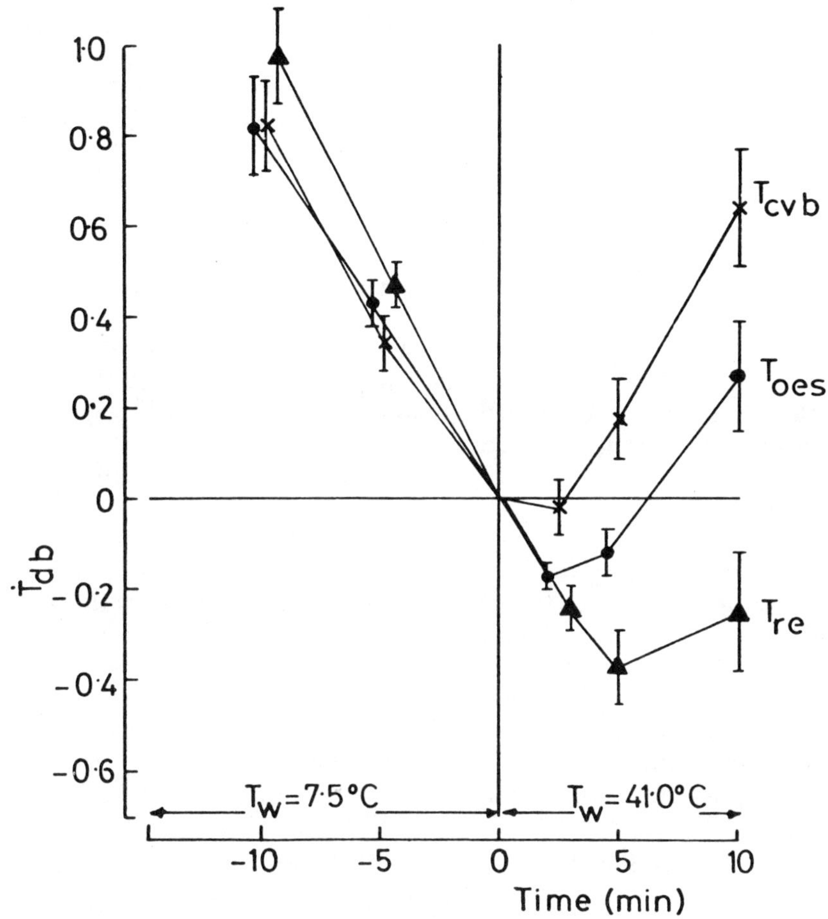

Figure 16-2. Mean (± standard error) changes in core temperature ($\dot{T}_{db}$) in three sites being monitored in 24 live pigs during the last 10 min of cooling in cold water (t_w 7.5°C) and the first 10 min in hot water (T_w 41.0°C). Changes are plotted relative to 0°C, the temperature at the end of cooling (mean = 31.5°C). (T_{cvb}: central venous blood temperature; T_{oes}: esophageal temperature; T_{re}: rectal temperature.)

What then is the nature of this beneficial mechanism, and in what way is it related to postimmersion collapse and death?

There is as yet no positive proof of any specific mechanism(s), but one can speculate as to a possible one(s). Rapidly rewarming the skin alters the firing rate of the cutaneous thermoreceptors and reduces shivering dramatically. This, in turn, reduces oxygen consumption and the demand on cardiac output with a consequent reduction in heart rate. Coronary filling improves because of the slowing heart rate (64) and the reduced viscosity of the warmed blood returning from the cutaneous circulation. Restoration of the "hydrostatic squeeze" results, with its consequent benefits on venous return and cardiac output (65) and systemic pressure.

It has been postulated (63) that on rescue from cold water it is the abrupt withdrawal of the "hydrostatic squeeze" (which may sometimes barely enable a viable cardiac output to be maintained during immersion in an individual who is hypovolemic) that is the most likely explanation of "postimmersion collapse and death." Such an explanation may account for postrescue collapse with loss of consciousness but eventual recovery, a pattern that is sometimes seen but is not readily explicable in terms of return of cold blood from the periphery.

The factual evidence supporting the use of the hot-water immersion technique for rewarming hypothermic victims relates solely to a cold-water immersion etiology (20) in which the major complication is "postrescue collapse." The possible mechanism of action speculated on in the discussion above suggests why this may be so.

In cases of chronic accidental hypothermia, the most important complication during treatment is "rewarming collapse." The benefit of hot-water immersion in preventing the onset of this condition is not known, but, considering its etiology (peripheral vasodilatation associated with hypovolemia), it is likely that this method of treatment would be dangerous, in addition to increasing the monitoring difficulties.

When to Rewarm

When to rewarm will remain a controversial aspect of the treatment of hypothermia for many years to come, but the following guidelines are offered for consideration.

1. Patients whose esophageal temperature continues to fall or remains stable after the surface of the body has been adequately insulated *must* be actively rewarmed.
2. Patients who have an undesirable cardiac arrhythmia *should* be actively rewarmed.
3. Patients whose temperature is below 28°C *should* be actively

rewarmed, and consideration should be given to rewarming all those below 30°C.

4. Known diabetics *should* be actively rewarmed until a body temperature of 31°C to 32°C is attained, at which time their diabetic state should be assessed and stabilized before the rewarming proceeds.
5. Acute hypothermia victims who are conscious and shivering *may* be rewarmed, but those who are unconscious should only be rewarmed in a properly equipped unit where any complications can be dealt with promptly.
6. Secondary hypothermia victims *may* be actively rewarmed in order to better assess the underlying pathology and to assist in overall stabilization.

How to Rewarm

The technique of rewarming adopted depends on the facilities and staff available. The recent results quoted by Ledingham and Mone (56) should dispel once and for all the fear that invasive monitoring and specific treatment maneuvers cannot be managed in a competent unit or indeed that such actions are in themselves harmful. However, such an aggressive approach to treatment is not possible in small outlying hospitals or in the field. In these situations, when it is not possible to transfer the patient to a larger central hospital, it may be safer to adopt the less aggressive passive approach (28) of maintaining the rate of rise of temperature around 0.5°C per hour while monitoring the cardiovascular state and blood gases and correcting both as necessary.

Rewarming Collapse

In the course of rewarming, there may be a sudden fall in peripheral resistance that is unmatched by an increase in cardiac output, resulting in severe hypotension. This is particularly likely to occur in the chronic forms of accidental hypothermia in which fluid depletion may be quite severe. Its etiology is probably related to the removal of the local peripheral vasoconstricting effect of cold while the hypothermic's vasomotor center is still malfunctioning (66). Prevention is best achieved by central venous and arterial pressure monitoring, prudent intravenous fluid therapy, and careful control of surface temperature in order to prevent overheating before the vasomotor center returns to full activity.

Conclusions

The method and rate of rewarming chosen for any particular hypothermic patient must depend on the etiological mechanisms of the individual case and the expertise and facilities available. There is no overall procedure that can be applied to every case. Whichever method of rewarming is selected, care must be exercised to safeguard against rewarming collapse.

References

1. Kelly B: The Forty Martyrs of Sebaste. *From* Butler's Lives of the Saints, vol. 1, pp. 254-257. London, Virtue and Company Ltd, 1936.
2. Naucler S: Berichte von einem Mannes welcher dem Anschein nach Efroren war denn aber wie der zum Leben verhollen war. K Schwed Akad Wiss *18*:107-112, 1757.
3. Lind J:An Essay on the Most Effective Means of Preserving the Health of Seamen in the Royal Navy. Plato's Head, London, D. Wilson, 1762.
4. Currie J: The effects of water, cold and warm, as a remedy in fever. *In*: Treatment of Shipwrecked Mariners, Appendix II. London, Cadell and Davies, 1798.
5. Franklin J: The Life of Sir John Richardson. London, Longman, Green and Company, 1868.
6. Richardson RG: Larrey: Surgeon to Napoleon's Imperial Guard. London, Murray, 1974.
7. Varigny H: Smithsonian Report 1890, 407-428.
8. Andjus RK, Locelock JE: Reanimation of rats from body temperatures between 0°C and 1°C by microwave diathermy. Jour Physiol *128*:541-546, 1955.
9. Smith AU: Studies on golden hamsters during cooling to, and rewarming from, body temperatures below 0°C. Proc Roy Soc Med *145*:391-426, 1956.
10. Walther. Virchow's Archiv. *25*:414. Cited by Britton SW, Can Med Assoc Jour *22*:257-261, 1950.
11. Laufman H: Profound accidental hypothermia. Jour Amer Med Assoc *147*:1201-1212, 1951.
12. Lapchinski FF: Treatment of frozen limbs. Vrach St Petersburg *87*:119-125, 1880.
13. Burton AC, Edholm OG: Man in a Cold Environment. London, Edward Arnold Publishers Ltd., 1955.
14. Britton SW: Extreme hypothermia in various animals and in man. Can Med Assoc Jour *22*:257-261, 1930.
15. Talbott HH, Consolazio WV, Pecora LJ: Hypothermia: Report of a case in which the patient died during therapeutic reduction of body temperature. Arch Intern Med *68*: 1120-1132, 1941.
16. Wayburn E: Immersion hypothermia. Arch Intern Med *79*:77-91, 1947.
17. Grosse-Brockoff F: Pathology, physiology, and therapy of hypothermia. *In*: German Aviation Medicine, World War II, pp. 828-842. Washington, D.C., Department of the Air Force (Surgeon General), 1946.
18. Matthes M: German airforce rescue services. *In*: German Aviation Medicine, World War II, p. 1148. Washington, D.C., Department of the Air Force (Surgeon General), 1946.
19. Weltz GA, Reiter R: Animal tests on chilling and warming in water. Combined intelligence Objective Subcommittee G-2 Division. SHAER APO143 C105 Target No. 24 Medical, 1945. (D.R.I.C. Translation 5183, December 1977, BR45934.)

20. Alexander L: The treatment of shock from prolonged exposure to cold, especially in water. Combined intelligence Objectives Subcommittee APO413 C10 105. Item No. 24. HMSO London, 1945.
21. Bigelow WG, Lindsay WK, Greenwood WF: Hypothermia: Its possible role in cardiac surgery, an investigation in dogs at low body temperature. Annals Surg *132*:849-860, 1949.
22. Drew CE, Anderson IM: Profound hypothermia in cardiac surgery. Lancet *1*:748-750, 1959.
23. Cooper KE, Ross DN: Hypothermia in Surgical Practice. London, Cassells, 1960.
24. Blair E: Clinical Hypothermia. New York, McGraw-Hill, 1964.
25. Niazi SA, Lewis FJ: Profound hypothermia in man. Annals Surg *147*:264-266, 1958.
26. Duiguid H, Simpson RG, Stowers JM: Accidental hypothermia. Lancet *2*:1213-1219, 1961.
27. Nicolas F, Nicolas G, Heurtel A, Baron D, Rodineau PL, De Larjartre AY: Vingt-quatre observations d'hypothermies accidentelles. Anaesthesie Analgesie Reanimation *31*:485-538, 1974.
28. MacLean D, Emslie-Smith D: Accidental Hypothermia. Oxford, Blackwell Scientific Publishing, 1977.
29. Behnke AR, Yaglou CP: Responses of human subjects to immersion in ice water and to slow and fast rewarming. Jour Appl Physiol *3*:591-602, 1950.
30. Hardwick RG: Two cases of accidental hypothermia. Brit Med Jour *1*:147-149, 1962.
31. Pugh LGC: Accidental hypothermia in walkers, climbers and campers: Report to the Medical Commission on Accident Prevention. Brit Med Jour *1*:123-129, 1966.
32. Keatinge, WR: Survival in Cold Water. Oxford, Blackwell Scientific Publishing, 1969.
33. Cooper KE, Baron DN, Compstan ND, Dawson AM (eds.), Recent Advances in Medicine, p. 343. London, Churchill, 1968.
34. Waddell WG, Fairley HB, Bigelow WG: Improved management of clinical hypothermia based upon related biochemical studies. Annals Surg *146*:542-559, 1951.
35. Ledingham I McA, Mone JG: Treatment after exposure to cold. Lancet *1*:534-535, 1972.
36. Bigelow WG, Hopps JA, Callaghan JC: Radio frequency rewarming in resuscitation from severe hypothermia. Can Jour Med Sci *30*:185-193, 1952.
37. Blair E, Swan H, Virtue R: Clinical hypothermia: A study of ice water surface immersion and shortwave diathermy techniques. Annals Surg *22*:869-879, 1956.
38. Lovelock JE, Smith AU: Heat transfer from and to animals in experimental hypothermia and freezing. Annals NY Acad Sci *80*:487-499, 1959.
39. Neureuther G: Die Waermepackung. *In*: Matter P, Braun P, de Quervain M, and Good Z (eds.), Symposium Forum Davos: Skiing and Safety III. Davos, Switzerland. Offsetdruck, 1979.
40. Cohen D, Hercus V: Controlled hypothermia in infants and children. Brit Med Jour *1*: 1435-1439, 1959.
41. Macus P: Laboratory comparison of techniques for rewarming hypothermic casualties. Av Spac Environ Med *49*:692-697, 1978.
42. Harnett RM, O'Brien EM, Sias FR, Pruitt JR: Initial treatment of profound accidental hypothermia. Av Spac Environ Med *51*:680-687, 1980.
43. Lloyd EL: Accidental hypothermia treated by central rewarming through the airway. Brit Jour Anaesth *45*:41-48, 1973.
44. Hayward JS, Steinman AM: Accidental hypothermia: An experimental study of inhalation rewarming. Av Spac Environ Med *46*:1236-1240, 1975.
45. Fernandez JP, O'Rourke RA, Ewy GA: Rapid active external rewarming in accidental hypothermia. Jour Amer Med Assoc *212*:153-156, 1970.

46. Davies DM, Millar J, Millar IA: Accidental hypothermia treated by extracorporeal blood rewarming. Lancet *1*:1036-1037, 1967.
47. Kugelberg J, Schuller H, Berg B, Kallum B: Treatment of accidental hypothermia. Scand Jour Thoracic Cardiovasc Surg *1*:142-146, 1967.
48. Towne WD, Geiss WP, Yanes HO, Rahimtoola SH: Intractable ventricular fibrillation associated with profound accidental hypothermia: Successful treatment with partial cardio-pulmonary by-pass. New Engl Jour Med *287*:1135-1136, 1972.
49. Turina M, Hosseli G: Successful rewarming with the heart-lung machine after accidental hypothermia. *In*: Matter P, Braun P, de Quervain M, and Good Z (eds.), Symposium Forum Davos: Skiing and Safety III. Davos, Switzerland. Offsetdruck, 1979.
50. Lash RF, Burdett JA, Ozdil T: Accidental profound hypothermia and barbiturate intoxication (a report of rapid "core" rewarming by peritoneal dialysis). Jour Amer Med Assoc *201*:269-270, 1967.
51. Grossheim RL: Hypothermia and frostbite treated with peritoneal dialysis. Alaska Med *15*:53-55, 1973.
52. Jessen K, Hagelston JO: Search and rescue services in Denmark with special reference to accidental hypothermia. Aerospace Med *43*:787-791, 1972.
53. Binhold: cited by Ungley CC *in*: Research and development of life-saving equipment: Medical aspects of shipwreck. British Intelligence Objectives Subcommittee Report No. 494, 1945.
54. Freeman J, Pugh LGC: Hypothermia in mountain accidents. Int Anaes Clin 7:997-1007, 1969.
55. Linton AL, Ledingham I McA: Severe hypothermia with barbiturate intoxication. Lancet *1*:25-26, 1966.
56. Ledingham I McA, Mone JG: Treatment of accidental hypothermia: A prospective clinical study. Brit Med Jour *280*:1102-1105, 1980.
57. Khalil HH: Hypothermia by internal cooling. Lancet *1*:1092-1094, 1958.
58. Exton-Smith AN: Accidental hypothermia. Brit Med Jour *4*:727-729, 1973.
59. Dill DB, Forbes WH: Respiratory and metabolic effects of hypothermia. Amer Jour Physiol *132*:685-697, 1941.
60. Bloch M: Cerebral effects of rewarming following prolonged hypothermia. Significance for the management of severe cranio-cerebral injury in acute pyrexia. Brain *90*:769-784, 1967.
61. Golden F St C: Why Rewarm? *In*: Matter P, Braun P, De Quervain M, and Good Z (eds.), Davos, Switzerland, Offsetdruck, 1979.
62. Golden F St C, Hervey GR: The mechanism of the afterdrop following immersion hypothermia in pigs. Jour Physiol *272*:26P-27P, 1977.
63. Golden F St C, Hervey GR: The after-drop. *In*: Adam JM (ed.), Proceedings of the Third International Action for Disaster Conference, 1979. Aberdeen University Press, Aberdeen, 1981.
64. Berne RM: The effect of immersion hypothermia on coronary blood flow. Circ Res *2*: 236-242, 1954.
65. Arborelius M, Ballidin UI, Lilja B, Lundgren GEC: Haemodynamic changes in man during immersion with head above water. Aerospace Med *43*:592-598, 1972.
66. Brendel W: Die Bedlutung der Hirntemperatur für die Kaltegenregulation im der Einfluss der Hirntemperatur auf den Kreislauf des Hundes. Arch Ges Physiol *270*:648-657, 1960.

CHAPTER SEVENTEEN

The Effect of Airway Warming on Severe Hypothermia

Donald E. Roberts, Ph.D., John F. Patton, Ph.D., and Donald W. Kerr, M.S.

The use of the lungs as a heat exchanger for rewarming hypothermia victims has been widely advocated. The proponents of this method suggest that it is noninvasive and expedient in the field and that it applies heat directly to the body's core. Other investigators have calculated that the quantity of heat that can be supplied by this method is insufficient to perform these tasks.

Hayward and Steinman (1) cooled humans to 35°C in a comparison of airway warming and bath warming. They reported that both tympanic and esophageal temperatures were higher in airway warming than observed in other methods, thus supporting the theory of targeting heat to the core. In a related study, Morrison and associates (2) reported that the temperature of hypothermic subjects (35°C) increased by 0.77°C after 30-min of hyperventilation (50 L per minute) with warmed, humidified air but improved by only 0.39°C after breathing room air normally for 30 min.

Lloyd and associates (3, 4, 5) designed portable resuscitation equipment that mixes CO_2 with soda lime to produce heat and then passes O_2 through the mixture to form a heated, humidified inspired gas mixture. This system allows the technique to be used in remote areas. Lloyd claimed that this device adds about 1.2 kcal per square meter per hour in addition to preventing the loss of 8 to 9 kcal per square meter per hour.

Harnett and associates (6) compared airway rewarming to trunk immersion and spontaneous rewarming in mildly cooled human

The views, opinions, and findings contained in this report are those of the authors and should not be construed as an official Department of the Army position, policy, or decision, unless so designated by other official documentation.

volunteers. They reported that airway rewarming showed the least amount of temperature afterdrop. This data was confirmed by Collis and associates (7), who compared the effects of airway warming to the effects of heating pads, hot whirlpool baths, and shivering.

A comparison of airway warming with bath warming, piped suit warming, and spontaneous rewarming was conducted by Marcus (8). He reported that hot baths were the most effective technique for raising deep-body temperature but that all methods produced an afterdrop in temperature.

Finally, Guild (9) concluded that central body rewarming via the airway has not been shown to be of sufficient value to warrant being adopted by rescue sources in the field.

In all of the published reports involving the use of airway warming in humans, the degree of hypothermia has been very mild. The authors of this chapter decided to compare the response to airway warming with the response to active external rewarming in an animal model with severe hypothermia (28°C). Active external rewarming was chosen because it is more reliable than passive external and because it could be controlled to a greater degree. One group of dogs was rewarmed through external means only, and a second group of animals was rewarmed through external means combined with airway warming.

Methods

Twelve healthy mongrel dogs were used for this study. The animals were lightly anesthetized with pentobarbitol (25 mg per kilogram BW), and an endotracheal tube was inserted.

Aerterial blood pressure was measured through a polyethylene catheter (P.E. 200) placed in the right femoral artery and connected to a Statham P-23 AA pressure transducer. The output was continuously recorded on a Brush 200 chart recorder. Cardiac output was determined by the cardiogreen dye dilution technique, with the dye being injected from a small catheter (P.E. 80) placed above the right heart via the external jugular vein. Blood was withdrawn from the left femoral artery and passed through a Lexington clinical densitometer and then returned to the animal. Lead II EKG was recorded on the Brush recorder.

Cardiac blood temperature was measured by means of a thermocouple placed above the right heart via the external jugular vein. The temperature was measured by a Leeds and Northrup Numatron and recorded on a Digital Equipment PDP-11 computer. Care was taken that neither the catheter nor the thermocouple was in contact with the heart.

Blood gases were measured on a Radiometry ABL-2 blood gas analyzer from free-flowing arterial samples taken from the left femoral artery. Blood gases were measured at the beginning of cooling, at maximum cooling (28°C), and after rewarming.

Cooling was accomplished by placing the animals between blankets filled with circulating cold fluid. External rewarming was obtained by heating the fluid to a temperature of 41°C.

Airway warming was by means of a Bennett model I cascade humidifier. Air was bubbled through warmed water, which was heated to supply air at 41°C. During severe hypothermia (less than 30°C), respiration was supplemented by positive-pressure ventilation when spontaneous respiration was not present.

Results

The control data for animals rewarmed by both methods is presented in Table 17-1. These values were obtained prior to cooling the dogs. All values were within normal ranges, and there was no difference between the two groups.

Table 17-1
Baseline Data

Parameter	ER Group	ERA Group
HR	133 ± 14 b/min	132 ± 12 b/min
CO	2.6 ± .91 L/min	2.14 ± .27 L/min
HCT	39 ± 3	40 ± 2
BP	119 ± 16 mm Hg	126 ± 14 mm Hg
pO_2	67 ± 7	75 ± 15
pCO_2	57 ± 1	51 ± 8
pH	7.143 ± .01	7.136 ± .01

Figure 17-1 shows the change in heart rate (HR), cardiac output (CO), arterial blood pressure (BP), and hematocrit (HCT). Each animal served as its own control. The data are presented as the percentage change from control.

The HR was depressed in the externally rewarmed (ER) group and the externally rewarmed with supplementary airway warming (ERA) group at 28°C and was still below control upon rewarming. There was no difference in the HR response of the two groups. The CO

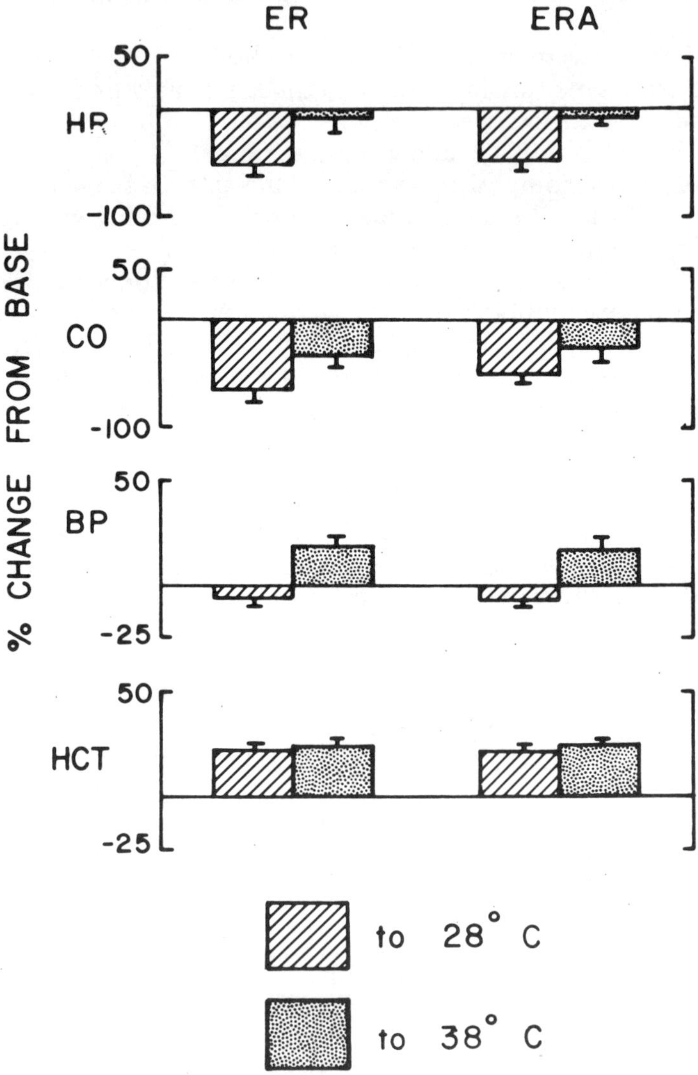

Figure 17-1. Changes in heart rate (HR), cardiac output (CO), arterial blood pressure (BP), and hematocrit (HCT) calculated as a percentage change from the control level.

was depressed during cooling and remained significantly depressed from control upon rewarming. Both groups responded similarly.

BP was depressed during cooling and elevated above control

following rewarming. There was no significant difference between the two groups. Total peripheral resistance (TPR) calculated by a standard formula (12) is shown in Table 17-2.

$$\text{TPR (dynes sec/cm}^5\text{)} = \frac{\text{Pressure head} \times 13.6 \times 980}{\text{Flow (ml/sec)}}$$

The data for Table 17-2 were calculated from the average values for each variable and not from individual values for blood pressure and cardiac output.

Table 17-2
Total Peripheral Resistance (dynes sec/cm^5)

State	ER Group	ERA Group
Control	36,600	47,083
Cold	95,260	81,408
Rewarmed	63,509	73,602

HCT increased similarly in both groups with cooling and remained elevated with rewarming. The increase in HCT was not unexpected, since these animals had an intact spleen and in the dog the spleen serves as a reservoir of red blood cells. However, the increase in HCT occurs even when the spleen is removed, but the magnitude of the increase is lower.

Figure 17-2 shows the values for pO_2, pCO_2, and pH. The pO_2 and pCO_2 were calculated as percentage change from control levels, while pH was plotted as real numbers. The pO_2 level was depressed during the cold phase of hypothermia for both groups. The most significant change occurred in the pO_2 upon rewarming. Airway warming resulted in an inhanced increase in the pO_2 level. This may have been partly achieved by the augmented breathing while the animal was cold. The ER group did not completely return to control upon rewarming. The pCO_2 response was similar in both groups of animals. Depressed pCO_2 on rewarming suggests that both groups were hyperventilated on rewarming.

The pH of both groups was low at the beginning of the experiment, and this may be due to the fact that it was taken at a temperature of 35°C. The pH of the airway group was improved significantly more than the external group.

Figure 17-3 shows the average cooling curves for the cardiac temperatures in each group of animals. External rewarming supplemented by airway warming is represented by the dotted line; the solid line

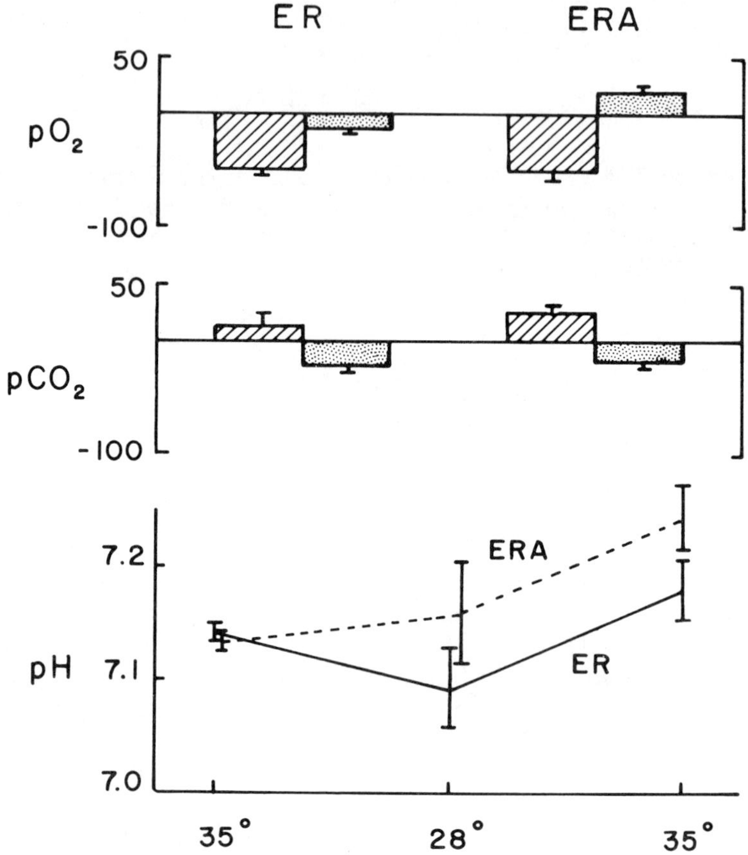

Figure 17-2. Changes in pO_2, pCO_2, and pH. The pO_2 and pCO_2 are shown as a percentage change from control.

represents data obtained from control animals receiving only external rewarming. The lines are not significantly different.

Figures 17-4 and 17-5 present tracings for two animals from the ERA group. In each of these, the upper trace is the blood pressure recording and the lower is the EKG trace for lead II. Both figures show the tracings at three different times in the experiment. The first trace was made during control before cooling was started. The second was made during the rewarming phase of the experiment. The third was taken near the end of the experiment. Abnormal EKGs were observed during rewarming in two-thirds of the ERA group. In animals receiving airway warming, a number of premature ventricular contractions

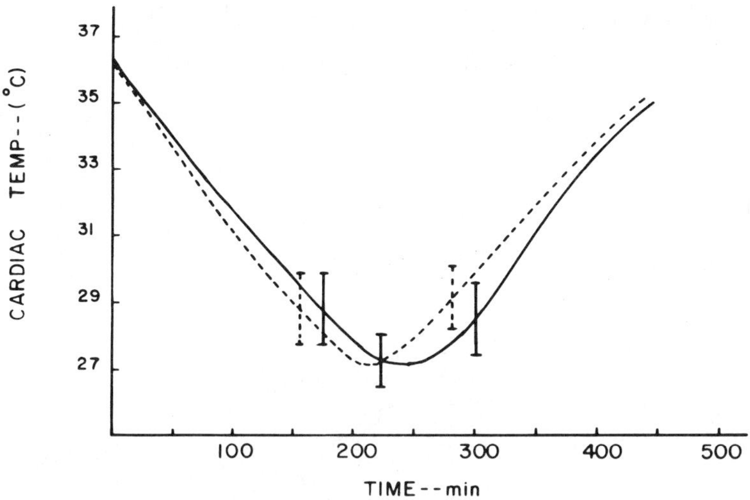

Figure 17-3. Cooling curves for both groups, with the externally rewarmed group represented by the solid line and the externally rewarmed group with airway warming represented by the dotted line.

occurred during the rewarming phase. These dysrhythmias began soon after rewarming was initiated and persisted until a temperature above 33.5°C was reached. No PVCs were observed in the ER group.

Discussion

There is disagreement concerning the use of airway warming for the resuscitation of hypothermia victims. The proponents of airway warming (1, 3, 10, 11) tend to favor the use of airway warming under field conditions over the use of external warming methods. In cases of mild hypothermia, airway warming plus passive external warming may be sufficient. Hayward and Steinmay (1) and Morrison and associates (2) felt that airway warming is an active therapy and that the heat flow is from the airways to the blood returning to the heart as well as structures in the mediastinum. Morrison and associates (2) reported that for each 10-L-per-minute increase in ventilation the rate of rewarming increases by 0.3°C per hour. At the reported rate of 1.54°C per hour in hyperventilating subjects, a hypothermia victim with a temperature of 30°C would still require almost 5 hr to reach normothermia.

Guild (9) reported that for the hypothermia victim breathing air at

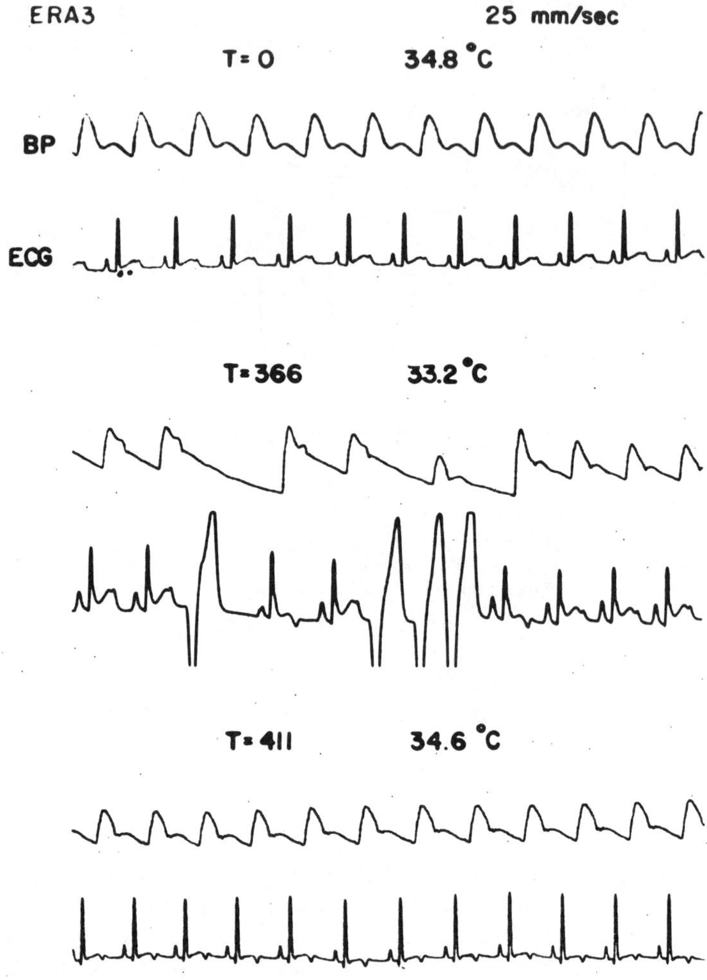

Figure 17-4. Arterial blood pressure and electrocardiogram tracings from dog ERA3, showing the responses at three different temperatures.

45°C: 100% RH the heat gained would be 9.4 Kcal per hour at a minute ventilation of 3 L per minute and 23.17 Kcal per hour at a minute ventilation of 10 L per minute.

A rise of 1°C in body temperature for a 70-kg man would require approximately 56 Kcal (specific heat of body tissue equaling 0.8 Kcal per kilogram). Assuming that the "core" of the body comprises

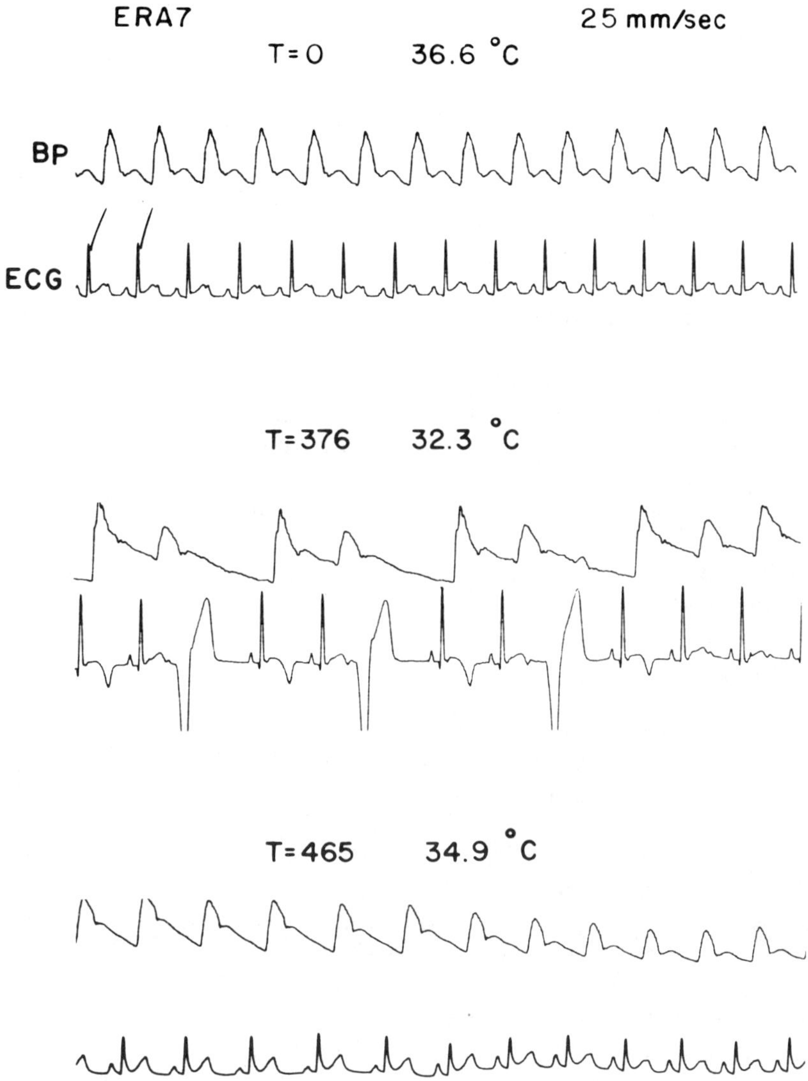

Figure 17-5. Arterial blood pressure and electrocardiogram tracings from dog ERA7, showing the responses at three different temperatures.

60% of the body mass, it would require 35.5 Kcal to raise the core body temperature by 1°C. At a minute ventilation of 3 L per minute, the whole body would be warmed at 0.17°C per hour and the core at

0.25°C per hour. On the basis of these considerations, Guild (9) concluded that the placement of airway-warming devices aboard rescue craft does not appear to be justified if the treatment of hypothermia victims is to be their only use. The use of warmed, humidified air in a rescue situation in which ventilation is required for other reasons could be justified.

The data obtained in this experiment support those investigations that have shown that airway warming is of minimal or no benefit. The use of airway warming in conjunction with active external rewarming did not rewarm the animals at a faster pace. It could be argued that variation within the experiment was significant and that a greater number of experiments would better answer the question. However, the benefits observed would still be relatively small.

A significant change observed was the improvement of the pO_2 to levels above control in animals supplemented with airway warming. This is possibly because the control levels were taken at a somewhat lowered level (35°C) at the beginning of the experiment. This increase would be sufficient reason to justify the use of ventilatory assistance at higher minute ventilation rates than would normally be found in a hypothermia victim.

As the animals were cooled, vasoconstriction occurred, and during rewarming there was some vasodilatation (Table 17-2). Since this was an active external rewarming, it might be expected that the total peripheral resistance would have decreased with rewarming. The fact that it did not probably suggests that the dog is not an appropriate model in this respect. Humans store more blood in their extremities, and external rewarming could be expected to change total peripheral resistance in humans to a greater extent than it did in dogs, possibly leading to a larger afterdrop in temperature.

Some reasons for the decreased cardiac output could have been the reduced venous return, the decreased cardiac contractility and the sludging of blood that occur with hypothermia. The continued decrement in CO after rewarming is probably due to the increased viscosity of blood upon exposure to cold (12). In subsequent studies involving cooling dogs without spleens, the CO was depressed in a similar fashion.

The EKG tracings presented in Figures 17-4 and 17-5 represent the most interesting aspect of this study. The EKGs of hypothermic patients usually show sinus bradycardia, atrial fibrillation, muscle tremor artifact, prolonged QRS duration with the Osborn wave present, and prolonged Q-T interval (13). The temperature threshold of greatest danger for ventricular fibrillation is considered to be 30°C (5).

Figure 17-4 and 17-5 show the characteristic EKG changes occurring with hypothermia, but they also demonstrate abnormal PVCs. Although a PVC is not considered to be very serious in itself, it can become important in a heart stressed by cold and when other circulatory problems are present. The fact that the PVCs were present below the threshold of 30°C and continued for several degrees above that makes the possibility of significant cardiac dysrhythmias even greater. The fact that this occurred only in those animals being treated with warmed, humidified air is even more cause for alarm. It is difficult to speculate what might be causing this problem, but it could be related to the condensation of fluid within the bronchial tree. Anesthesiologists using warmed, humidified air to maintain patients during surgery have noted an increase in bronchospasms. This increased bronchospastic activity may influence a heart that is already irritable because of cold stress. The literature has not reported this finding in humans in situations in which airway warming was used, but there are few data on the use of airway warming in humans except in cases of mild hypothermia.

In conclusion, airway warming, when used by itself, does little to rewarm the hypothermic patient. When used with other means of warming, either active or passive, airway warming can be useful in decreasing the heat lost from the airway. The benefits observed in the blood gases also support the use of warmed, humidifed air/O_2 as an adjunct to other forms of rewarming. However, airway warming should be used cautiously until the significance of dysrhythmias observed in the present experiments can be evaluated.

References

1. Hayward JS, Steinman AM: Accidental hypothermia: An experimental study of inhalation rewarming. Av Spac Environ Med *46*:1236-1240, 1975.
2. Morrison JB, Conn ML, Hayward JS: Thermal increment provided by inhalation rewarming from hypothermia. Jour Appl Physiol *46*:1061-1065, 1979.
3. Lloyd EL: Accidental hypothermia treated by central rewarming through the airway. Brit Jour Anaesth *45*:41-48, 1973.
4. Lloyd EL, Conliffe NA, Orgel H, Walker PN: Accidental hypothermia: an apparatus for central rewarming as a first aid measure. Scot Med Jour *17*:83-90, 1972.
5. Lloyd EL, Mitchell B: Factors affecting the onset of ventricular fibrillation in hypothermia. Lancet *2*:1294-1296, 1974.
6. Harnett RM, O'Brien EM, Sias FR, Pruitt JR: Initial treatment of profound accidental hypothermia. Av Spac Environ Med *51*:680-687, 1980.
7. Collis ML, Steinman AM, Chaney RD: Accidental hypothermia: An experimental study of practical rewarming methods. Av Space Environ Med *48*:625-632, 1977.
8. Marcus P. Laboratory comparison of techniques for rewarming hypothermic casualties. Av Space Environ Med *49*:692-697, 1978.

9. Guild WJ: Rewarming via the airway (CBRW) for hypothermia in the field? Jour Roy Nav Med *64*:186-193, 1978.
10. Johnson LA: Accidental hypothermia: Peritoneal dialysis. Jour Amer Coll Emer Phys *6*:556-561, 1977.
11. Shanks CA, Marsh HM: Simple core rewarming in accidental hypothermia. Brit Jour Anaesth *45*:522-525, 1973.
12. Folkow B, Neil E: Circulation. New York, Oxford University Press, 1971.
13. Clements SD, Hurst JW: Diagnostic value of electrocardiographic abnormalities observed in subjects accidentally exposed to cold. Amer Jour Card *29*:729-734, 1972.

CHAPTER EIGHTEEN

Near-Drowning and Its Treatment

Barbara B. Tabeling, M.D.

Recreational activities involving water have become increasingly popular. Many homes now have swimming pools, and public facilities include indoor as well as outdoor pools. Boating is a major form of recreation. Scuba diving has enjoyed an enormous increase in popularity, and, unfortunately, many scuba enthusiasts have inadequate training. The ability to travel long distances rapidly allows many to pursue such recreational water activities year-round. The increase in leisure time available to the general population and the relative affluence of Americans contribute to their ability to pursue such recreational activities.

With these activities, there is always a risk of drowning or near-drowning. Approximately 6,000 persons drown in the United States each year. This number has not decreased in recent years in spite of an increased awareness of the need for recreational safety and the widespread knowledge of resuscitation techniques. Half the victims are less than 20 yr old, and the majority are male (1). It has been estimated that 8 persons nearly drown for every 1 who does drown (2). Thus, water-related accidents have significant impact on the population of the United States.

Definitions

The distinction between drowning and near-drowning is important in understanding the literature related to these injuries. Modell offered a classification system that considers this distinction (3). "Drown," as defined by Webster's dictionary, means "to suffocate by submersion, especially in water" (4). Modell's classification of drowning includes the subcategories with aspiration and without aspiration. Although the vast majority of drowned persons aspirate water or gastric contents, 10% to 12% do not aspirate but instead die from hypoxia due to laryngospasm, or breath holding (5).

"Near-drowned" describes those persons who survive submersion, at least temporarily. This category is also divided into those who aspirate and those who do not. A clinical series has demonstrated that 10% to 12% of victims of near drowning do not aspirate (6).

"Delayed death subsequent to near-drowning" describes those persons who survive the accident but who die later as a result of the injury or secondary complications. Frequently, such deaths are due to central nervous system hypoxia, unrecognized pulmonary insufficiency, or septicemia. It is difficult to determine the number of delayed deaths after near-drowning because of variations in the reporting of primary and secondary causes of death.

Many factors influence the severity of the injury in near-drowned humans. Besides the effects of the volume and the tonicity of the water aspirated, materials contaminating the water can lead to chemical injury or bacterial infection (7). Even when no water has been aspirated, the severity of hypoxemia due to lack of ventilation can be enough to cause irreversible central nervous system damage before resuscitation is instituted (8).

The temperature of the water can also affect the degree of injury (9, 10). Very cold water can cause rapid cooling of the body, particularly in children who have a large body surface area relative to their body mass. Resuscitation with complete recovery after 40 min of submersion in icy water has been reported (11). Other case reports have documented similar results after prolonged submersion in cold water. The potential for functional survival should prompt the aggressive resuscitation of these victims.

The "diving reflex" appears to be another protective mechanism during submersion (12, 13, 14). The reflex occurs in humans. although the intensity varies with individuals. The reflex is initiated by the immersion of the face in water, particularly cold water. It is believed that the reflex is initiated by stimulation of the third division of the trigeminal nerve and is intensified by a deep inspiration simultaneous with facial immersion. The efferent nerve is in the vagus, which causes intense bradycardia and vasoconstriction. These effects cause blood to be delivered primarily to the heart and brain and, thus, protect crucial organs.

Pathophysiology

Oxygenation and Acid-Base Balance

The primary injury in drowning and near-drowning is to the lungs, and it results in hypoxia and respiratory and metabolic acidosis (3, 7). Even when water is not aspirated, hypoxemia occurs rapidly (8) and can result in central nervous system damage or death. Approximately 12% of drowned and near-drowned victims do not demonstrate evidence of aspiration (5, 6). The effects of airway obstruction, such as would occur from laryngospasm, were demonstrated by Modell and associates in experimental animals (8). With tracheal obstruction, arterial pH decreased an average of .05 units per minute and arterial carbon dioxide tension ($PaCO_2$) increased an average of 6 torr per minute. However, arterial oxygen tension (PaO_2) decreased dramatically from a baseline average of 92 torr to 40 torr after 1 min and 4 torr after 5 min. In spite of the severe hypoxemia, 80% of the animals were resuscitated after 5 min of tracheal obstruction by a brief period of positive-pressure ventilation and, in some cases, closed chest cardiac massage.

Craig demonstrated the effects of hyperventilation and breath holding on alveolar gas tensions (15). He found that, after hyperventilation, exercise performed during breath holding resulted in profound alveolar hypoxia while carbon dioxide tension did not increase to a level necessary to stimulate respiration. He postulated that this phenomenon may be responsible for "underwater blackout," which occurs in competent swimmers during underwater swimming and results in drowning or near-drowning.

The aspiration of water may result in severe hypoxemia that is not readily reversed. In an experimental animal study (16), the aspiration of 22 ml per kilogram of fresh water or saline caused PaO_2 to decrease to an average of 40 torr within 1 min. The PaO_2 did not improve in untreated animals during the 1-hr-long study. In the same study, transient respiratory acidosis occurred but resolved spontaneously within 1 hr, while metabolic acidosis also occurred but did not completely resolve during this time. Similar degrees of hypoxemia and acidosis have been described in humans (6, 17).

The severity of hypoxemia or acidosis determined with the initial analysis of arterial blood does not allow the clinician to predict the victim's outcome (6, 17, 18, 19). Although patients with severe hypoxemia at the time of admission to a hospital have lived, others with nearly normal blood gas tensions have died. The respiratory component of the acidosis may resolve spontaneously or with the institution of mechanical ventilation. The metabolic acidosis may require the intravenous administration of sodium bicarbonate until arterial oxygenation and cardiovascular stability are restored (6).

Although hypoxemia results from the aspiration of either fresh water or seawater, the cause of the hypoxemia differs. After freshwater aspiration by experimental animals, water is absorbed into the circulation and none can be drained from the lungs after 5 min (20). Ventilation-perfusion abnormalities after freshwater aspiration result from the alteration of the surface-tension properties of pulmonary surfactant (21). Damage to surfactant allows the alveoli to become unstable and to collapse, causing absolute right-to-left intrapulmonary shunting of blood and arterial hypoxemia. In addition, areas with low but finite ventilation-to-perfusion ratios coexist and contribute to hypoxemia (22). After seawater aspiration, the hypertonic fluid remains in the alveoli and the volume is further increased by the movement of body fluid into the alveoli because of the osmotic gradient (22, 23). The perfusion of these fluid-filled, unventilated alveoli results in absolute right-to-left intrapulmonary shunting of blood and arterial hypoxemia. Since the amount of pulmonary surfactant is reduced by seawater aspiration but the surface-tension properties of the remaining surfactant are unchanged, there is little relative intrapulmonary shunting (areas with low but finite ventilation-to-perfusion ratios) after seawater aspiration (21). Pulmonary edema is caused by the fluid contained in the lung. In experimental animal studies, 1.5 times more fluid than the volume of seawater aspirated could be drained from the lung 5 min after aspiration (24).

Therapy for the pulmonary injury of near drowning is directed toward the reversal of intrapulmonary shunting (24, 25). After freshwater aspiration, it is necessary to maintain alveolar inflation mechanically until pulmonary surfactant regenerates. Both human case series (6) and experimental animal studies (25, 26) have demonstrated that continuous positive-airway pressure (CPAP) and positive end-expiratory pressure (PEEP) improve ventilation-to-perfusion ratios and, thus, reduce intrapulmonary shunting and improve arterial oxygenation after frewshwater near-drowning. Controlled mechanical ventilation (CMV) with PEEP provided the greatest improvement in intrapulmonary shunting in animals that aspirated fresh water. Spontaneous breathing with CPAP produced similar results, although not as consistently as CMB with PEEP. CMV without PEEP caused little improvement in the same study. CMV with PEEP is seldom necessary for near-drowned humans, because intrapulmonary shunting can usually be reduced satisfactorily with CPAP and, when necessary, intermittent mandatory ventilation (IMV). Although not as yet confirmed in the laboratory, clinical experience suggests that IMV at a rate of two to four breaths per minute may help reinflate alveoli so that CPAP can maintain alveolar inflaction.

After seawater aspiration, CPAP or PEEP improves intrapulmonary shunting by redistributing fluid and reexpanding fluid-filled alveoli (6, 24). Supplemental oxygen alone is generally not beneficial because there is little relative intrapulmonary shunting. Mechanical ventilation is usually unnecessary after seawater aspiration.

Cardiovascular System

Cardiovascular abnormalities found soon after near-drowning include hypotension and arrhythmias and are usually due to hypoxemia and acidosis (6, 20, 23). Studies have shown that near-drowned humans rarely aspirate enough water to cause changes in serum electrolyte concentrations severe enough to affect cardiac function (27). Although water is absorbed into the circulation after freshwater aspiration and lost from the circulation after seawater aspiration, (20, 23, 28, 29), redistribution of body fluids initially serves to maintain intravascular volume. During the course of treatment, most near-drowned patients suffer absolute hypovolemia as a result of fluid loss or relative hypovolemia as a result of the effects of positive-airway pressure on venous return to the heart and so require supplemental fluid therapy to maintain cardiac output. Thus, cardiovascular stability after near-drowning is achieved by the reversal of hypoxemia and acidosis and by the maintenance of intravascular volume.

Other Systems

Central nervous system damage is the major secondary injury after near-drowning, and it is due to cerebral hypoxia and edema (7, 30, 31). Varying degrees of brain damage, ranging from 0% to 21%, have been reported in near-drowned survivors (30-33), and so this matter is extremely important in current investigations on the subject of therapy for victims of near-drowning.

The occurrence of other organ damage after near-drowning is unusual, but reported cases suggest that injury occurring to other systems is usually due to hypoxia and hypotension (7, 34). Multisystem organ failure may also be the consequence of overwhelming infection.

Treatment

The primary goal of therapy must be to provide adequate oxygenation as rapidly as possible. Thus, prompt restoration of ventilation and circulation are the cornerstones of therapy. The victim must be removed from the water as quickly as possible and assessed for evidence of spontaneous ventilation. If none is found, artificial ventilation using the mouth-to-mouth technique should be instituted. After the institution of ventilation, circulation must be evaluated. If a pulse is not palpable, closed chest cardiac massage should be started. The basic technique for cardiopulmonary resuscitation, as described by the American Heart Association (35), is continued until spontaneous ventilation and circulation are restored or until the responsibility has been transferred to a physician in the emergency room.

Occasionally, it is impossible to remove the victim from the water immediately. In such a case, artificial ventilation can be instituted while the victim remains in the water. A technique has been described that provides both artificial ventilation through the utilization of a scuba regulator and closed chest massage (36). Such techniques are difficult to perform, and their effectiveness is difficult to evaluate. Therefore, they should not be used when the victim can be removed from the water.

All near-drowned victims should be taken to a hospital for further evaluation and observation, regardless of the degree to which recovery is successful at the scene of the accident. If the emergency transportation service is capable of providing supplemental oxygen, the victim should receive oxygen in the highest concentration available during transfer. Those victims who continue to suffer cardiopulmonary arrest or who are unconscious at the time of transport should undergo endotracheal intubation for airway protection and for mechanical ventilation with a high inspired oxygen concentration (F_IO_2) whenever the emergency technicians can provide this procedure. Other techniques for advanced life support, such as the monitoring of the electrocardiogram and the establishment of intravenous access and fluid therapy, should be performed whenever possible. Drug therapy, such as the administration of sodium bicarbonate, or cardiac defibrillation can be directed by the physician in charge through radio communication with the emergency technicians.

In the emergency room, any of the previously described procedures that are deemed necessary but have not yet been performed take priority. In addition, the assessment of arterial oxygenation and acid-base status is critical for the determination of further therapy, and so arterial blood must be obtained for the analysis of pH and carbon dioxide ($PaCO_2$) and oxygen (PaO_2) tensions. Supplemental oxygen therapy is continued until analysis of arterial blood-gas tensions indicates that oxygen therapy is no longer needed.

A complete physical examination, with specific attention to the heart, lungs, and central nervous system, must be performed rapidly. Since other life-threatening injuries may have been sustained at the time of the accident, a thorough examination is mandatory. Such possible injuries include decompression sickness and cerebral air embolism in a near-drowned scuba diver or traumatic quadriplegia due to diving in shallow water.

Initial laboratory tests should include a complete blood-cell count, a determination of serum electrolyte concentrations, and urinalysis. The results of these tests are frequently normal, but they provide baseline values and may indicate necessary changes in intravenous fluid therapy. An electrocardiogram should be obtained in order to determine whether arrhythmias or hypoxic myocardial damage are present.

A chest X ray is obtained regardless of the apparent severity of the injury and usually reveals pulmonary edema, infiltrates, or atelectasis (6, 7). However, the X ray should never be used in lieu of arterial blood gas analysis to evaluate the severity of the injury or the results of therapy, because the X ray can appear normal even when arterial hypoxemia is severe. The X ray may be used further to evaluate the position of an endotracheal tube or a central venous catheter or to determine the presence of barotrauma or injuries secondary to closed chest massage.

The patient who is neurologically intact and who has normal arterial blood gases and chest X ray at the time of admission should be observed in the hospital for 12 to 24 hours. If a repeat evaluation shows no evidence of deterioration, he or she may be discharged after the observation. A follow-up evaluation within a few days is recommended.

The patient with mild hypoxemia necessitating low concentrations of supplemental oxygen requires more intense observation, since pulmonary function may deteriorate and hypoxemia may worsen. This patient is best monitored in the emergency room or the intensive care unit. If further deterioration does not occur within 24 hr, the patient may be transferred to the ward for further therapy and may be discharged when supplemental oxygen is no longer needed. In general, arterial blood gases should be normal or nearly so while the patient is breathing room air, the chest X ray should show no evidence of infection, and the patient should be afebrile for at least 24 hr before discharge. Again, follow-up evaluation within several days is recommended.

The patient with central nervous system damage or moderate-to-severe hypoxemia requires prompt admission to an intensive care unit for invasive monitoring and intensive respiratory support. Aggressive respiratory therapy begins in the emergency room and continues in the intensive care unit.

CPAP is the therapy of choice for reducing intrapulmonary shunting and improving arterial oxygenation after near-drowning (6, 24, 25). If the patient is alert and cooperative and does not require mechanical ventilation to maintain normocarbia, up to 12 torr of CPAP can be applied through a tight-fitting anesthesia mask. If the patient is unconscious or requires mechanical ventilation or greater than 12 torr of CPAP, endotracheal intubation is necessary. The CPAP is increased in increments of 2 to 5 torr, and respiratory rate and arterial oxygenation or intrapulmonary shunting (Qsp/Qt) are monitored with each increment. Appropriate levels of CPAP result in normalization of the respiratory rate, improvement in PaO_2, and reduction in Qsp/Qt (37). As the PaO_2 improves, the F_IO_2 should be reduced to 0.4 or less in order to avoid absorption atelectasis and the toxic effects of oxygen. An F_IO_2 of 0.3 or less allows for the evaluation of any relative intrapulmonary shunting that may be present (38). Once the patient has stabilized, CPAP is gradually reduced in decrements of 1 to 2 torr and PaO_2 or Osp/Qt is monitored frequently for evidence of deterioration. If PaO_2 decreases or Qsp/Qt increases after a reduction in CPAP, the previous level of CPAP is still necessary.

When a high level of CPAP is required, it must not be interrupted unless absolutely necessary, because pulmonary edema may recur within seconds and the resulting hypoxemia may persist for some time after CPAP is reinstituted. Therefore, suctioning is not performed routinely and is only allowed when essential for airway patency.

CMV is rarely needed for near-drowned humans. If the patient has inadequate alveolar ventilation, the addition of IMV allows the patient to continue to breathe spontaneously while receiving only the number of mechanical breaths necessary to normalize arterial pH (39). The use of IMV allows for better venous return to the heart because intrathoracic pressure is less than when CMV is used and because spontaneous ventilation facilitates venous return as well as better matching of ventilation and perfusion. Although not proven in a controlled fashion, the addition of 2 to 4 IMV breaths per minute may improve arterial oxygenation at a given level of CPAP by reinflating collapsed alveoli that may then remain inflated by CPAP.

Standard monitoring in the intensive care unit includes continuous monitoring of the electrocardiogram and frequent observation of blood pressure, respiratory rate, temperature, and urinary output. Many near-drowned patients also require invasive hemodynamic monitoring for optimal therapy. An indwelling arterial catheter allows constant observation of blood pressure and provides access for repeated sampling of arterial blood. The placement of a balloon-tipped thermodilution pulmonary artery (Swan Ganz) catheter facilitates the treatment of patients who are unstable or who require relatively high levels of CPAP by allowing the measurement of cardiac output and central venous, pulmonary arterial, and pulmonary arterial occlusion pressures (of which the latter reflects left-heart filling pressure) and the calculation of systemic and pulmonary vascular resistances and Qsp/Qt. Through the use of such information, the effects of changes in CPAP on Qsp/Qt and cardiac output can be evaluated. Since many near-drowned patients are hypovolemic and since CPAP reduces venous return to the heart, fluid therapy is also guided by the information obtained from the pulmonary arterial catheter.

Although many victims of near drowning aspirate substances other than water, few suffer pulmonary infection (6). For this reason, prophylactic antibiotic therapy is not recommended. Still, near-drowned patients should be carefully observed for evidence of infection, such as fever, increased white blood cell count, a new infiltrate on the chest X ray, or deterioration of PaO_2. If pulmonary infection develops, it frequently is evident 24 to 48 hr after injury, and therapeutic antibiotics are instituted at that time. Frequent gram stains and sputum cultures facilitate the appropriate choice of antibiotics.

All victims of near drowning should receive aggressive therapy regardless of their apparent neurological status at the time of admission, since numerous patients with marked neurological deficits have recovered with normal function. Methods for cerebral resuscitation should be determined by local standards. Current investigations may soon provide insight into the risks and benefits of techniques for cerebral resuscitation.

Summary

When resuscitation is prompt and therapy aggressive, the rate of survival after near-drowning is excellent (31). The primary injury to the lung results in hypoxemia. Any other organ damage that occurs is usually due to hypoxia, and so the reversal of the pulmonary lesion is paramount in therapy. Specific measures for the maintenance of cardiovascular stability or cerebral resuscitation may be necessary. Although infection is uncommon, unrecognized infection may result in death and so the possibility must be constantly considered.

References

1. Vital Statistics of the United States, vol. 2, Mortality, Part A, pp. 1-245. U.S. Department of Health and Human Services. Hyattsville, Md., National Center for Health Statistics, 1980.
2. Schuman SH, Rowe JR, Glazer HM, Redding JS: The iceberg phenomenon of near drowning. Crit Care Med *4*:127-128, 1976.
3. Modell JH: Pathophysiology and Treatment of Drowning and Near-Drowning. Springfield, Ill., Charles C. Thomas, 1971.
4. Webster's Eighth New Collegiate Dictionary. Springfield, Mass., G. and C. Merriam Company, 1980.
5. Cot C: Les Asphyxies Accidentelles (submersion, electrocution, intoxication, oxycarbonique) Etude clinique, therapeutique, et preventive. Editions medicales N. Paris, Maloine, 1931.
6. Modell JH, Graves SA, Ketover A: Clinical course of 91 consecutive near-drowning victims. Chest *70*:231-238, 1976.
7. Fuller RH: The 1962 Wellcome prize essay: Drowning and the postimmersion syndrome: A clinocopathologic study. Milit Med *128*:22-36, 1963.
8. Modell JH, Kuck EJ, Ruiz BC, Heinitsch H: Effect of intravenous vs. aspirated distilled water on serum electrolytes and blood gas tensions. Jour Appl Physiol *32*:579-584, 1972.
9. Fleetham JA, Munt PW: Near-drowning in Canadian waters. Can Med Assoc Jour *68*: 914-917, 1978.
10. Conn AW, Edmonds JF, Barker GA: Near-drowning in cold fresh water: Current treatment regimen. Can Anaesth Soc Jour *25*:259-265, 1978.
11. Siebke H, Breivek H, Rod T, Lind B: Survival after 40 minutes' submersion without cerebral sequelae. Lancet *1*:1275-1277, 1975.
12. Gooden BA: Drowning and the diving reflex in man. Med Jour Aust *2*:583-587, 1972.
13. Hunt PK: Effect and treatment of the "diving reflex." Can Med Assoc Jour *111*:1330-1331, 1974.
14. Campbell LB, Gooden BA, Horowitz JD: Cardiovascular responses to partial and total immersion in man. Jour Physiol *202*:239-250, 1969.
15. Craig AB, Jr: Causes of loss of consciousness during underwater swimming. Jour Appl Physiol *16*:583-586, 1961.
16. Modell JH, Gaub M, Moya F, Vestal B, Swartz H: Physiologic effects of near drowning with chlorinated fresh water, distilled water and isotonic saline. Anesthesiology *27*:33-41, 1966.
17. Fandel I, Bancalari E: Near-drowning in children: Clinical aspects. Pediatrics *58*:573-579, 1976.
18. Orlowski JP: Prognostic factors in pediatric cases of drowning and near-drowning. Jour Amer Coll Emer Phys *8*:176-179, 1979.

19. Kruus S, Bergstrom L, Suutarinen T, Hyvonen R: The prognosis of near-drowned children. Acta Paediatr Scand *68*:315-322, 1979.
20. Modell JH, Moya F: Effects of volume of aspirated fluid during chlorinated fresh water drowning. Anesthesiology *27*:662-672, 1966.
21. Giammona ST, Modell JH: Drowning by total immersion: Effects on pulmonary surfactant of distilled water, isotonic saline, and sea water. Amer Jour Dis Child *114*:612-616, 1967.
22. Modell JH, Moya F, Williams HD, Weibley TC: Changes in blood gases and A-aDO2 during near-drowning. Anesthesiology *29*:456-465, 1968.
23. Modell JH, Moya F, Newby EJ, Ruiz BC, Showers AV: The effects of fluid volume in seawater drowning. Ann Intern Med *67*:68-80, 1967.
24. Modell JH, Calderwood HW, Ruiz BC, Downs JB, Chapman R: Effects of ventilatory patterns on arterial oxygenation after near-drowning in sea water. Anesthesiology *40*: 376-384, 1974.
25. Bergquist RE, Vogelhut MM, Modell JH, Sloan SJ, Ruiz BC: Comparison of ventilatory patterns in the treatment of freshwater near-drowning in dogs. Anesthesiology *52*:142-148, 1980.
26. Ruiz BC, Calderwood HW, Modell JH, Brogdon JE: Effect of ventilatory patterns on arterial oxygenation after near-drowning with fresh water: A comparative study in dogs. Anesth Analg *52*:570-576, 1973.
27. Modell JH, Davis JH: Electrolyte changes in human drowning victims. Anesthesiology *30*:414-420, 1969.
28. Swann HG, Brucer M: The cardiorespiratory and biochemical events during rapid anoxic death: VI. Freshwater and sea water drowning. Texas Rep Biol Med 7:604-618, 1949.
29. Swann HG, Brucer M, Moore C, Vezien BL: Freshwater and sea water drowning: A study of the terminal cardiac and biochemical events. Texas Rep Biol Med *5*:423-437, 1947.
30. Conn AW, Montes JE, Barker GA, Edmonds JF: Cerebral "salvage" in near-drowning following neurological classification. Can Anaesth Soc Jour *27*:201-210, 1980.
31. Modell JH, Graves SA, Kuck EJ: Near-drowning: Correlation of level of consciousness and survival. Can Anaesth Soc Jour *27*:211-215, 1980.
32. Pearn JH, Bart RD, Jr, Yamaoka R: Neurologic sequelae after childhood near-drowning: A total population study from Hawaii. Pediatrics *64*:187-191, 1979.
33. Peterson B: Morbidity of childhood near-drowning. Pediatrics *59*:364-370, 1977.
34. Fuller RH: The clinical pathology of human near-drowning. Proc Roy Soc Med *56*:33-38, 1963.
35. American Heart Association: Standards and guidelines for cardiopulmonary resuscitation (CPR) and emergency cardiac care (ECC). Jour Amer Med Assoc *244*:453-512, 1980.
36. March NF, Matthews RC: New techniques in external cardiac compressions: Aquatic cardiopulmonary resuscitation. Jour Amer Med Assoc *244*:1229-1232, 1980.
37. Downs JB, Klein EF, Jr, Modell JH: The effect of incremental PEEP on PaO_2 in patients with respiratory failure. Anesth Analg *52*:210-215, 1973.
38. Douglas ME, Downs JB, Dannemiller FJ, Hodges MR, Munson ES: Change in pulmonary venous admixture with varying inspired oxygen. Anesth Analg *55*:688-695, 1976.
39. Downs JB, Modell JH: Patterns of respiratory support aimed at pathophysiologic conditions. ASA Refresher Courses in Anesthesiology 5:71-85, 1977.

Additional Commentary on Hypothermia

APPENDIX A

Urban Hypothermia in the United Kingdom

K. J. Collins, M.B., B.S., D.Phil.

The problem of hypothermia in the elderly, which has been particularly well reviewed in this volume by Dr. Keith Cooper, is one that has become increasingly familiar in the United Kingdom since the early 1960s, when population studies on the prevalence of urban hypothermia first gave rise to serious concern (1). Claims were made at that time that there were possibly more than 20,000 deaths from hypothermia annually and that many elderly bedridden people died in their homes without the condition having been diagnosed. Though these figures can now be disputed on the grounds that the earlier surveys were not national or random and had mostly relied on oral temperature measurements, there is still no satisfactory answer to the problem of accurately estimating the prevalence of urban hypothermia. One of the main difficulties comes in drawing conclusions from statistics on the incidence of low deep-body temperatures in the elderly and on mortality due to hypothermia registered on death certificates. The Registrar General's returns from 1970 to 1978 show that the number of certificates that register hypothermia as a cause of death has remained constant in spite of the increasing publicity about and awareness of the condition and the widespread use in the United Kingdom of low-reading clinical thermometers.

The failure to maintain the constancy of the internal environment and of thermostasis is implicit in the act of dying, and so it may be impossible to distinguish between the primary and secondary roles of environmentally induced low deep-body temperature and existing disease. It is not surprising, therefore, that "pressure groups" find it difficult to reconcile the Registrar General's statistics (in 1978 a total of 708 death certificates mentioned hypothermia, of which only 21 registered hypothermia as an underlying cause) with the findings of the 1972 national survey (2) that 0.5% of the elderly sample (30,000 people when projected on a national scale) had a deep-body (urine) temperature of 35.0°C or below. It is often not appreciated that the description of urban hypothermia in the 1972 national survey in the elderly embodied three important caveats: (a) that hypothermia was identified only in morning measurements and that no one was hypothermic in the afternoon, (b) that the lowest urine temperature in the total sample of 2,000 was 34.2°C, and (c) that the authors advised against making firm projections of hypothermia for the population as a whole.

The incidence of hypothermia in the elderly, as pointed out by Dr. Cooper, appears to be higher in the United Kingdom than in other countries. This may be due to the fact that special attention is focused on the incidence and prevention of hypothermia in the elderly in the United Kingdom during the winter months, but it may also be a reflection of the traditional old and cold housing stock in the country. It is of relevance that recorded monthly deaths in the United Kingdom show a close association between death rates and external temperature for most diseases (particularly myocardial infarction, stroke, and pneumonia) and that this association is stronger in the elderly (3). Low indoor ambient temperatures may well play a part in increased mortality, but the causal relationship has not been established. Acute changes in ambient temperature within a day or between days are not, however, associated with significant changes in national mortality figures. Two or more days of temperature change are required, and it seems clear that longer-term (1 wk or more) temperature changes are much more important. Information from Scandinavia and Canada, where winter temperatures are very much lower than in the United Kingdom, suggest that deaths caused from being cold indoors are practically unknown. In Toronto it is claimed that there is no increase in winter death rates because of Toronto's well-built and warm houses.

If contributory medical disorders for the most part determine the prognosis in patients with hypothermia, then it would appear that secondary hypothermia as the result of disease is likely to be underdiagnosed in the elderly and may not be registered on death certificates. In order to help clarify the notification of hypothermia, a simple general classification can be suggested: *primary* hypothermia due to an inherent impairment or dysfunction of the thermoregulatory system: this would apply, for example, to the failure of thermoregulatory processes in some elderly people and to immature development of these processes in the premature infant; *secondary* hypothermia associated with medical conditions predisposing to modifications in temperature regulation, including drug abuse and the effects of alcohol; *accidental* hypothermia in which the condition occurs unintentionally in a healthy individual at any age as the direct result of cold exposure; and *therapeutic* (artificial) hypothermia induced for clinical or surgical purposes.

References

1. Collins KJ, Exton-Smith AN: Urban hypothermia: Thermoregulation, thermal perception and thermal comfort in the elderly. *In*: Adam JM (ed.), Hypothermia: Ashore and Afloat, pp, 158-176. (Proceedings of the 1979 Conference on Disasters Caused by Cold) Aberdeen, Aberdeen University Press, 1981.
2. Fox RH, Woodward PM, Exton-Smith AN, Green MF, Donnison DV, Wicks MH: Body temperatures in the elderly: A national study of physiological, social and environmental conditions. Brit Med Jour *1*:200-206, 1973.
3. Bull GM, Morton J: Environment, temperature and death rates. Age and Ageing 7:210, 224, 1978.

APPENDIX B

Discussion

Monday A.M., June 1 (Drs. Hayward, Paton, and Lilja)

Q. The level of potassium in the last patient was 3.5 meq/L? Could you comment on potassium in some of your cold patients and what you've done about it?

A. Dr. Lilja: The problem with hypokalemia certainly is seen in these patients, but by in large we have not done a lot. One of the advantages of putting them on bypass is that we can start giving the potassium slowly and maintain their blood pressure through utilizing the pump. But by in large I don't think we've done anything particular in terms of trying to rapidly correct either hypo- or hyperkalemia, and I would certainly be interested in what other people have attempted, but we just have not done anything too rapidly. Maybe Dr. Paton could comment.

A. Dr. Paton: I would agree, and I would think that 3.5 meq/L is in the dangerous zone. I would think that anywhere between 3.5 or 5.0 or 5.2 meq/L is probably not going to be all that dangerous.

Q. I'm a physician's assistant. I am concerned about the fact that everyone is talking about the acute effects and treatment, but it seems apparent that there can be some long-term problems with neurologic deficits following severe acute hypothermia. Could you comment on that please?

A. Dr. Lilja: I agree that this is one of the real problems that we have, not only in treatment of hypothermia, but in all the patients that we have to resuscitate that are profoundly ill. Oftentimes, because of hypoxia or other reasons, they end up with a long-term neurologic deficit. I'm not sure what the answer is, quite honestly. Because a number of these patients do make good recoveries, I think it behooves us to try to resuscitate them. I really don't have an answer though, and I don't think that at this time we are in a position to predict which patients will do well and which patients won't. Hopefully, with more research in the area we may be able to develop some predictive factors so we can tell early on who we should work on and who we shouldn't. But I at least am not aware of any good prognostic indicators in eventual neurological outcome at this time.

A. Dr. Paton: And I don't think that even if we went to the extent of monitoring the patient with an EEG, assuming that you were in sophisticated surroundings, that would help you because as the patient gets colder, the EEG flattens out too, so that doesn't help you and you can also get peripheral neurologic defects which, I think, are sometimes ignored or are thought to be due to frostbite or whatever. Early in the days of hypothermia for cardiac surgery, it was recognized that, if adults were immersed for about an hour or so, a number of them developed peripheral neurologic defects in their hands and their feet. And it was then that the peripheral temperatures started to be measured in our institution and it was found that, if you had a peripheral temperature of skin or subcutaneous tissue of 3 or 4°C for more than about 45 min, there was significant incidence of peripheral neurologic defect, some of which recovered given time, so there are not only central defects, but there are peripheral defects which you should look for.

Q. Diathermy was not mentioned. Can that be used in raising core temperature?

A. Dr. Paton: Yes, it can be used. There has been a fairly extensive use of that technique in the operating room. However, it has some dangers, and the greatest being burns. If the coils are not wrapped around the patient very carefully and very carefully insulated from the patient, you can get terrible burns, so that while it is a fairly effective means of warming somebody up it is also, I think, a potentially dangerous method. And I think it is worth mentioning that all hypothermic patients are very easily burned and that's why the ranges of external warming which you should use are limited.

Q. I have a couple of questions. First one is for Dr. Paton. You mentioned the use of digitalis for the patient with pulmonary edema.

We haven't used digitalis in our emergency room and I'm wondering about problems with digitalis toxicity. It seems to me that this is a good setting for problems with digitalis and there are other, it seems to me probably safer methods to treat pulmonary edema. I was wondering if other people have had experience with digitalis toxicity in this setting.

A. Dr. Paton: Not that I'm aware of. I would think that the metabolic breakdown rate is going to be slower, but in terms of the number of hours that you will be treating the hypothermia patient I'm not sure how important that is going to be. But I would certainly use digitalis in smaller doses than you would in an uthermic patient. But I think, in general, the indications for using digitalis are probably going to be the same, but I would use smaller doses and probably space the doses wider apart if the person remains hypothermic.

Q. OK, I have another question for Dr. Lilja. Have you ever used warm blood in treating hypothermia patients who were severely anemic?

A. Dr. Lilja: No, we haven't and I don't think that we really would. We just use warm fluids. I think that the only indication for giving blood that I would use would be if the patient had a concomitant hemorrhage of some kind and we were having to keep up with blood loss. I would not use it just for anemia though.

Q. Dr. Paton, on your slides, I noticed that your patients with sinus bradycardia and your patients with bradycardia and normal sinus rhythm combined had the highest mortality. Your patients with sinus tachycardia had literally none. Are there any advantages of implanting a temporary pacemaker as long as you're probably putting in a Swan-Ganze or something? Has this ever been done to convert the slower rhythms to a tachycardia?

A. Dr. Paton: I wouldn't advise that for this reason: that the cardiac output of a paced heart is not nearly as good as the cardiac output of a slower heart that's unpaced. And so, I think that if you really want to set into some sophisticated investigation of this, you would have to measure cardiac output, because I don't think either heart rate or blood pressure is the critical factor. What you're really interested in is how much that heart is putting out.

Q. Does Dr. Lilja have any views as to where these patients should be treated, particularly those with moderate or severe hypothermia?

Should they be taken to the nearest medical facility, maybe a local, small community hospital, or does he feel that the benefits of being transferred to a tertiary care unit where cardiopulmonary bypass and invasive monitoring are more freely available?

A. Dr. Lilja: I think that's a rather difficult question, a loaded question as a matter of fact, but I think the majority of hypothermic patients probably can be managed safely and effectively at a local hospital because I think most of the warming techniques available can be utilized there (other than bypass). I think the only real advantage of bypass would be in the arrested patient. Now whether the risk of transportation is greater than using peritoneal lavage at the local hospital, certainly we've had a couple instances that I know of, one or two very recently in this area, where patients in cardiac arrest were treated very successfully at small hospitals near Duluth with good results. And I think it is more important if you know how to manage fluids and can adequately monitor the cardiac output or at least get an idea of what is going on. I think that this is probably more important than the means that you utilize for rewarming. I think that if bypass is available then obviously that is the way to go, but I don't know if I would transport long distances.

Q. I would like to ask a question of Dr. Hayward. I have no personal experience at all with these survival suits that you showed, but it did cross my mind that maybe these are things that could be useful for mountain rescue teams or paramedic teams in areas as an insulating mechanism for the hypothermic victim. Do you have any experience? Do you think it would be good?

A. Dr. Hayward: Well, I think it is a good idea. It is certainly a convenient insulative system that could be superior to sleeping bags and blankets when you were in a cold, wet situation where many of the usual devices can lose their insulating effectiveness. A problem would be getting an unconscious victim into such a suit, especially when gentle handling is required. In response to one of the other points you made about survival suits, I feel that one of the features of survival suits that needs improvement in the future is face protection. There are a number of examples of people who have floated around in cold water with potential hypothermia survival time of many, many hours, yet who seem to have died in short periods of time, particularly in choppy or very rough water. My experience with lying in these suits is that after a short time it becomes very difficult to keep water out of the airway.

So, I think that some type of face shield would be an important addition to a survival suit in order that its thermal protection potential can be realized.

Q. While I have the microphone, I wanted to ask my colleagues a question too that relates to CPR. It seems that they both suggested that CPR, in a prehospital care situation for the hypothermic patient that's arrested, should be provided. I wanted to ask do you have any advice as to whether or not CPR should be maintained, and the normal procedures used for uthermic people. That is, would you maintain a rate that is normal; is there any evidence or suggestion that the procedure should be amended at all in terms of rate or force for hypothermic patients?

A. Dr. Paton: My answer to that would be I think you should use the normally prescribed rate. The implication behind your question is that because the person is hypothermic and their oxygen requirement is not as great that therefore they're protected to some extent and that therefore they don't need quite the same cardiac output. And this is a theory that is being put forward. The reason I would disagree with that is that the cardiac output that you can achieve with CPR is so lousy in the first place that you've got to take advantage of every little bit of cardiac output that you can generate, and I would strongly advise that you not modify the rate of CPR in accordance with the temperature because that's implying that you're really clever and that you can figure out how slow to do it in relation to the reduced oxygen demand and I don't think that we are that clever. We should give the patient the advantage of whatever cardiac output that we can give them.

A. Lilja: I'll agree.

Q. I have, in fact, three questions. One for each of the speakers, if I may. Dr. Hayward, first of all. You talked about the difference between the cooling rates of juveniles and adults. Is there any evidence of differences of cooling rates with increasing age after adulthood is reached?

A. Dr. Hayward: Not that I've been involved with elderly hypothermia. I would very much like to study that question to compare basic thermoregulatory responses of the elderly with the data we presently have. We've only used subjects up to the age of about 52 or 53 yr in our studies. Up to that age, we have not seen significant differences in cooling rates that we can ascribe to any age-induced alterations in vasoconstriction or shivering thermogenesis. The only effect has been through age-related differences in fatness. Middle-age adults tend to have more fat than university students and consequent slower cooling rates. I would very much like to obtain approval from our Human Subjects Committee to be able to study people in the 65-to-75 yr age-group. We need better understanding of their basic thermoregulatory performance.

Q. The second question which is directed to Dr. Paton and also relates to the age problem. I noticed that in defining the arrhythmia present on admission to his hospital you have seen in five out of the seven patients, as I recall, in asystole as opposed to ventricular fibrillation. Now, it so happened that all of these five were in age 12 and under, and I wondered if in fact this is not telling us something about the incidence of ventricular fibrillation in larger hearts, which would fit with the physiology of hypothermia and stress.

A. Dr. Paton: Those figures were actually taken from the literature and that struck me also that it may be related, and it is certainly true that in the operating room, as you cool down kids with congenital heart disease, the usual sequence of events is just to become slower and slower and slower and so into asystole and when they've rewarmed just to reverse it, whereas with the adults the usual sequence of events is to go from a relatively slow rate into ventricular fibrillation.

Q. The last, in fact, is two small questions, to Dr. Lilja. The first comment that he made, I think referred to advice about pre-hospital management and this question of CPR when you see ventricular fibrillation or asystole in the cold situation. Now, in my experience of doing ECGs in such patients one of the big problems is actually telling whether a patient has ventricular fibrillation as opposed to having interference due to shivering in sinus rhythm. Comment about that, because that is a very important practical issue and perhaps you can solve that one for us.

A. Dr. Lilja: I think again the one thing that we have to keep in mind is that as clinicians I think you have to pay attention to the rest of the patient and if they're breathing I guess you would assume that they are not in ventricular fibrillation; if they're not breathing, on the other hand, and you cannot feel a pulse, then I think you can assume ventricular fibrillation now. In the awake, shivering patient, generally I don't think that's a problem. . . . I wouldn't even worry about the cardiac function that much, if they are awake enough so that they're shivering. If they're profoundly hypothermic and not shivering, whether or not you're seeing ventricular fibrillation, asystole, or heart attack, if they're not breathing and you can't feel a pulse, I don't think that it makes a big difference. I would go ahead and do CPR.

Q. I think what I was really trying to provoke you into saying is that in the situation, which you described as a nice cut-and-dried issue, prehospital attaching ECG leads and trying to make any interpretation on the basis of that outside the hospital must be almost impossible.

A. Dr. Lilja: I think that in the shivering patient, you are right, and you can't do it. There's just too much interference from the shivering and the ECG is almost worthless.

Q. The second question relates to the evidence that you have for the efficacy of interperitoneal lavage rewarming. Have you in fact any real evidence that to add this to the other techniques that you used significantly changes things? The only evidence that I know of in the literature is the study by Leon Ames, who showed the rewarming rates using interperitoneal lavage were no better than external surface rewarming in the patient who is otherwise being properly treated.

A. Dr. Lilja: We have not done in humans a comparison between external and the peritoneal lavage. There was a recent paper presented a few weeks ago in San Antonio that would indicate that peritoneal lavage does significantly increase the core temperature. Whether that is any faster than suface rewarming I really don't think there is good evidence. I agree with you. I do think, however, that peritoneal lavage may help in combination with other modalities to increase the rate even more. And the other thing which I think is very important is that it is a diagnostic test, and I think that if you don't know what's going on with these patients I do think it should be done for diagnostic purposes as well. And since you have the catheter in there you might as well keep running the warm fluid in and the cold out, I guess. I can't see that it's going to increase your morbidity at all.

R. Well, I would take issue on that point. The advantages are there as you describe, and that's a very useful pointer, but particularly if you're going to persist with peritoneal lavage there's no doubt that you will produce stasis more quickly than you would simply because in the very patient who's got a reason for hypoventilation and alveolar collapse you're adding another factor which is restricting diaphramatic movement and that will undoubtedly increase, as we know from peritoneal lavage for other reasons, the risk of respiratory problems.

Q. This is to Dr. Lilja and Dr. Hayward. You mentioned in the blood workup of patients when they initially presented in the emergency room you get CPK and then CPK isoenzymes on patients. I'm interested if you could summarize your experience with that. The reason I'm raising the question is we've retrospectively looked at about 51 patients that came to our emergency room and noticed that patients with high CPKs seem to do better in terms of survival and we postulated that maybe these are people who are "better shiverers." And to Dr. Hayward I wonder if you have ever looked at CPK in normal subjects and seen if in fact people who warm up more quickly have higher muscle, not heart, but muscle CPK isoenzyme levels.

A. Dr. Lilja: I must admit that I haven't looked at our data in that regard. I really can't give you a good answer. It's something that we'll have to do.

A. Dr. Hayward: I have not measured CPK.

Q. Dr. Paton, I have a little kind of problem with your right recommendation on CPR for a couple of reasons. I think it's pretty well accepted that CO_2 production is halved with every 8°C drop in core temperature. Thus, unless you can adjust the fixed inspirator CO_2 to maintain normcapnia in a patient who is hyperventilating, I think you're going to clinically see hypocapnia in its undesirable sequelae if you're going to ventilate with 100% oxygen. If you have carbon available, I could see going at normal rates.

A. Dr. Paton: I think that the question was related to the speed with which external cardiac massage was done. I don't think it was directed towards ventilation.

Q. I think there are some references that suggest that half-normal rate in compressions also might be desirable, but I didn't want to get into that. But separating that out from the respiratory recommendation, what would your respiratory recommendation be?

A. Dr. Paton: I thought that I made it clear that my recommendation is not to hyperventilate people but to keep the ventilatory rate down.

Q. But if you're going at 5 to 1 or 15 to 2, which is the normal thermic recommendation, I would think that that would be hyperventilating the hypothermic patient using 100% oxygen.

A. Dr. Paton: I can't argue with you one way or the other because I have no data to go on, but that's what I said. I think that if you try and intellectually adjust your rates without having any specific data to go on, I think you're going to end up trying to be more clever than you actually are. Now, this is the advantage, of course, of having an arterial line in and taking acid-base measurements and then you modify what you're going to do according to your measurements. But in terms of the rate of external massage, I would stick to my guns that I wouldn't reduce that rate at all, for the reasons that I gave.

Q. But as a practical point for prehospital personnel with no blood gases?

A. Dr. Paton: I'd tell them to go on including the ventilation because I don't think the sort of ventilation that you're going to get will result in hyperventilation. I would tell them to go at the normal rate.

Monday P.M., June 1 (Drs. Conn, Young, and Hernández)

Q. The question to you, sir, is related to the comment that you made about the effects of hypothermia at 30° or below on the immune system, and I think you just gave us a comment that you've felt that there was some evidence which suggested that at that temperature the immune mechanism was depressed. I wonder if you would care to amplify that statement.

A. Dr. Conn: I have information on this subject which I have yet to read in depth. I believe that some people when exposed to acute hypothermia have this immune response with a formation of immunocomplex which makes the white cells diapedesis and come out of the circulation. Now that is said to occur not only with hypothermia, but with severe acidosis, asepsis, and sometimes with any type of stress. This is the work of H. S. Jacob [JCI: *60*: 260, 1977] and he has been writing on this now for 7 yr. Nobody asked me this, but I wonder why nobody wanted to know whether we used Dacadron® for brain swelling. We did for 5 or 6 yr even though it's reported to work only on brain tumors and brain abscesses. The neutropenia has been observed after we stopped using decadron and perhaps we were masking this effect from cold-water drowning. I have many more questions myself than I have answers, and I really can't tell you much more except we're studying this with our pathology department right now.

Q. Would you summarize again for me the factors that make a healthy newborn at risk for hypothermia, and a premature baby? Could you go over that again? What are the factors that make kids at risk? If we took a kid and put him in a cold environment, what are the things that would make them more at risk than a normal adult? For both healthy and premature kids?

A. Dr. Young: This is a question of considerable importance. For example, children who are brought in by helicopter frequently arrive with a considerable degree of cold injury. It is important to remember that the full-term infant, at 37°C, should be completely capable of maintaining his own body temperature when fully clothed. The premature infant is at greater risk of developing hypothermia either acutely or chronically because his surface-volume ratio is greater than that of the full-term infant. Secondly, he has smaller amounts of body fat with very thin skin. Finally, acidosis, peripheral vasoconstriction, infections, and other types of drugs may lower their resistance to hypothermia. These are the major risk factors which affect the premature infant.

Q. I would like to ask Dr. Conn what success he's had treating disseminated intravascular coagulation [DIC] in those children with severe multiorgan failure that have been drowned.

A. Dr. Conn: None. We start to correct DIC by the usual methods, but it hasn't made any difference. If they have DIC, it's a pretty serious prognostic factor.

Q. We recently had a patient that we could correct the DIC with the usual things—fibrogen, a replacement with the cryoprecipitate, fresh-plasma platelets, but we found out we could not correct the DIC until we got the temperature up around 32°C. Between 28 and 30°C we were not successful. I wondered if anyone else has had a similar experience.

A. Dr. Conn: Very interesting, because that's quite new to me. . . . I'm very interested in that.

Q. Dr. Conn, in your Reye's syndrome study, you use a lot of ventricular catheters to control the ICP [intracranial pressure], but you're using bolts for your drowners, category C3.

A. Dr. Conn: There are two problems. That statement is we have used intraventricular catheters, but very rarely in Reye's syndrome and the reason is the Reye's brain swelling occurs so rapidly that when you do a quick CAT scan prior to being sure that the brain is swollen there is no ventricle to put an intraventricular drain in. We've used the intraventricular drains primarily under the age of 6 mo because the thickness of the skull is too small to hold a Richmond bolt. There are good points and bad points of an intraventricular drain. One is that it is very simple for you or the nurse to let off a quarter or a half a CC and watch the ICP come down. Anyone [who] can do this instantaneously relieves any wave or pressure, and that's easy to insert if the brain isn't already swollen. The problem is that the neurosurgeons in particular are very concerned about a foreign body in the ventricle for more than 2 or 3 days, because they develop a ventriculitis and cerebritis that may be worse than the disease. Therefore, we have limited ourselves primarily to a bolt for the initial measurements of intracranial pressure.

Q. I also have a question for Dr. Young. Your three patients who died all died with signs of cerebral edema. In your series and in your other series that you reported on, all of which had a poor outcome who required CPR on arrival—were any particular measures taken to control cerebral edema with these patients?

A. Dr. Young: Three of the four children whom we reported in our article on hypothermia and drowning had measurements of their intracranial pressure (ICP). The first boy, a survivor, did not develop increased ICP; the second child did have evidence of a swollen brain on postmortem examination, although his Richmond bolt failed to document this. There are many theories about why the intracranial bolt may fail to accurately measure ICP. First, the intracranial bolt samples a very small area of the brain. Second, the brain, which has the consistency of firm pudding, may herniate into the bolt and prevent accurate measurement. Although the direct measurement of ICP has been a very useful technique, there are many associated mechanical problems. The third child did not have an intracranial monitoring device. The fourth child had malignant intracranial pressure, which we treated unsuccessfully with hypothermia, hyperventilation, and diuretics. We were completely unable to control the increased intracranial pressure.

A. Dr. Conn: I think I'd have to agree with those comments. I've suggested that the insertion of a bolt very simple, and then simply we don't believe in epidural or extradural bolts because of the low dural compliance. And when I talk about putting a bolt in there's always a nick made through the dura at the time, so there's direct continuity of CSF through to the fluid in your conducting tubing. But I can also agree we've great difficulties at times. We have had as many as three bolts in one patient trying to decide which one was reading correctly, and you can be grossly misled if there is a wedge of brain tissue in the lumen of the Richmond bolt. So you're quite right. But without it you really don't know what's going on, and we found that after losing a drowned child, after 2 days of HYPER, he woke up and then became comatose and died. From then on, we put bolts in everybody.

Q. For Dr. Conn, I'd like to go back to the treatment of the immune suppressant or the C 5 problem. You mentioned that you weren't using Decadron® or used to use decadron and then stopped, and I believe in one of your case histories I noticed that you said you stopped giving Solumedrol®. Are you now routinely using methylprednisolone in the treatment of these patients?

A. Dr. Conn: We are studying it. We have considered using 30 mg per kilo of methylprednisolone. We use it. . . . The problem that you're stuck with, basically, is this: you have a study going on where blood samples are being taken all the time and we're looking for C 5. It takes us 48 to 72 hr to get the answer at the present time. Some units can get it within an hour and know as that starts to go up before your white cells fall that you can inject a large dose of methylprednisolone; so we're working blindly. That's what we've been doing within at least 8 to 12 hr. But it's only been used on two or three cases. It's very recent. Prior to that we had stopped using Decadron® because of the problem of infection 2 or 3 days down the road and stress ulcers, and it didn't seem to make any difference and theoretically it shouldn't make any difference to actual brain swelling of this type. But we may have been hiding the development of subsequent neutropenia.

Q. If I may, I would just like to ask Dr. Conn what are his thoughts about the conclusions of Kruse in Finland that a low temperature correlated positively with a poor outcome, at least as far as his 30 patients were concerned.

A. Dr. Conn: I don't think you can draw conclusions from that. I know, in fact I'm going to be seeing him next week, that his brain incidence overall results were something like 21%, if I remember his series of last year, and the problem is that we're trying to combine apples and lemons and everything else. My first thought would be that the lack of correlation between severe hypothermia and successful results was simply that they were in the cold too long, and the second point may be whether they've offered any kind of CPR courses for their ambulance people.

C. I'd like to make a comment in relation to some remarks that Dr. Young made about the differences or similarities, whichever way you look at it, between what we do in the operating room with children and what occurs with accidents. And there's one major difference which is not being commented on and that is the child in the operating room is totally heparinized and the blood is completely incapable of clotting. And I think that is a very important consideration probably in the possible development of both cerebral damage and damage to the myocardium. I think we'd have massive myocardial infarcts in the people whose hearts are stopped for 3 hr if they were not herparinized to the point that their blood is totally incoagulable.

Q. I would like to ask both Dr. Young and Dr. Conn if there's any evidence histologically that some of the damage that occurs in these children is related to intravascular coagulation on a microscopic level. I don't mean gross coagulation but diffuse microscopic coagulation.

A. Dr. Young: Many of these children at postmortem examination have "respirator" brain; that is, the brain has become necrotic and it is not possible to recognize intravascular coagulation (fibrin aggregation within the blood vessels). Some of the children have had clinical evidence of coagulopathy with abnormal clotting parameters. I am in complete agreement with you that there is a great deal of difference between the artificial environment of hypothermia as it is used in the operating room versus the accidental drowning victim.

C. One other brief comment. He referred to the children in the early experience in cardiac surgery. You did have cerebral damage. I think the reason for that is very clear, that the people who were using that technique at that time, and I think the first paper was published by Dr. Bjork in Sweden. And I've discussed this with him at some detail that he was using an extremely efficient heat exchanger. And what happened was he was able to cool the blood down very rapidly, and I referred to this this morning, and shift the hemoglobin dissociation curve away over to the left so that the warm brain was being perfused by extremely cold blood, which could not give up adequate amounts of oxygen.

Tuesday A.M., June 2 (Drs. Tabeling, Mager, and Lomax)

Q. It's apparent that more information is needed in regards to the incidence of sepsis in these near-drowning cases, and I would like to find out if possible if there is anything known about the organisms involved; what parts of the body perhaps lung, it sounds like, but perhaps other areas, and what is the source. Is it felt to be occurring prehospital as the example of falling into a contaminated water, or is it perhaps related to technique of tracheal tube placement enroute or somebody carrying their intratracheal tube around in their back pocket for a while, or is it occurring within the hospital with all the invasive techniques for monitoring and so forth? Certainly this appears to be a disease of progress, as are many of the infections we see in hospital patients today. . . . Many of these patients perhaps would not have survived to this point without the invasive work that's being carried out, but I think we need to critically evaluate each and every of the modalities utilized, and it appears that at the present time the topic of this conference, hypothermia, at least as utilized in that instance may in fact be detrimental rather than beneficial. Any comments about the specific organisms and/or source, Dr. Tabeling?

A. Dr. Tabeling: In the three patients who died, one patient had an overwhelming staph infection with severe pulmonary damage and also had small staph abscesses in the kidneys; one patient had *Pseudomonias*; one patient had *Klebsiella*. We've also noticed several instances in which blood cultures grew *Aeromones hydrophilia*, which is a common water organism. We've also grown streptococcal pneumonia from patients, so I think the source could be many places. I was also interested in Dr. Conn's remarks yesterday, particularly regarding the effects of hypothermia on complement activation and whether or not there may be something in that area that's causing some of the severe multiorgan failure that we see because two of the three patients in our series who died were the scuba divers. Diving accidents can cause a syndrome with DIC and cardiovascular collapse that we saw in these patients. And I wonder very much if there was not some effect on the complement-activating system that may have made them more susceptible to sepsis.

Q. One perhaps related question is have you observed in your series a hypothermic on arrival or, say, have you looked at that aspect and have you observed the alternate pathway mediated leukopenia which was cited as perhaps a complication of that treatment? Certainly, that phenomenon is known to occur with a number of invasive procedures—heart, lung bypass, hemodialysis, etc.—and has it at least in the past been felt to be rather a transient phenomenon of some of those instances, and I was not aware until yesterday of its association with hypothermia, and did you see that in your series, or have you looked at that?

A. Dr. Tabeling: I reviewed, as I mentioned earlier, 58 of these cases. None of them had a remarkable hypothermia at the time of admission, but I must comment that frequently the temperature was not taken in the emergency room, which I see as a problem. Of course, in Florida we don't see quite as much hypothermia. No, I did not notice any leukopenias early on. We only noticed leukopenia in the patients who developed sepsis, and they did develop a decrease in white blood cell count.

A. Dr. Conn: In answer to your question about infection in these cases, we have been doing automatically and routinely blood cultures, urine cultures, tracheal cultures, everything from the time they hit ICU. And almost invariably for 72 to 96 hr we can't grow anything. Our policy is that if the patient seems to be getting worse, we start antibiotics blindly. At postmortem—for example that case I showed you that died 12 to 14 days following with a severe lung problem; cultures had never grown anything in the hospital of any kind, but at postmortem there was a very weird organism found in the sewage. We've also found this organism that Barbara just mentioned on several occasions, but by that time the patient was getting better, and it's very difficult to interpret how much of the lung problem, which is a major consideration, is due to aspiration of vomitus at the time of resuscitation (aspiration of water—with collapse and secondary infection), or whether it's a primary pneumonia, but if it's *Pseudomonas* we're pretty sure. And occasionally we've had *Pseudomonas* grow and quickly stamp that out. But that, we believe, is a hospital-born infection. We haven't got hard data on infection. . . It's one thing we've looked at, but we have been so busy looking at the brain we haven't looked at that aspect, . . . but it's coming.

Q. I'd like to make two comments rather than ask two questions to Dr. Mager concerning hypoglycemia and hypothermia. He did not mention perhaps a rather more important effect of diabetes in inducing hypothermia. Now I'm not sure whether you have any data on this, but hypothermia and diabetes sometimes go together, and one of the effects, of course, that one has to consider is the autonomic neuropathy that develops with some diabetic patients. I wonder whether you have any observations on the relationship between the lack of utilization of glucose, on the one hand, and the autonomic neuropathy of diabetes, on the other. That's one question. The other comment which perhaps covers a very broad problem is that of brown adipose tissue, which you mentioned in passing at the beginning. Now, to my knowledge there's very little evidence that brown adipose tissue plays any part in thermogenesis of the adult man. I've tried to look for brown adipose tissue in postmortem autopsies and have failed to find it in older people. So these two questions about diabetes and brown adipose tissue, please.

A. Dr. Mager: I believe there have been several recent literature reports concerning hypothermia in diabetics while on various medications. However, I am not familiar with the specific details. Regarding your second question of why we don't find brown fat in humans, the classical response is that, if you look hard enough, you will find it. Additionally, there is some evidence that in the elderly there may be either a decrease in the total brown fat content or a decreased sensitivity of the brown fat to norepinephrine.

C. Thank you. I just wanted to say, for example, that in the adult human the work that has been done in which catecholamines are given to people in order to stimulate these hot areas in the intrascapular regions look very nice on paper. But the methods used, the thermography, for example, certainly leave a lot to be desired. And the most important experiment of all, which is to plunge a needle biopsy into the area to see whether you've got brown fat, was never done, so I still think we're a bit in the dark as to whether brown fat plays an active part in the adult or not.

C. Dr. Mager: Yes. I think it's a very important question. While we have a moment's pause, I'd like to comment, if I may, on some things that Dr. Lomax mentioned. One, there were several investigations by Drs. Freinkel and Arky in the early 1960s on alcohol hypoglycemia and hypothermia, which led to some of the work which I reported today, and they demonstrated that alcohol per se does induce a hypothermic response. Secondly, there is no strong evidence of cold acclimatization in man. Primarily, man does not show increased thermogenesis as the rat does, nor does he show increased circulating levels of thyroid hormone. We did demonstrate, years ago, an increased thyroid turnover in the cold. Thus, in answer to Dr. Lomax's question, although you can observe small peripheral changes in the vasodilatation and constriction patterns . . . in the hands of fishermen who work in very cold climates, full documentation of acclimatization of man to cold is lacking.

Tuesday P.M., June 2 (Drs. Cooper, Ledingham, and Collins)

Q. The biggest question I have is when is CPR done, and do we not do CPR on a patient who appears to be lifeless, he's found in the alley behind a saloon and he's cold. Do we not do CPR on him because he may be hypothermic and because we may cause his heart, which may possibly be functioning (although we can't detect it clinically) to go into ventricular fibrillation?

A. Dr. Ledingham: I would like to say that I can only refer to the situation that I have described in the industrial centers of big cities, and as far as I'm concerned, if you get a patient of the sort we've been describing in our experience in the UK and I realize that what I'm going to say is controversial . . . almost anything that I would say in response to this would be controversial. . . . But my own feeling is that more harm would be done by doing CPR, certainly more harm would be done in our country if CPR were carried out than if a great care and attention were taken to getting that patient to hospital as rapidly as possible. I'm inclined to share the view that was expressed by Dr. Mills that it's likely that you will do more harm to such patients who, in our experience, don't actually die in transit from the site to hospital. They do die from time to time after they reach hospital even under the best conditions, but not many of them die coming from the scene to hospital, and so for a whole lot of reasons, some of which are pertinent in this country, others of which are not, we would certainly not advocate CPR in this situation that I described.

A. Dr. Collins: I must say that I'm on the spot on this one too. It's clear, I think, that if you're dealing with a submersion hypothermia from all that we've heard that probably you'll have to do some form of CPR before you get in the hospital. That seems to improve a very vital part of the survival. The second thing is that, if you start CPR, then you clearly have got to keep it up. There's no point in stopping it again, and if anyone's ever tried doing CPR for 6 or 7 hr [they know that] it's a horrendous procedure. I'm always faced with the one of what to do if . . . it's going to take you 5 hr to get out and get some help and then another 3 or 4 hr to get the patient to the hospital. And I don't honestly know how to answer that one. And certainly if you do start a fibrillation, you can't convert them to a normal rhythm until the temperature is brought up a little bit. So, I guess that this is another instance where we're going to require a lot more information before we can decide what is the correct answer. If there is a correct answer.

A. Dr. Ledingham: The only additional information that I can contribute to this one concerns the Scottish mountain rescue services, and I realize that's a low-key kind of thing by comparison with Dr. Mills's experiences in Alaska, but in the last 10 yr, and I will before this is written down anywhere check chapter and verse, but I think I'm right in saying that [at] a similar symposium held in Aberdeen in Scotland 2 yr ago their principal spokesman reported that no one who had been found alive on the Scottish hills and had been then brought down had died in transit. Now that is without CPR. And for us, that's pretty good evidence that to do something else is clearly not going to improve on that.

A. Dr. Mills: I do feel that there should be more known about the cold heart. I don't feel that a normothermic heart, for which CPR originally was designed, is the same as the hypothermic heart. I do think that we should know more about the physiology of the heart in its cold state and at various levels of cold.

C. I think that if you emphasize to the lay public that it's normal to have a very low respiratory rate, exceedingly low respiratory rate, in hypothermia and that if they have any spontaneous respirations, you assume cardiac output to the brain stem and you tell them you do not start CPR. If you establish there is no breathing, you start your ventilations. We have our theories that the rate should be adjusted to maintain normocapnia, but whatever that might be, you would start ventilation. After you start ventilation, you check for a pulse. I think you have to think what is going to cause the most harm. In our setting, which is an urban setting, we have a lot of drunks, and a lot of myocardial infarcts. We have a lot of medical problems and people fall out on the street; somebody looks at them and says, "Well, it's cold today, there's snow on the ground, it must be hypothermia, I'm not going to start CPR on this patient." I think that you'll kill off more people than if you take the other approach of assuming that the public can be educated to the point of check for a long time for a pulse, check a long time for respirations, start CPR, whether it's modified CPR which we would prefer over regular CPR is arguable, but certainly initiate CPR. The only difference on the flow chart which alters that for the normal American Heart Association flow chart, which right now recognizes the problem that you've addressed which says ABC, continue resuscitation until arrival at a facility or danger to yourself exists. So I would say to you that under normothermic circumstances if I arrive and find you fibrillating out in the woods and I can scream as loud as I want but the nearest person is 10 miles; I'm going to do it for a while until I get tired. I think that common sense should hold in a hypothermic situation.

C. Dr. Ledingham: Yes, I think there's no fundamental difference between us, apart from the fact that I worry a little bit about inadvertently commencing CPR on a patient who actually has a perfectly reasonable blood pressure, but in the hypothermic situation the pulse is impalable.

C. Dr. Golden: I would like to make a comment on this. It's a question I'm very often asked as well. . . . What should one do if you're out sailing in a yacht or in a fishing boat and you come across some survivors, . . . or some individuals I should say, floating in the water following an immersion accident of some sort, a boating accident. Should you do cardiac massage on these people? Well, I think most of the answers have already been given by others, but basically my rationale for the advice of saying no, don't start it, is that if the individual is a drowning victim and therefore, one normally advocates doing CPR in drowning victims, well then, if he is already in arrest by the time you rescue him and you're not sure how long he has been in the water, well then he was probably arrested for some time and there is little point in starting the CPR. If, on the other hand, you know he has been in the water for a very short period of time, then by all means, if you want to, you can start CPR then. But, if you come across some survivors in the water that have been there for some period of time, you're not sure whether they're suffering from hypothermic cardiac arrest or whether they are, in fact, just extremely bradycardiac. I think the individual stands a better chance if you do nothing about cardiac massage but just take them aboard, insulate them, and if he's alive, well then he'll start re-warming and if he isn't, he won't. And if he was dead when you got him, he was dead anyway.

Q. I have a three-part question which I'd like to address to Dr. Collins, Dr. Cooper, Dr. Ledingham. The first part is can elderly people get cold at home? And the second part of the question is, if this is true, which I think it is, are there public policy implications here? Let me give an example. I'm from the state of Michigan, which has a relatively retrogressive law concerning utility shutoffs in the winter, and this winter we had two elderly people who were brought in hypothermic to our emergency room who had experienced utility shutoffs. And the third part of the question is can we define a dangerous environment for certain subpopulations of people, like the elderly or people with certain diseases, or people who are taking certain medications?

A. Dr. Collins: I think as chairman, I might start off. Certainly, we have studied urban hypothermia in UK and found that people can get hypothermic at home and perhaps, not necessarily suffering from any [other] medical complaint. We find people who are hypothermic in bed quite often with apparently enough insulation to keep them warm, so it's not simply a social problem, the problem of clothing and adequate heating in the home. As far as defining what are safe temperatures in the home, this is an extremely difficult one, and we've tried to tackle that in UK by assuming that there might be two temperatures—the first one a temperature which is adequate for comfort for most people, elderly people, and a temperature that would be dangerous for people with a certain amount of clothing and a certain amount of activity to continue in. I think one can get a reasonable idea from a clo level of about 1.0 clo of insulation and sitting as an activity for 3 or 4 hr. I think that seems to be an adequate level of insulation and activity to maintain comfort in a temperature of about 21°C (that's the sort of temperature we have to really look at). The computerized work that's been done at the Pierce Laboratory where one can predict the rate at which deep-body temperature falls, providing you've got no shivering, and this can be done and perhaps a little vasomotor activity. And I think one might say that in a temperature of say 5°C with no shivering an elderly person might be able to survive without getting into a hypothermic state for about 5 hours.

C. Dr. Cooper: The only other comment that I would add to that is, yes, my experience when I was in Oxford was that people certainly can go cold in their own homes and that those who do are not restricted to any one socioeconomic group.

A. Dr. Ledingham: If I could address myself briefly to the second part of the question, . . . which is the public policy component. The system, I think I'm correct in saying, has changed within the last 2 yr in the UK. It used to be that the services were cut off as you described. In the UK now people are allowed to go into debt and they argue the loss afterwards as to the need for having gotten into debt. And elderly, older patients are allowed to get themselves out of that situation after the anxiety is over. That is the first point. The second is that I think there will be a percentage of older people who know they're about to go into debt and prefer not to, and so we have felt that it's important, as others have said at this meeting, that prevention is a lot better than cure here, and we're addressing ourselves to this problem by designing a special chair for these people because we have already determined from our surveys that many of them spend 5 to 8 hr of their waking hours in one single chair. And the device that we've got fitted pretty well on with just now, I think, may be least the first step as an answer to that problem.

Q. Right now it stands as four very distinguished gentleman saying to not start CPR in the field, to . . . our second and third speakers yesterday, Dr. Paton and Dr. Lilja, who specifically indicated that in the presence of asystole, if a patient wasn't breathing and had no heart beat, that it should be started. I'm just wondering is there any possibility of a meeting of the minds? Or did I misinterpret what the gentlemen yesterday were saying, or is there more thought that you want on this? I have to go back and carry some work back, along with Bill, to people in Alaska.

A. Dr. Cooper: I didn't say that you shouldn't start it in the field. I said that we don't really know that the evidence is really very clear about this. Now, and I stick my neck out, if you've got someone a little knowledgeable out on the trail and it's going to take you 8 hr to get somebody to proper care, if there has been a recognized heart beat and it suddenly stops, I think you've got to do something about it. The second thing is that I think it's possible to start rewarming in the field, for example. You can build a shelter, a huge fire and radiate to the victim, and start warming him up, in which case you stand a chance of his surviving. If you're talking to first-aid groups about this, for goodness sakes, tell them if they try and do something, the chances of success may not be very high so don't go off with a great big guilt trip if you don't win.

Wednesday, A.M., June 3 (Drs. Ledingham, Golden, Mills, Danzl)

C. Dr. Ledingham: I'd like to preface my remarks with just one or two comments. The first will have been obvious to many of you already and that is that we may not come to a formal conclusion on this issue today because it is a very difficult issue and perhaps the best, wisest, comment that I could make at this stage is that I would suspect that the best way of tackling this is not under the circumstances that we find ourselves in today, or indeed in the last two or three days, but to have a small group of individuals informed in the area to get together and really contrive all the various situations that would seem to be likely in the field and then see how many times this requirement for CPR would arise. The other comment I would make at this stage is that anything we say at this stage must be regarded as a group of interim suggestions. So, with these preliminary comments, what I feel is that if we're talking in terms of hypothermia of possible hypothermic victims, and with the qualification that I'm talking exclusively about land-based accidents, I think the best thing that I could say is that under usual circumstances obtaining in most industrial cities I think that the usual standard criteria for instituting CPR should obtain. I personally don't see any particular reason why we should separate out hypothermia victims from any other of the collapsed and inverted coma types of individuals that we might be likely to find. Perhaps, adding to that, but if there is any doubt in your mind under these circumstances that if you feel the individual is hypothermic I'd be more likely to put these doubts aside because of the increased likelihood of success of CPR under these circumstances. I feel less unhappy about saying that in the urban situation, CPR should be started using the conventional criteria for instituting CPR. Once the patient has arrived in the hospital, then the question of differentiating between hypothermia and death can be made, but even there it is obviously going to be a tricky situation when you remember that it has been said many times before that the only way you can distinguish between these two is to warm the hypothermic individual and then only when his temperature is normal can you really distinguish between life and death.

Now, in the exposure situation, obviously again this is a very personal opinion, I feel that if one comes upon an individual who is not breathing, has no pulse, and in whom one sees dilated pupils, then I personally would leave that individual alone. . . . I wouldn't start CPR. Now, you may say that's not a very revolutionary thought, but, in fact, you will regrettably leave one or two people that might theoretically be resuscitated because these same factors obtain in the urban situation and you might have some success. But, having said that, my own feeling is that if we're talking about the mountainside or some of the other exposure situations that we've been describing in the last couple of days, that kind of grouping together of factors, for me, that would constitute an indication for leaving alone. Secondly, if the patient, individual, is breathing and has no pulse under these circumstances I would also leave them alone, I would not institute CPR. What I would do, and not too many people have commented on what I consider to be very much more important under these circumstances, is concentrating like mad on reducing the risk factors. Now the risk factors in this situation are maintaining a patent airway. If we're talking about a paramedic team arriving, then the question of giving oxygen and giving some fluids is a very, very much more important issue than the question of whether CPR should be started under these circumstances. Reducing risk elements, like making sure that aspiration doesn't occur, stabilizing fractures, because many of these individuals will have associated trauma, and, consequent on some of the comments that have been made, making sure that whatever else, we don't have a head-up tilt if that can possibly be avoided because certainly in our experience that's a circumstance to avoid.

And then, finally, the only other group that's left then is the patient who falls into the second category, who is breathing when first seen, has no pulses but then stops breathing. Now this is the situation where I think CPR may be considered, but in my view it should only be started if there are reasonable chances of that being taken to a logical conclusion. Now, when I saw that I mean without increasing the risk to other members of that group, so that if you're talking about associates of a group that have already been out on the mountainside, exposed to the same risks as the person who's become hypothermic, I would regard that as an indication for starting CPR, but if you're talking about paramedic team that's dropped in out of the blue and picked up such an individual, then that's a different situation and I think CPR could reasonably be started under these circumstances. But the other factors that bear upon this are essentially not medical issues; they are lay issues that the circumstances around the scene will dictate. I think that summarizes briefly what I had to say on that.

C. Dr. Danzl: It should be assumed that responsive patients have adequate cardiopulmonary function for their degree of hypothermia. In establishing unresponsiveness, the traditional shake and shout is clearly not indicated. Perhaps it should just be a shouting match while checking A, the airway. Assume the patient has a spinal injury and do a jaw thrust or chin lift. Check for a prolapsed tongue, vomitus, aspirated dentures, etc., and be sure that you have a patent airway. Moving to B, you check for breathing. We emphasize to rescuers that profound hypothermia causes significant depression of respiratory minute volume, and the patient may appear apneic. Attempt to take 2 full minutes to check for any spontaneous respirations, being aware that if you stare at your watch you get impatient if the patient doesn't breathe for 2 minutes. We'll hope that rescuers take at least a minute or longer to check for spontaneous respiration. Looking, listening, and feeling for respiration may be aided in a cold, ambient temperature where you may see mist but not see any thoracic excursions if the patient's rigid. If you're convinced that the patient has any spontaneous respirations, assume the patient has a positive cardiac output. We are not aware of any patient who had persistent spontaneous respirations in hypothermia who had no cardiac output; so these patients are insulated and gently transported, with available rewarming techniques. If there are no spontaneous ventilations, four quick breaths are given. Finding a peripheral pulse in a severely vasoconstricted patient is difficult. We'll assume that you have no stethoscope, so check for central pulses or put your ear right over the apex and listen for any audible heart tones. At this point, if there are no audible heart tones and there are no respirations, you decide whether to begin CPR. Rescuers are encouraged to begin CPR unless there's a danger to the rescuer or there's no possibility of rewarming in the field or getting to a facility to rewarm the patient. In discussing compressions and ventilations, ideally you would be using 95% oxygen with 5% carbon dioxide. If unavailable, initially use 100% oxygen. Pre-hospital ventilation is at half-normothermic rates. We've had some trouble with hypocapnia and induced ventricular irritability. For initial IVs we prefer D5 normal saline to rehydrate the patient. After gentle extrication, gurneys are preferably carried not rolled, and transportation is not code 3 with sirens and the lights. We attempt to eliminate all the possible mechanical factors which are known to precipitate ventricular fibrillation.

C. Dr. Golden: I think there's very little I can add, in fact, I entirely support the two previous speakers. I think, to go back to very simple terms, our aim should be to keep people alive who are alive at time of rescue; in other words, as Dr. Ledingham says, to reduce the risk factors we should really clearly differentiate between effective cardiac massage and attempted cardiac massage. It's all very well to talk about cardiac massage here and to teach it in the hospital, but when you're out in a boat on the sea and it's difficult to find a level surface and the boat is rocking around, you have difficulty keeping your own balance. Now when you start thinking of doing cardiac massage under these circumstances, it's an entirely different kettle of fish, so it's a question of whether you can keep an effective cardiac massage going because, once you've started it, you are not permitted to stop. That raises the next question—the feasibility of keeping it going for protracted periods. So basically what we're teaching is that on a ship or in a small boat, yacht, or something, when you're not within easy access of a hospital unit where supportive therapy can be maintained and the individual can be defibrillated, etc., well then one doesn't start cardiac massage. But if on a helicopter when you rescue someone from the sea and you're now trying to take him to a hospital which may be an hour or 2 hr away, well then by all means you can do it under those circumstances. So that really is the only opinion I have.

C. Dr. Mills: Perhaps some accord may come of this. You have heard a good summary of what should probably be done. The situation I would like to describe, as could many of you in the western and northeastern states also, is a little more harsh and brutal. In many cases, the duration of the hypothermic state is longer, usually 24 to 36 hr or more. It would seem that, if after a reasonable length of time of examination of the victim, there is some, any, evidence of life (breathing, moaning, motion, pulse) or evidence of life on more sophisticated instruments (EKG or Doppler, in the rescue vehicle), then I would recommend no CPR. The cases in which the above signs are present may total 80% to 85% of the victims discovered. It is important to keep the stethoscope in place for at least a minute and a half or two minutes for evidence of heartbeat or pulse, and if an EKG strip is available, you'll be surprised how much time elapses before there is any evidence of electrical activity of the heart. We're now left with the 15% to 20% of victims with no sign of life at the time of discovery. If the victim is found in an urban area, an hour or so away from a hospital, even with an estimated or recorded temperature of 65° to 70°F (18° to 21°C), I would not give CPR but would carefully move the patient to an emergency room, where under physiological control, regardless of the method of warming, he might be under the monitor care and be brought to a normal state. This method has been described. If I were in an isolated area but had a patient who was cold and conscious, I would think that tub warming might be adequate, but any type of rapid rewarming in an unconscious patient where one is unable to follow up with other methods of care, particularly fluid care and the utilization of inspired air and oxygen, makes such methods hazardous. If you have a situation that we often find, where the victim cannot be rescued for one reason or another and they cannot be cared for immediately and are found in a cold state, conscious or unconscious, then many decisions must be made. At this point, I think you should go along with whatever the state of the victim is at the time and make sure that you avoid further loss of heat. If the patient is without signs of life and you have good evidence to believe that you're going to be there with him without the ability to move him or continue rescue for 1, 2, 3, or 4 days, then a further decision must be made. If you institute CPR, and a severe arrhythmia develops which you would attempt to diagnose and probably couldn't, unless the rescue personnel happened to be paramedics, then as a result of CPR, at least from some present thought, the patient may develop very marked ventricular fibrillation. Does that mean the patient was in cardiac arrest, literally lifeless and you brought him to life, or does it mean that the patient was alive, in a metabolic ice box, and, as a result of CPR, then developed the severe and dangerous arrhythmia? With the patient then in ventricular fibrillation, something must be done immediately, and, in the situation in which you find yourself, it might be most difficult to begin care to eliminate the ventricular fibrillation. It is possible that a heart that is barely perfusing may become almost nonfunctional as a result of the altered state and severe arrhythmia. Dr. Templin and I have discussed this for Alaska, and it is our feeling that this meeting should recognize this rather gray, even black area. It is felt that the rescuer should be given an alternative of making up his own mind at the time whether CPR should be done and, if CPR is performed, whether it can be continued or whether, if CPR isn't done, that there is sufficient method and time available to bring the individual into an area where his immediate needs and resuscitation care can be applied.

C. Dr. Hamlet: At least in normothermia there's good evidence. I've heard the argument that if you do CPR in a cold heart you're going to cause a myocardial contusion and I think there's good evidence against that from two different points of view. One is that manual CPR in normothermia and therefore in hypothermia probably does not cause the flow of blood by mechanical compression on the heart between the sternum and the vertebral bodies. Rather it's by changes in the negative interthoracic pressure, which really shouldn't be altered by the core temperature. So, whether the blood moves in the cardiac output which is 45% of the normal at 28°C is not 20% of normal. I think there's going to be [a] linear graph that's developed that shows that you can still be able to generate changes in the negative interthoracic pressure with compressions.

C. Dr. Ledingham: Far be it for me to dampen the enthusiasm of any research group in this field, but I don't think that is an issue. I agree with what's just been said. I think there's actually a handful, albeit a small number, but very solid evidence that external cardiac massage in the hypothermic heart right down to 18°C is a perfectly reliable maneuver and people have been recovered after 2 or 3 hr of such maneuvers. Quite happily the patient I reported on in 1964 was massaged for 2½ hr and woke up as soon as his temperature reached normal. So I don't think there's any problem about that.

C. Dr. Mills: It's possible that the problem of CPR and the resultant difficulties that have come from its use in hypothermia, or apparently have been thought to be a result of its use, are a result of incomplete studies. I don't believe much has been done in all aspects of the hypothermic heart itself in advising us of what we might expect of a cold heart. This is particularly so in the area of massage and compression. But from our experience in the field, in Alaska, of the eight deaths reports this meeting, five had obtained CPR at the time of rescue, followed by ventricular fibrillation. I think one of the possibilities that exists that has given CPR a bad name is the fact that when we say CPR, we're not discussing the usual mouth-to-mouth respiration. I think that now we're discussing thoracic compression, and there is certainly a lot of difference in the method and amount of compression and the way it's delivered. I have heard it taught that one compresses the heart and can do the various maneuvers so that if a few ribs break that is not important compared to the person's life. It may well be that some of the problems we have are a result of aggressive cardiac compression that might damage a cold heart but may permit survival of a normothermic myocardium.

Q. I have a question for anyone on the panel, and it relates to the point that both Dr. Mills and Dr. Golden have made that once you start CPR, you must maintain it. Now I understand that's true in the normothermic heart, and I wonder what evidence there is that this is true on the heart at 27°C, especially in view of the fact that at the same time we advocate we don't even have to do CPR while we transport them. Is it possible to give 5 minutes of adequate CPR, if that is possible infuse the brain and the other tissues with a little bit of oxygen because you don't know how long it's been hypoxic and then be able to take the strain off if you're in a transport situation the urgency of having the fatigue of having to keep it up. So the question is, is there any evidence that once started on the hypothermic heart, you have to maintain it?

A. Dr. Mills: I'll give you some interesting evidence that is anecdotal. We know of three cases wherein CPR was instituted where the patient went immediately into ventricular fibrillation, measured by a sophisticated rescue crew. Now would you be willing to stop CPR in that victim? It is most likely that without aggressive CPR (as in controlled cardiac surgery or in the physiological control of a hypothermic patient after rescue) the warming heart might avoid (I think it most often does) the complication of ventricular fibrillation. Once ventricular fibrillation occurs, CPR with or without xylocaine bolus and at the proper time electrical cardioversion may be required until a normal rhythm is gained.

C. Some of us treat the urban hypothermic; Dr. Mills treats the exposure hypothermic; Dr. Nimeroff teaches on how to resuscitate the immersion or submersion hypothermic. Dr. Nimeroff has gotten just fantastic results from his hyperacute induction cases where the child has been under water, usually a young person but some of his later ones up to 43 yr old, of people who have been immersed and submersed for periods of around 40 minutes with good neurologic return. Would any of you not start CPR on a submersion case when [there is] the possibility [that] longer transportation would be necessary?

A. Dr. Golden: I think you're talking about a drowning case rather than a pure hypothermic victim. In near drowning, always give CPR if indicated; there is no controversy about that. If the victim you are treating has been submerged, or waves have been breaking over his face, then near drowning is the most obvious explanation for any cardiopulmonary problems that may be present, and you must give CPR as indicated. That's the teaching of the American Heart Association and every other similar national authority, and I don't think anybody would dispute that.

Index

Index